CLINICAL PRACTICE OF COGNITIVE THERAPY
WITH CHILDREN AND ADOLESCENTS

Clinical Practice of Cognitive Therapy with Children and Adolescents

❖

The Nuts and Bolts

ROBERT D. FRIEDBERG
JESSICA M. McCLURE

THE GUILFORD PRESS
New York   London

Library of Congress Cataloging-in-Publication Data

Friedberg, Robert D., 1955–
   Clinical practice of cognitive therapy with children and adolescents:
the nuts and bolts / Robert D. Friedberg, Jessica M. McClure.
      p. ; cm.
   Includes bibliographical references and index.
   ISBN 1-57230-723-4 (hardcover : alk. paper)
   1. Cognitive therapy for children. 2. Cognitive therapy for
teenagers. I. McClure, Jessica M. II. Title.
   [DNLM: 1. Cognitive Therapy—methods. WM 425.5.C6 F899c 2002]
RJ505.C63 F75 2002
618.92′89142—dc21

                                                              2001054319

About the Authors

Robert D. Friedberg, PhD, is a clinical psychologist on the faculty of the Wright State University School of Professional Psychology. He is an Associate Professor and directs the Predoctoral Internship Program and the Preventing Anxiety and Depression in Youth Program (PANDY). Dr. Friedberg is the author of three other books on children and adolescents: *Switching Channels* (with Carolyn Mason and Raymond Fidaleo), *Therapeutic Exercises for Children* (with Barbara Friedberg and Rebecca Friedberg), and *A Professional Guide to Therapeutic Exercises for Children* (with Lori Crosby). He has authored numerous articles in scholarly journals and delivered presentations on cognitive therapy with children and adolescents to professional audiences. Dr. Friedberg is a Founding Fellow in the Academy of Cognitive Therapy.

Jessica M. McClure, PsyD, works as a clinical psychologist specializing in the assessment and treatment of children and adolescents for the Children's Hospital Medical Center in Cincinnati, Ohio. She is an adjunct faculty member at the Wright State University School of Professional Psychology, where she teaches several child-focused courses. Dr. McClure has coauthored presentations and articles on the treatment of children and adolescents and currently serves children and adolescents experiencing depression, anxiety, behavior problems, and developmental delays.

Acknowledgments

Thank you to my wife, Barbara, and daughter, Rebecca, whose love and support inspired me throughout this project. I value the collaboration and collegiality with my coauthor, Jessica McClure, whose attention to detail is peerless. Kitty Moore, our editor, was an exceptional guide, shepherding us through this project with creative and insightful comments. The many clinical trainees I supervised deserve mention, as our lively discussions led me to refine many ideas. I want to acknowledge the many young clients and families my trainees and I served and thank them for entrusting their care to us. I am grateful to the Wright State University School of Professional Psychology for giving me the opportunity to pursue my clinical service and research. Finally, special thanks goes to Carol Smart, who typed and retyped earlier versions of the manuscript with professionalism and good humor.

ROBERT D. FRIEDBERG

I would like to acknowledge the invaluable support that my family and friends provided me throughout this endeavor. I express my deepest appreciation to my husband, Jim McClure, for all of his patience and encouragement over the countless hours of work. Thanks to my coauthor, Robert Friedberg, for his great sense of humor and collaboration on this project. I am grateful to my colleague Denise Price, who endured numerous questions and provided endless encouragement throughout the process. Finally, Carol Smart's clerical skills were much appreciated throughout the writing of this book.

JESSICA M. MCCLURE

Contents

CLINICAL PRACTICE OF COGNITIVE THERAPY WITH CHILDREN AND ADOLESCENTS

1

❖

Introduction

When we began writing this book, we thought about "How do we be-gin?" As cognitive therapists, we found it natural to begin with a series of questions to introduce the purpose of the book, its content, and its for-mat, as well as ourselves to you.

WHO ARE WE?

We are cognitive therapists at different stages in our careers. Robert Friedberg is a clinical psychologist who is in the middle stages of his ca-reer, while Jessica McClure is beginning her professional career. Dr. Friedberg has worked with children and their families in a variety of out-patient and inpatient settings. His work is fundamentally shaped by the writings of Aaron Beck and Martin Seligman, as well as by his mentors Christine Padesky and Raymond Fidaleo. Dr. McClure has had clinical experience with children and adolescents in a variety of settings, includ-ing inpatient psychiatric hospitals, pediatric medical centers, outpatient clinics, and innovative prevention programs.

We began writing this text together when Dr. McClure trained under Dr. Friedberg's supervision in the Preventing Anxiety and Depression in Youth program at Wright State University School of Professional Psychol-ogy. We thought that a book written by two psychologists at different points in their careers would speak to professionals with different levels of experience.

WHY WRITE A BOOK ON COGNITIVE THERAPY
WITH CHILDREN AND ADOLESCENTS?

We wanted to write a book that makes use of cognitive therapy principles and offers a coherent theoretical framework. Cognitive therapy as developed by Aaron T. Beck is a robust clinical and theoretical system that has been applied to many adult problems and populations (A. T. Beck, 1976, 1985, 1993; A. T. Beck, Emery, & Greenberg, 1985; A. T. Beck, Rush, Shaw, & Emery, 1979), but few cognitive therapy texts on children apply Beck's approach to youngsters (Knell, 1993; Ronen, 1997). In addition, child psychotherapy often lacks a coherent theoretical focus (Ronen, 1997).

WHAT WILL THIS BOOK TEACH YOU?

This book offers a complete guide on how to do cognitive therapy with schoolchildren and adolescents. In addition to teaching many techniques, the book will also emphasize the guiding principles that shape Beck's cognitive therapy. Collaborative empiricism and guided discovery, the leitmotifs of cognitive therapy, are defined in Chapter 3 and subsequently illustrated throughout the text. The session structure that characterizes cognitive therapy is described in Chapter 4. Applying cognitive-behavioral techniques in the absence of a case conceptualization is a major clinical error (J. S. Beck, 1995). Furthermore, techniques disembodied from theory fall flat. Accordingly, case conceptualization is a basic blueprint for success in cognitive therapy (J. S. Beck, 1995; Persons, 1989); the nuts and bolts we use to build a case formulation are presented in Chapter 2.

This book also takes into consideration developmental and multicultural issues throughout the text. Developmental sensitivity is crucial for successful cognitive-behavioral work with children (Ronen, 1997; Silverman & Ollendick, 1999). Accordingly, social developmental issues are delineated at the end of this introductory chapter. Further, we explain how you might modify different techniques for younger children and adolescents. Chapter 2 discusses the incorporation of multicultural considerations and familial factors into a comprehensive case conceptualization.

Chapters 5 through 14 describe various cognitive-behavioral treatment strategies, ranging from problem identification to techniques for crafting a Socratic dialogue with children to child-friendly forms of cognitive-behavioral intervention. Each chapter deals with the application of these methods with young children and adolescents. Moreover, cognitive-behavioral approaches for depressed, anxious, and aggressive youth are addressed in individual chapters.

WHAT IS COGNITIVE THERAPY?

Cognitive therapy is based on social learning theory and uses a blend of techniques, many of which are based on operant and classical conditioning models (Hart & Morgan, 1993). In brief, social learning theory (Bandura, 1977; Rotter, 1982) is based on the assumption that a person's environment, personal dispositional characteristics, and situational behavior reciprocally determine each other and that behavior is an evolving, dynamic phenomenon. Contexts influence behavior and behavior in turn shapes contexts; sometimes the contexts may have the most powerful influence over a person's behavior and at other times personal preferences, dispositions, and characteristics will determine behavior.

Imagine that a child must select an instrument to play in the school band. If all instruments are available as options, the child's choice (e.g., saxophone) will predominantly be a function of his/her individual characteristics. However, if only a few instruments are available (e.g., trumpets, flutes, and clarinets), and many students are competing for each instrument, contextual factors will predominate. The child's appraisal of each situation will shape his/her subsequent behavior. For instance, his/her participation in school music activities may increase or decrease (e.g., "This school sucks. They don't have saxophones."; or "Wow, I get to play the trumpet!"). This behavior will subsequently further shape the context in which the musical instruments are presented. Clearly, social learning theory explicitly and implicitly encourages clinicians to examine the dynamic mutual influence between individuals and the larger context in which they behave. Moreover, social learning theory examines the way subsequent behavior impacts current circumstances.

Cognitive therapy holds that five interrelated elements are involved in conceptualizing human psychological difficulties (A. T. Beck, 1985; J. S. Beck, 1995; Padesky & Greenberger, 1995). These elements include interpersonal/environmental context as well as individuals' physiology, emotional functioning, behavior, and cognition. All these separate features change and mutually interact with each other, creating a dynamic and complex system. The cognitive model has been graphically illustrated in many other publications (J. S. Beck, 1995; Padesky & Greenberger, 1995).

Cognitive, behavioral, emotional, and physiological symptoms occur in an interpersonal/environmental context. Thus, the model explicitly incorporates the systemic, interpersonal, and cultural context issues that are so pivotal to child psychotherapy. The symptoms do not occur in a vacuum, so clinicians should consider a child's particular circumstances when assessing and treating youngsters. In general, while considering context, cognitive therapists intervene at the cognitive-behavioral level to influence thinking, acting, feelings, and bodily reaction patterns (Alford & Beck, 1997).

For example, Alice is a 16-year-old Caucasian girl who lives with her biological mother and stepfather in a poor neighborhood with inadequate schools. She is the product of an unwanted pregnancy and is overtly rejected and scapegoated by her parents. Within this context, she is experiencing physiological (stomachaches, excessive sleeping), mood (depression, hopeless feelings), behavioral (passivity, avoidance, withdrawal), and cognitive symptoms ("I'm worthless."). While this example is severe, it nevertheless illustrates that the child's symptoms need to be considered in the context of environmental circumstances and personal dispositions that initiate, exacerbate, and maintain the distress.

How children interpret their experiences profoundly shapes their emotional functioning. Their view is a major focus of treatment. The way youngsters construct "mental packages" about themselves, relationships with other people, experiences, and the future influences their emotional reactions. Children do not passively receive or respond to environmental stimuli. Rather, they actively construct information by selecting, encoding, and explaining the things that happen to themselves and others.

This information-processing system is hierarchically layered, consisting of cognitive products, cognitive operations, and cognitive structures (A. T. Beck & Clark, 1988; Dattilio & Padesky, 1990; Ingram & Kendall, 1986; Padesky, 1994). Automatic thoughts are the cognitive products in this model (A. T. Beck & Clark, 1988). They are the stream-of-consciousness thoughts or images that are situationally specific and pass through people's minds during a mood shift. Thus, Barbara may ask a friend to play during recess and the friend may refuse, saying she wants to play with another child (situation). Barbara feels sad (emotion) and interprets the situation by telling herself, "Judy is not my friend anymore. She doesn't like me" (automatic thought). Automatic thoughts, which are relatively easy to identify, have received a great deal of attention in the cognitive therapy literature. However, they represent only one element in the cognitive model.

Cognitive distortions have also received considerable attention (J. S. Beck, 1995; Burns, 1980). Cognitive distortions reflect cognitive processes in this model (A. T. Beck & Clark, 1988). Distortions transform incoming information so that cognitive schemata remain intact. Cognitive distortions work through assimilation processes and maintain homeostasis. For instance, Susan's schema reflects a perception of incompetence: she believes that she can't do anything right or well. Consequently, she feels anxious (emotion) in performance situations. Accordingly, Susan may earn a high mark in a school math test (situation) and believe the grade does not matter because the test was too easy (automatic thought). Thus, the child is discounting her success (cognitive distortion). The information that is discrepant with her core belief is nullified. In this way, the cognitive schema remains intact, perpetrating itself through the distortion process. Susan is unable to extract disconfirming data from the environment. School is likely to remain a situation that exposes her to performance pressure and self-devaluation. In turn, she will likely continue to dread performance pressures.

The cognitive schemata represent core meaning structures that direct attention encoding and recall (Fiske & Taylor, 1991; Guidano & Liotti, 1983, 1985; Hammen, 1988; Hammen & Zupan, 1984). Schemata drive cognitive products and operations. These cognitive structures reflect the most basic beliefs individuals hold. Kagan (1986) described the schema as "the cognitive unit that will store experience in a form so faithful a person can recognize a past event" (p. 121).

Imagine a 15-year-old youngster with social anxiety who recalls being humiliated at a Cub Scout meeting when he was 6. Each time he enters a new social situation, his schema brings him back to his original humiliation such that he feels like he is reexperiencing the event. Perhaps this explains the clinical phenomenon in which clients seem so regressed and immature when they are severely distressed. In the case of this 15-year-old boy, whenever his schematic buttons were pushed, he saw himself and the world through the eyes of a scorned 6-year-old Cub Scout.

Schematic material is relatively unaccessible and often lies latent until activated by a stressor (Hammen & Goodman-Brown, 1990; Zupan, Hammen, & Jaenicke, 1987). In cognitive theory, schemata may represent a vulnerability factor that predisposes children to emotional distress (A. T. Beck et al., 1979; Young, 1990). Conceptually, a pessimistic attributional style may be considered a diathesis for childhood depression (Gillham, Reivich, Jaycox, & Seligman, 1995; Jaycox, Reivich, Gillham, & Seligman, 1994; Nolen-Hoeksema & Girgus, 1995; Nolen-Hoeksema, Girgus, & Seligman, 1996; Seligman, Reivich, Jaycox, & Gillham, 1995).

Schemata develop early in life, become reinforced over time, and as a consequence of repeated learning experiences become consolidated by adolescence and young adulthood (Guidano & Liotti, 1983; Hammen & Zupan, 1984; Young, 1990). Early schematic material may be encoded at the preverbal level and accordingly may contain nonverbal images in addition to verbal material (Guidano & Liotti, 1983; Young, 1990). Children's schemata tend not to be consolidated as well as adult schemata. For instance, Nolen-Hoeksema and Girgus (1995) concluded that the pessimistic attributional style is in place by 9 years of age, but the deleterious effects of this style may not emerge until several years later. In fact, Turner and Cole (1994) found that cognitive diathesis was more striking in eighth graders than in either fourth or sixth graders.

As most therapists realize, recognizing when meaningful cognitions have been identified is not as simple as it superficially seems. You need a guide or map. Cognitive therapy provides us with a useful template through an understanding of the *content-specificity hypothesis*, which posits that different emotional states are characterized by distinct cognitions (Alford & Beck, 1997; A. T. Beck, 1976; Clark & Beck, 1988; Clark, Beck, & Alford, 1999; Laurent & Stark, 1993). Aspects of the content-specificity hypothesis have been subjected to empirical investigation that support it (Jolly, 1993; Jolly & Dykman, 1994; Jolly & Kramer, 1994; Laurent & Stark, 1993; Messer, Kempton, Van Hasselt, Null, & Bukstein, 1994).

According to the content-specificity hypothesis, depression is characterized by the classic *negative cognitive triad* (A. T. Beck et al., 1979). Depressed individuals tend to explain unfavorable events through a self-critical view of themselves ("I'm an idiot."), a negative view of their experiences/other people ("Everything is ruined. No one is going to like me."), and a pessimistic view of the future ("It's going to stay this way forever."). A depressed person's thoughts tend to be past-oriented and represent themes reflecting loss (A. T. Beck, 1976; Clark et al., 1999).

Anxiety is characterized by different clusters of cognitions than depression (A. T. Beck & Clark, 1988; Bell-Dolan & Wessler, 1994; Kendall, Chansky, Friedman, & Siqueland, 1991). In anxiety, *catastrophizing* is common: anxious individuals' thoughts tend to be future-oriented and characterized by predictions of danger (A. T. Beck, 1976). Chapter 6, on identifying thoughts and feelings, further elaborates on the content-specificity hypothesis and its clinical application.

Overall, these tenets of cognitive therapy are well researched and theoretically sound. Consequently, cognitive theory provides a solid foundation for working with children and directs you to theoretically driven interventions based on the case conceptualization. For instance, we focus on the child's information-processing systems as a way of identifying the child's automatic thoughts and cognitive schemata. The content-specificity hypothesis provides a framework for recognizing the automatic thoughts that maintain and perpetuate maladaptive schemata as well as a method for determining their relationship to the child's negative affective arousal. By understanding cognitive theory, processes, and appropriate intervention strategies, you can develop the basic knowledge, and skills necessary for conducting effective cognitive therapy with children.

WHAT ARE THE SIMILARITIES BETWEEN COGNITIVE THERAPY WITH ADULTS AND COGNITIVE THERAPY WITH CHILDREN AND ADOLESCENTS?

While cognitive therapy must be adapted to suit the unique characteristics of children, several tenets originally established through adult work still apply (Knell, 1993). For instance, collaborative empiricism and guided discovery are useful with children. In addition, the session structure can also be flexibly applied with children. Accordingly, agenda setting and eliciting feedback are central tenets that guide cognitive therapy with children. Spiegler and Guevremont (1995) rightly note that homework is a core construct in cognitive-behavioral therapies, one that allows children to experiment with skills in real-life contexts. Cognitive therapy with children remains problem-focused, active, and goal-oriented (Knell, 1993), just as it does with adults.

WHAT ARE THE DIFFERENCES BETWEEN COGNITIVE THERAPY WITH ADULTS AND COGNITIVE THERAPY WITH CHILDREN AND ADOLESCENTS?

At the same time, cognitive therapy with children differs from cognitive therapy with adults. First, very few children come to therapy on their own volition (Leve, 1995). They are brought to treatment, usually by their caregivers, due to problems they may or may not admit having. Moreover, clinical experience suggests that most frequently children are referred to therapy because their psychological difficulties create problems for some system (e.g., family, school).

Children rarely initiate treatment nor do they usually have a choice about when it ends. In some cases, children may enjoy therapy and make significant progress yet for various reasons their parents terminate treatment. In other cases, children may avoid the therapeutic process and even dread therapy, yet external circumstances (e.g., juvenile court stipulations, school requirements, parents) may force them to continue. In neither case do these children control the process.

Although many children may welcome the opportunity to disclose their thoughts and feelings to an adult, for others the experience of going to psychotherapy to talk with an adult in an authority position creates a substantial amount of anxiety. Not surprisingly, children often voice a realistic sense of uncontrollability. Thus, you must work assiduously to engage the child in the treatment process and increase his/her motivation for treatment.

Cognitive therapy with children is generally based on an experiential, here-and-now approach (Knell, 1993). Since children are action-oriented, they readily learn by doing. Connecting coping skills to concrete actions is likely to help children attend to, recall, and perform the desired behavior. Additionally, action in therapy is enlivening. Children's motivation will increase when they are having fun.

Children function within systems such as families and schools (Ronen, 1998). Ronen aptly noted that "the focus of CBT [cognitive-behavioral therapy] lies with treating children within their own natural environment whether referring to the family, school, or peer group" (p. 3). Accordingly, therapists must appreciate the complex systemic issues that surround children's problems and design treatment plans accordingly. Without a consideration of systemic issues, therapists are "flying blind." The systems in which children function can reinforce or extinguish adaptive coping skills. Family involvement and school consultation are critical for successful initiation, maintenance, and generalization of therapeutic gains.

Children have different capabilities, limitations, preferences, and interests than adults. Sitting in a chair facing another person talking about psychological problems can feel foreign and unsettling to youngsters. Since cognitive therapy with children relies on verbal and cognitive capacities, you must carefully consider children's ages as well as their social-cognitive skills (Kimball, Nelson, & Politano, 1993; Ronen, 1997) and adapt the level of intervention to the child's age and developmental capacities. Younger children tend to profit from simple cognitive techniques such as self-instruction and behavioral interventions whereas adolescents will likely benefit from more sophisticated techniques requiring rational analyses (Ronen, 1998).

Age, while important, is a nonspecific variable (Daleiden, Vasey, & Brown, 1999). Therefore, we must remain mindful of various social-cognitive variables such as language, perspective-taking ability, reasoning capacity, and verbal regulation skills (Hart & Morgan, 1993; Kimball et al., 1993; Ronen, 1997, 1998). When therapeutic task demands exceed children's social-cognitive capacities, they may mistakenly appear resistant, avoidant, and even incompetent (Friedberg & Dalenberg, 1991). Mischel (1981) rightly contended that "children are potentially sophisticated (albeit fallible) intuitive psychologists who come to know and use psychological principles for understanding social behavior, for regulating their own conduct, and for achieving mastery and control over their environments" (p. 240). Simple, meaningful therapeutic tasks that are developmentally sensitive successfully engage even young children in cognitive-behavioral therapy (Friedberg & Dalenberg, 1991; Knell, 1993; Ronen, 1997). For instance, thought diaries that include thought bubbles are readily understood by young children (Wellman, Hollander, & Schult,

1996). Thus, social-cognitive variables direct what, how, and when various cognitive-behavioral procedures are used.

Language ability will influence how much children will profit from direct verbal interventions (Ronen, 1997, 1998). With less verbally facile children, drawing, puppet play, toy play, games, craft work, and other tasks that require less verbal mediation may be indicated. Reading and storytelling with these children may be ways by which we may be able to increase their verbal sophistication. Moreover, movies, music, and television shows are media that could facilitate greater verbal mediation. Shaping tasks to match children's language skills is a crucial clinical challenge.

Several authors have delineated important developmental variables and tasks for cognitive therapists to consider (Kimball et al., 1993; Ronen, 1997). Ronen (1998) aptly notes that determining whether a child's behavior is problematic requires an understanding of the requisite developmental tasks that children confront: "As children grow up, they are expected to gain control of their bladders, they are expected to learn that their parents always come back and to stop crying when they leave; and they are expected to gradually gain self-control skills, develop assertiveness, and an ability for self-evaluation, and learn to conduct verbal communication and negotiation instead of crying whenever they wish for something" (p. 7). When children's behavior significantly deviates from developmental expectations, clinicians work to correct these derailed developmental processes. In fact, guiding children and their families through these developmental detours is often a major treatment focus.

In this book, we try to show a way of working with children that is playful and fun. While many of the psychological issues that challenge children are painful and distressing to them, uncomfortable topics can be dealt with in an imaginative, creative, and engaging manner. In our experience, it appears that when children are more engaged and invested in therapy, the less it seems like work.

Explicit reinforcement is a central part of working with youngsters (Knell, 1993). Children are reinforced for cleaning up their toys in the playroom, completing homework, disclosing their thoughts and feelings, and the like. Rewards communicate expectations and serve motivation, attention, and retention functions (Bandura, 1977; Rotter, 1982). Put simply, rewards engage children, direct them to what is important, and teach them what to remember.

A WORD ABOUT OUR TRANSCRIPTS AND EXAMPLES

All of the case examples and transcripts are fictionalized or disguised clinical accounts. They represent a combination of our cases and experiences as ways to simply illustrate concepts. We realize that in your real clinical world, issues are rarely this clear and simple. Finally, while we have treated numerous children of color, most of the clinical examples presented are with Caucasian, European American children and adolescents. Moreover, most of the existing empirical and theoretical research is based on Caucasian, European American children. Therefore, we encourage you to cautiously generalize our concepts and practices to your work with children of color. The sections on cultural-context issues throughout the book should alert you to possible ethnocultural issues and prompt culturally responsive modifications where necessary.

2

❖

Case Conceptualization

The first step when working with a child is to develop a case conceptualization. Case conceptualization facilitates the therapist's task of tailoring techniques to custom fit a youngster's circumstances. The individual case conceptualization guides the choice of techniques, their pacing and implementation, as well as the evaluation of progress. Each case you face is different. Our task is to create a general conceptual framework that allows for maximum flexibility. In this chapter, we define case conceptualization, compare it with diagnosis and treatment planning, explore the various domains we consider important, and discuss the relationship among these domains.

When we supervise trainees, we find that case conceptualization is a hard sell. Many new therapists want a "bag of tricks" and dismiss case conceptualization as an abstract exercise. Yet case conceptualization is one of the most practical tools they can have in their tool kit. Case conceptualization tells therapists when and how to use their tools.

CASE CONCEPTUALIZATION: ONCE IS NEVER ENOUGH

The case formulation is a dynamic and fluid process that requires you to generate and test hypotheses (J. S. Beck, 1995; Persons, 1989). You must continually revise and refine your picture of the child throughout the treatment process.

A hypothesis-testing attitude toward case conceptualization necessitates good data analysis skills. First, simply constructed conceptualizations are generally the best approach (Persons, 1995). You will be weighing multiple variables—ranging from objective test scores to cultural context variables—and will be pulled to complex formulations. Yet we urge you to keep it simple.

Second, effective case conceptualization is propelled by open-mindedness. Rather than single-mindedly adhering to one perspective, we continually ask, "What's another interpretation of these data we have obtained?" You also need to hold onto explanations supported by data obtained from the client and be ready to discard hypothesis that are unsupported. Collaboration with the client facilitates case conceptualization. Sharing the conceptualization with children and their families provides a valuable sounding board for you; their reactions to the formulation likely will provide you with useful data.

CASE CONCEPTUALIZATION
AND TREATMENT PLANNING

Treatment planning provides direction and specifies a path for clinical progress. *Treatment plans* detail the sequence and timing of interventions. Not surprisingly, effective treatment planning should be based on case conceptualization. As Persons (1989) rightly argued, case conceptualization drives intervention strategies, predicts obstacles to treatment, provides a way to negotiate therapeutic dilemmas, and troubleshoots unsuccessful treatment efforts.

Shirk (1999) lamented that treatment packages are often ingredients in search of a recipe. The case conceptualization process offers a recipe for putting together the various ingredients included in a treatment plan. For example, self-monitoring and self-instructional methods may be indicated in treating an aggressive child. The case conceptualization will not only tell the therapist what techniques to use at a particular time, but also guide him/her in adapting the techniques to fit the individual child. If the child is more concrete in his/her thinking, a visual aid such as an Anger Thermometer may be used. If the child is more abstract, a traditional rating scale might be used. Psychoeducational materials should be selected on the basis of a case conceptualization. For instance, for youngsters who have good reading skills, printed materials are indicated. On the other hand, for children whose reading skills are poor, videotapes are useful.

CASE CONCEPTUALIZATION AND DIAGNOSIS

Case conceptualization clearly differs from diagnosis. Diagnostic classification systems summarize the symptoms in general terms. Case conceptualizations are personalized psychological portraits. Diagnostic classifications are atheoretical, whereas case conceptualizations are theoretically derived. Accordingly, diagnostic classifications tend to be descriptions rather than explanations. Case conceptualization offers a more explanatory hypothesis, explaining why symptoms emerge; how various environmental, interpersonal, and intrapersonal factors shape these symptom patterns; and what the relationship is between ostensibly discordant symptoms. Finally, case conceptualization is a broader clinical task than diagnosis. In fact, case conceptualization subsumes diagnosis, including it as a component but not overly weighting its importance.

CASE CONCEPTUALIZATION: "DRESSING UP" THE CLIENT PICTURE

The following section offers the multiple components that constitute a case conceptualization. If you simply review the parts, you may neglect the whole picture. As a way to simplify the case conceptualization process, we offer a "wardrobe" metaphor. Each component in the case conceptualization system is like a separate article of clothing. There are socks, shirts, skirts, shoes, hats, pants, and so on. When dressing, a person takes care to make sure a hat goes on the head and shoes are properly placed on feet. Moreover, coordination of the separate clothing articles is commonplace. Synthesizing the various components of the case conceptualization process requires similar coordination. Each variable is matched with other aspects so that a coherent whole is formed from its parts.

Once the wardrobe components are sorted and categorized, a system for applying these concepts can be implemented. You have to know how to put on the clothes—for example, you have to put pants on one leg at a time. In this way, a theoretical model shapes a case conceptualization.

In cognitive therapy, relationships exist between the various elements in a case conceptualization. Clearly, the information-processing variables are pivotal. As articulated by the cognitive model, a child's behavior patterns are learned responses shaped by the interaction of environmental, intrapersonal, interpersonal, and biological factors. Moreover, the behaviors are embedded within a cultural and developmental context. Case conceptualization addresses all these aspects.

Synthesizing the various components into a coherent whole is difficult. Children and adolescents are complex human beings whose behaviors are multiply determined. Figure 2.1 presents the components and hypothesizes relationships between the variables. The presenting problem is at the center of the conceptualization. The case conceptualization begins with the presenting problem. The cognitive model addresses five symptom clusters (physiological, mood, behavioral, cognitive, and interpersonal).

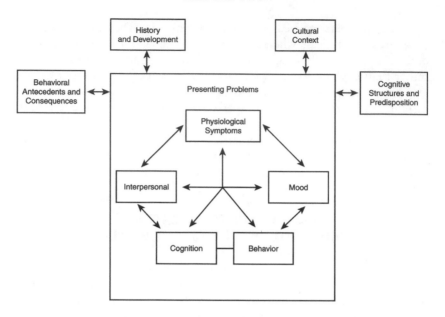

FIGURE 2.1. The relationship between the components of a case formulation.

The four variables (history/developmental, cultural context, cognitive structures, behavioral antecedents and consequences) surrounding these core problems are interrelated and influence one another.

For example, a youngster's developmental and learning history clearly has an impact on his/her presenting problem, and this in turn shapes his/her development and history. Suppose Andy is a shy, anxious child who avoids friends, school, and clubs. He fears rejection and believes he will only be safe if he stays near Mom and Dad. As a preschooler, he was behaviorally inhibited and had bad experiences at daycare. When he first started kindergarten, his mother and father became extremely anxious. All these elements contribute to his current problem. Additionally, due to his current anxiety and withdrawal, he is missing out on some important developmental opportunities like going to birthday parties and hanging out with buddies. In this way, the presenting problems and developmental history interact.

The other variables (cultural context, cognitive structures, behavioral antecedents/consequences) interact with the presenting problem in similar ways. Andy's escape response is negatively reinforced by his avoidance of anxiety. The continued escape and avoidance further supports his beliefs that anxiety is dangerous, that he can't cope without his mother's constant support, and that avoidance is the antidote to anxiety. His familial cultural context and environment may also support his anxiety. Suppose he lives in a violent neighborhood where safety is secured by close attachment to parents and home. Further, cultural beliefs regarding parenting (e.g., "A parent's job is to ensure the safety of the child. This safety is best achieved by keeping the child close by your side.") also determine behaviors.

COMPONENTS OF THE CASE FORMULATION

Presenting Problems

The first step is to define the presenting problem in a way that reflects the unique situation of the child and his/her family. We recommend being as specific as possible. Persons (1989) has suggested ways to transform general problems into discrete ones by dividing problems into their cognitive, physiological, behavioral, emotional, and interpersonal components. In this way, a personalized picture can be drawn.

For example, an 8-year-old girl presents with low self-esteem. "Low self-esteem" is a very vague, general term that does not give you a clear understanding of the specific difficulties this child faces. Through the interview and her self-report measures, your understanding of her experience of low self-esteem becomes clearer. The *behavioral* aspects included shying away from novel tasks and new people, crying, difficulty persisting with a frustrating task, and passivity. The *emotional* components included sadness, anxiety, and some irritability. Having one or two friends and being repeatedly criticized by her father represents the *interpersonal* aspects of her low self-esteem. When the child experienced these circumstances, she suffered several *physiological* reactions such as stomach cramps, headaches, and sweating. Finally, the youngster's *cognitive components* included thoughts such as "I'm no good at most things"; "People think I'm a jerk"; and "My dad thinks I'm no good." As Figure 2.2 illustrates, the vague presenting complaint has been transformed into more viable therapeutic issues. Treatment can now specifically target problem areas.

Test Data

Assessment is a key component in cognitive therapy. Many cognitive therapists rely on both interview data and information gleaned from assessment instruments. Most cognitive therapists use objective self-report measures and checklists. These instruments provide data on the presence of symptoms, as well as data on their frequency, intensity, and duration. The

GENERAL PRESENTING PROBLEM

Low self-esteem

PARTICULAR COMPONENTS

Behavioral: Shying away from novel tasks and new people, crying, difficulty persisting in a frustrating task, and passivity

Emotional: Sadness, anxiety, irritability

Interpersonal: One or two friends, repeated criticism by father

Physiological: Stomach cramps, headaches, and sweating

Cognitive: "I'm no good at most things. People think I'm a jerk. My dad thinks I'm no good."

FIGURE 2.2. Operationalizing low self-esteem.

information culled from test data may be integrated with the client's verbal report and the therapist's clinical impressions.

Typical objective self-report instruments include the Children's Depression Inventory (CDI; Kovacs, 1992), the Revised Manifest Anxiety Scale for Children (RCMAS; Reynolds & Richmond, 1985), the Multidimensional Anxiety Scale for Children (MASC; March, 1997), the Children's Behavioral Checklist (CBCL; Achenbach & Edelbrock, 1983), the Hopelessness Scale for Children (Kazdin, Rodgers, & Colbus, 1986), and the Fear Survey Schedule (Scherer & Nakamura, 1968). The Beck Depression Inventory–II (BDI-II; Beck, 1996), Beck Hopelessness Scales (BHS; Beck, 1978), and Beck Anxiety Inventory (BAI; Beck, 1990) may be used with adolescents. The Beck Scales for Children are interesting measures which are currently being constructed (J. S. Beck, personal communication, 1998).

Some cognitive therapists may elect to use the Minnesota Multiphasic Personality Inventory for Adolescents (MMPI-A; Butcher et al., 1992) to assess personality dimensions. Projective techniques such as the Thematic Apperception Test (TAT; Murray, 1943), Children's Apperception Test (CAT; Bellak & Bellak, 1949), Roberts Apperception Test for Children (RATC; McArthur & Roberts, 1982), and the Rorschach inkblot test (Exner, 1986) are used by some cognitive-behavioral clinicians.

Regardless of the instrument employed, the initial test data provide a baseline for therapeutic work. Self-report measures may be periodically readministered to evaluate treatment progress. The scores reflect severity of distress, acuity, and functionality. Accordingly, the test data augments interview data and clinical impressions. Decisions regarding initial treatment targets and future intervention strategies can be enhanced through the use of test data.

Cultural Context Variables

A major influence on family practices is ethnocultural background (Cartledge & Feng, 1996b). Since ethnocultural context shapes family socialization processes, and since these family practices influence symptom expression, you should expect a child's clinical presentation and response to treatment to be influenced by his/her cultural background (Sue, 1998).

Carter, Sbrocco, and Carter (1996) offer a useful theoretical framework for conceptualizing the way ethnicity influences symptom expression, treatment response, and help-seeking behavior. Although the model was developed for adult African American clients with anxiety disorders, the paradigm has implications for children and adolescents.

Carter et al. (1996) conceptualized clients along the dimensions of racial identity and level of acculturation. African Americans with a high level of racial identity who are highly acculturated have a firm sense of their own ethnic identity yet also accept the values of the dominant culture. Clinically, these individuals present with a high perception of personal control and an active problem-solving stance. Their symptom presentation will likely approximate the symptoms shown by their Caucasian counterparts. Carter et al. (1996) hypothesized that once these clients connect with a therapist who understands their symptoms and appreciates their ethnicity, they will stay in treatment and profit from clinical interventions.

African American clients who have a strong racial identity but low levels of acculturation will respond to treatment quite differently. These individuals have well-developed ethnic identities but ascribe to relatively few values embedded within the dominant culture. Carter and her colleagues claimed that these clients will recognize symptoms differently, attribute these symptoms to physical or spiritual causes, and likely manifest different symptoms than anxious Caucasian clients. Not surprisingly, these clients will initially seek assistance from medical professionals or clergy. Finally, Carter et al. (1996) concluded that although these clients may perceive anxious symptoms as signs that they are going crazy, they tend not to trust Caucasian mental health professionals. Accordingly, these individuals are likely to drop out of treatment early in the process.

"Culture," Cartledge and Feng (1996b) wrote, "is like a webbed system in which various aspects of life are interconnected. The various components of culture are not discrete but interactive. Kinship, economic, and religious subsystems, for example, all affect one another and cannot be understood in isolation" (p. 14). Like other history and developmental variables, there are several domains you will want to sample in your case conceptualization (Brems, 1993; Sue, 1998). Considering the child's and his/her family's level of ethnic identity and acculturation is a pivotal first step. Attitudes toward affective expression are also robust clinical variables (Brems, 1993).

Unique environmental circumstances may punctuate the lives of culturally diverse children. For example, poverty, oppression, marginalization, prejudice, and institutional racism/sexism differentially affect children from nonmajority cultures (Sanders, Merrell, & Cobb, 1999). Indeed, institutional prejudices will affect children's educational experiences. These attitudes and practices may contribute to inferior teaching, low expectations, and denigration of various individuals (Bernal, Saenz, & Knight, 1991). Indeed, minority status itself may represent a stressor (Carter et al., 1996; Tharp, 1991). These conditions may contribute to particular thoughts, feelings, and behavior patterns that are embedded in the problem expression. Forehand and Kotchick (1996) wrote that "because ethnic minority families of lower socioeconomic status experience stressors in their lives not typically present in the lives of middle-class European families, they may not respond in the same manner to established treatment techniques or maintain the gains for as long as families in the middle income range" (p. 200). For example, it is an unfortunately common occurrence that children of color are frequently "tracked" by clerks in retail stores. Greater levels of irritability and anxiety would be natural accompaniments to this stressful experience. Zayas and Solari (1994) wrote, "The cumulative effects of socioeconomic disadvantage and negative stereotypes felt by racial and ethnic minority families lead them to develop adaptive strategies based on their beliefs about what it means to be a member of an ethnic minority or racial minority group" (p. 201).

Consider the following example. Alex, the only Latino boy in his sixth-grade class in a suburban school, felt excluded and uneasy all year. One day a classmate reported that his collection of gel pens was missing. For no apparent reason, many children blamed Alex. Although he was later exonerated, Alex withdrew more into himself, his schoolwork suffered, and he ended up being referred to your clinical practice. Upon presentation, Alex seems quiet, sullen, emotionally restricted, and withdrawn; he avoids eye contact, appears suspicious, and acts like he has a chip on his shoulder. It would be easy to label this child as resistant. However, considering the hassles he has been experiencing in school, his behavior is totally understandable. He likely equates therapy with punishment and expects the therapist to blame, reject, and perhaps pigeonhole him into a biased stereotype.

Language clearly mediates attitudes, behaviors, and emotional expression. Tharp (1991) rightly noted that culture shapes linguistic courtesies and conventions. For instance, length of pauses, rhythm of speech, and rules for turn taking in conversation are culturally defined. For example, white children tell stories that are topic-centered and thematically cohesive with temporal references (Michaels, 1984, as cited by Tharp, 1991). African American children tell less topic-centered stories that were more anecdotal and topic-associative. Interestingly, the Caucasian audience saw the African American story as incoherent whereas the African American audience viewed the story as interesting and detailed. This finding suggests that youngsters will tell their "stories" in various ways and we, as therapists, need to shape our interventions accordingly.

Different cultural groups may hold varying beliefs regarding obedience to authority (Johnson, 1993). The way these families react to the therapist's "authority" shapes their response to therapy. For instance, for individuals whose culture dictates relative deference to authority figures, collaborating with and giving negative feedback to the therapist will be unsettling. Conversely, the therapist's direction will be expected and welcomed. Additionally, children may be expected to dutifully comply with all parental requests.

As you can see, cultural context issues can impact a youngster's clinical presentation and response to treatment. In Table 2.1, we provide a sample list of questions to highlight important issues. While this list is not exhaustive, it may direct your attention to some heretofore neglected areas and alert you to other points worth considering. Regardless of the question asked, an appreciation of the youngster's cultural context should be integrated within the case conceptualization.

TABLE 2.1. Sample Questions Addressing Cultural Context Issues

- What is the level of acculturation in the family?
- How does the level of acculturation shape symptom expression?
- What characterizes the child's ethnocultural identity?
- How does this identity influence symptom expression?
- What are the child and family thinking and feeling as a member of this culture?
- How do ethnocultural beliefs, values, and practices shape problem expression?
- How representative or typical is this family of the culture?
- What feelings and thoughts are proscribed as taboo?
- What feelings and thoughts are facilitated and promoted as a function of ethnocultural context?
- What ethnocultural specific socialization processes selectively reinforce some thoughts, feelings, and behaviors but not others?
- What types of prejudice and marginalization has the child/family encountered?
- How have these experiences shaped symptom expression?
- What beliefs about oneself, the world, and the future have developed as a result of these experiences?

History and Developmental Milestones

Obtaining a personal and developmental history is standard clinical fare for most mental health professionals. Historical or background information yields data regarding the youngster's past learning. Historical data place the present complaints into an appropriate context. The frequency, duration, and intensity of the child's problems can be more soundly established.

Knowing how a child navigates developmental milestones also provides key information for case conceptualization. Typically, developmental delays will make a child more vulnerable to perceived criticism and lead to intolerance of negative affective states and possibly to depression. If the delays affect cognitive, emotional, and/or behavioral processing, the therapeutic approach may need to be modified. For instance, a child who has significant language and reading problems is unlikely to profit from sophisticated reading materials. Accordingly, simplification of the materials may be indicated.

Patterns of emotional and behavioral dysregulation are amplified through considering developmental milestones and learning history. For instance, a pattern of behavioral and emotional dysregulation may be revealed by a child's chronic sleeping, eating, and toileting problems; by aggressive behavior with peers; or by poor adjustment to changes in routine. Constitutional or temperamental vulnerability factors likely interact with environmental factors to produce children's behavior.

Developmental and historical data provides information regarding the child's caretakers as well as the child him/herself. For example, the accuracy and completeness of the caretakers' recall of developmental information is revealing. What might it mean if a mother is virtually clueless regarding the child's developmental achievements? Perhaps the mother has a poor memory for events, but she also might be inattentive and/or lacking in concern. You might then inquire what was going on during these times. Was the mother depressed or drinking? Was she suffering through marital conflict? Therapists might also develop hypotheses regarding parents who recall the minute details of a child's life (e.g., day, time, and year of first pooping in potty). Are these parents simply detail-oriented or do they tend to be so overattentive and overinvolved that they psychologically "crowd" their child?

Work and relationships are generally major history-taking foci in adult interviews. Children's "work" is play and school. A youngster's play activities, clubs, sports, and hobbies are quite revealing. Does the child enjoy solitary, isolative activities? Competitive games? Fantasy games? Additionally, examining a child's peer relationships is fruitful. Who are the child's friends? Does the child have friends who are his/her own age? Are they younger or older? How long do his/her friendships last? Are his/her friendships arduously made but easily lost?

Gathering information on the youngster's adjustment to and performance in school is a key task. School is a place where children respond to demands, demonstrate productivity, and interact with others. How is the youngster's academic performance? What factors compromise academic functioning (e.g., learning disabilities)? Has performance declined? How does he/she get along with others? How does he/she regulate his/her behavior in the classroom? How does the child respond to teachers' directives/commands? Has he/she ever been suspended or expelled?

Family relationships and attachment processes also convey meaningful information. Knowing how the different family members interact and get along gives the therapist more information about the child's functioning. Moreover, it places the child's behavior within a family context, allowing the therapist to discuss the similarities and differences in the child's functioning in various circumstances. For example, is the child aggressive at school but not at home? Is the child clingy at home but not at school? Does the child respond more compliantly to mother's directives than to father's commands?

Collecting information on the disciplinary practices employed by parents is a vital task for clinicians. Therapists will need to know how desirable behavior is promoted and undesirable behavior is discouraged. What parenting or child behavior management strategies are employed? What are the parents' styles? Are they overcontrolling, indulgent, authoritarian, authoritative, permissive, unattuned, or inattentive? How consistently do they apply consequences? Do parents/caretakers agree on the behavior to be promoted or discouraged? Do they agree on disciplinary methods?

We also suggest checking on the youngster's previous treatment experiences. The type, duration, and response to treatment are useful data points. Similarly, family and personal medical information is critical in uncovering medical conditions that may exacerbate psychological problems or psychological disorders that may exacerbate medical conditions. For instance, any chronic medical condition will be a stressor for children and their families. Psychological issues regarding control and autonomy may affect compliance with medical regimens. Family illness may also be a significant issue for children. Children understandably worry about ill caretakers. Not surprisingly, medical consultation is recommended in all these cases.

Substance use is also a major area for history taking. Illegal drugs, prescription medications, over-the-counter medicines, alcohol, household products (e.g., glue, aerosol products), cigarettes, laxatives, and even food items are just a few of the potential sources of substance abuse. Substance use and abuse clearly complicates symptom presentation. Moreover, youngsters tend not to be particularly forthcoming about their substance use. Nonetheless, therapists are strongly encouraged to examine possible substance abuse in the children and adolescents they treat.

The child's involvement with the legal system should also be considered. Involvement with the juvenile court system or law enforcement agencies should be noted. Clearly, a youth's legal problems reflect overall problem severity. Additionally, consultation with legal authorities may be indicated.

We realize that while this is not an exhaustive list of clinical considerations, it is nonetheless a great deal to think about. We summarize some of the pivotal questions in Table 2.2 as an organizational guide.

Cognitive Variables

The cognitive variables in the case conceptualization process were briefly noted in Chapter 1. Case conceptualization should consider cognitive processes, cognitive structure, and cognitive content. Not surprisingly, a case conceptualization addresses automatic thoughts, underlying assumptions, schemata, and cognitive distortions.

As previously mentioned, automatic thoughts reflect the explanations or predictions that accompany events and represent cognitive content. Automatic thoughts tend to be relatively easily accessible and can be readily identified through standard interventions. The automatic thought content often serves as the initial treatment target and provides clues regarding the core schema.

As mentioned in Chapter 1, schemata represent core organizing beliefs or personal meaning structures (A. T. Beck et al., 1979; A. T. Beck & Freeman, 1990) and are considered cognitive structures. Schemata exist out of awareness, yet profoundly influence cognitive processes and content. Understanding youngsters' schemata provides insight regarding multiple clinical variables such as the changeability of automatic thoughts, interpersonal behavior, responsiveness to treatment, and probability of relapse.

Schemata work to maintain homeostasis (Guidano & Liotti, 1983; Padesky, 1994). Information that is consistent with the meaning structure is assimilated, whereas discrepant information is rejected or transformed so that it matches the schema. As Liotti (1987) aptly noted regarding this process, "Novelty is actively reduced to what is already known" (p. 93).

Schemata are self-perpetuating. Young (1990) proposed three mechanisms that serve this self-perpetuating tendency. Schema maintenance processes preserve the cognitive structure through cognitive distortions and self-defeating behavior patterns. Recognizing the cognitive distor-

TABLE 2.2. Important Areas in History Taking

Developmental milestones

- Were there remarkable delays in developmental milestone?
- Are there language and speech problems?
- How well does the child read?
- How well does the child write?
- When did the child sleep through the night? How would you characterize the child's sleeping patterns and habits?
- When was the child toilet trained? How did it go? What were the difficulties? Have there been many toileting accidents?
- How would you describe the child's eating patterns?
- How does this child characteristically respond to changes in his/her routine?
- What type of baby was he/she? Fussy? Colicky? Sweet disposition? Etc.
- Who has taken care of this child? Has there been disruptions or inconsistency in the caretaking?
- Has he/she ever been a victim of sexual or physical abuse?

School

- What is the child's academic performance like? Has there been a decline in performance?
- How does he/she get along with classmates? Teachers?
- What was his/her adjustment to school like? How are his/her mornings before school? How are his/her afternoons after school?
- Has the child ever been expelled? Suspended? Received detention?
- How is the child's school attendance?

Peers and activities

- What are the child's activities?
- Who are the child's friends?
- How long do the child's friendships last?
- Are the child's friendships arduously made but easily lost?

Family relationships

- What is the child's relationship with each caretaker? Sibling?
- What is the household climate like? Conflictual? Warm? Permissive?
- What is the relationship like between major caretakers?
- Has the child ever witnessed domestic violence?
- How is the child's behavior similar and different with each family member?
- How does the child's family relationships differ from his/her relationships with others?

Disciplinary practices

- What disciplinary techniques are used?
- What techniques work well and/or don't work well?
- What are the parents' styles?
- Do the parents agree on discipline?

Medical conditions and previous treatment

- What medical/physical conditions are present?
- How do these medical conditions influence psychological functioning?
- How do the psychological conditions influence the medical condition?
- What has been the child's and family's response to past treatment?

Substance use and legal involvement

- What is the child's substance use?
- What is the child's use of laxatives, food, over-the-counter medicines? Household products?
- What is the extent of legal involvement?

tions embedded in youngsters' automatic thoughts facilitates more complete case conceptualization and intervention. For instance, personalization is well suited to the Responsibility Pie intervention discussed in Chapters 8 and 9. Time projection works well with emotional reasoning. Additionally, cognitive distortions mediate the way children view therapy and the therapist. For example, a child who frequently uses discounting may dismiss success in therapy and find it difficult to internalize treatment gains.

Young (1990) hypothesized that schemata also operate through schema avoidance. Schema avoidance can take three forms: cognitive avoidance, emotional avoidance, and behavioral avoidance. The purpose of schema avoidance is to prevent experiences that would question the schema's accuracy. In *cognitive avoidance*, the thoughts that trigger the schema are blocked. A good example is when you ask a distressed youngster what is going through his/her mind at the moment of an intense mood shift and he/she responds with an "I don't know." Sometimes cognitive avoidance is indicated by the youngster's sense that his/her mind is blank (e.g., "Nothing is going through my mind."). For such clients, their thoughts are too painful, embarrassing, or shameful to identify.

With *emotional avoidance*, instead of blocking the thoughts connected to the schema, the individual blocks the feelings associated with his/her thoughts. Young (1990) astutely remarked that self-mutilation (i.e., cutting or burning oneself) is often a function of emotional avoidance. The youngster may experience a prohibited feeling (e.g., anger) and then try to avoid the feeling by burning him/herself with a cigarette lighter.

Social isolation, agoraphobia, and procrastination are examples of *behavioral avoidance* (Young, 1990). In such cases, children do not perform behaviors that are related to the schema content. Since they avoid the behaviors, the schema content remains unquestioned.

Schema compensation is the last schema process. In *schema compensation*, the child acts in ways that are opposite to the schema content. For example, a boy may bully and mercilessly tease other children as a way to compensate for a schema reflecting weakness and a fragile sense of self. In the bully example, the boy does not have to deal with his perceived weakness and sense of inadequacy thanks to his threatening behavior. However, if the bullying and belittling fails, the youngster is ill equipped to manage his fragility.

A recent study by Taylor and Ingram (1999) suggests that negative cognitive schemata may contribute to children's depression in children as young as 8 years old. They concluded that "each time a negative mood state is encountered, high risk children may be developing, accumulating, strengthening, and consolidating the reservoir of information in the dysfunctional self-referent cognitive structures that will guide their views of themselves and how information is processed when adverse events evoke these structures in the future" (p. 208). Thus, schematic influence on children's psychological functioning may begin in children of elementary school age. However, schemata may not consolidate until adolescence (Hammen & Zupan, 1984). Therefore, appreciation of schema processes may be most pivotal in cognitive therapy with adolescents.

Behavioral Antecedents and Consequences

Behavioral responses are molded by stimuli that both precede and follow the behavior (Bandura, 1977, 1986). The classic A (antecedent), B (behavior), and C (consequences) behavioral paradigm nicely illustrates this process (Barkley, Edwards, & Robin, 1999; Feindler & Ecton, 1986). Antecedent and consequent determinants may be learned either vicariously (e.g., through observation) or by direct experience (Bandura, 1977, 1986).

Depending on the learning circumstance, antecedent stimuli may either directly elicit the behavior or simply set the stage for the behavior to occur. If the behavior is acquired through classical conditioning, certain stimuli have come to elicit emotionally charged behavior. In these instances, stimuli acquire the capacity to pull out an emotional response from the child. For example, suppose a demanding fifth-grade teacher slams his book closed every time he is about to announce a pop quiz. Suppose too that any quiz or test generates a variety of aversive physiological, emotional, and cognitive stimuli in a youth. Over time, through repeated pairings, the teacher's slamming of the book can elicit the same anticipatory anxiety in the youth as the quiz itself.

Antecedent stimuli "trigger" children's behavior. "Stressors" in children's lives are generally antecedent stimuli (e.g., parents' divorce, teacher's criticisms, peer's taunts). For example, antecedent stimuli are often recorded in the event column in a thought diary (described in Chapter 6), in subjective ratings of distress scales (described in Chapter 12), and on an ABC worksheet (described in Chapter 13).

Parental commands represent antecedent stimuli. Vague, indirect, hostile, and confusing parental directives rarely produce the desired behavior in a child. Rather, they often set the stage for noncompliance and contribute to coercive power struggles. Antecedent cues that set the stage for behavior are often called discriminative stimuli. Discriminative stimuli signal the child that the situation is right for reinforcement. When children selectively respond in the presence of discriminative stimuli and inhibit behavior in their absence, the behavior comes under stimulus control.

Behavioral consequences refer to the stimuli that follow a behavior. Consequences determine whether the specific behavior is strengthened or weakened. Consequent stimuli that strengthen a behavior or cause it to occur more frequently or enduringly are called *reinforcers*. There are two basic reinforcement processes: positive reinforcement (adding something pleasant to increase the rate of behavior) and negative reinforcement (removing something unpleasant to increase the rate of behavior). A father who praises and hugs his son for getting a good grade is using positive reinforcement. A teacher who removes a penalty like extra homework due to her students' improved performance is using negative reinforcement to increase study habits.

Punishment decreases the rate of behavior. For example, a father who responds to his son's tantrums by giving him a time-out, denying him rewards and privileges, or ignoring him is using punishment. Take the case of a mother who ignores her daughter's emotional expression thereby punishing this affective expressiveness. Not surprisingly, the child learns feelings are bad and becomes emotionally constricted. Basic reinforcement and punishment procedures are described in greater detail in Chapter 14.

Reinforcers and punishers occur on schedules. Schedules of reinforcement set the arrangement for contingencies. Stipulating how much behavior is required, how long the behavior is required to persist, or how often the behavior must occur before it merits reinforcement are reinforcement schedules. It is well known that behaviors established under intermittent schedules of reinforcement are quite enduring.

PLANNING AND THINKING AHEAD: PROVISIONAL FORMULATION, TREATMENT PLAN, AND EXPECTED OBSTACLES

Provisional Formulation

The provisional formulation coordinates the components in a dynamic and interrelated way. The formulation paints a picture of the youngster's external environment and inner world. The presenting problems, test data, cultural context, history and developmental data, behavioral variables, and cognitive variables are analyzed and integrated. In this way, you create an individualized psychological portrait that allows you to tailor the interventions to each child's unique circumstances and styles.

Anticipated Treatment Plan

The provisional formulation guides your treatment plan. Treatment plans vary from child to child since they must take into account each child's unique characteristics and circumstances. For instance, an anxious child who blushes, sweats, and has lots of muscle tension would probably benefit from relaxation training, whereas a worried child with ruminations and self-critical thoughts would not benefit from this kind of training. The formulation will inform you about when to use the conventional cognitive-behavioral techniques and when to creatively modify the traditional procedures. For example, a depressed child who has more developed verbal skills would profit from a reattribution done with paper and pencil whereas a less verbally sophisticated child may gain from a reattribution techniques done with arts and crafts.

Expected Obstacles

The route toward therapeutic progress is often bumpy. If you can anticipate the bumps or potholes on the road, you can swerve to avoid them or brace yourself for impact. The formulation helps you see the road ahead and predict obstacles. In this way, you can shape your treatment plan so you can negotiate therapeutic impasses.

For instance, if a child is perfectionistic, you might expect the child to procrastinate or avoid doing homework due to fears of failure. Or suppose you are treating an oppositional youngster whose parents are very inconsistent in their care. This child comes to therapy very irregularly. Since you know the parents inconsistently follow through on their own assignments, you will have advance warning to get plans in place to manage these difficulties.

CASE CONCEPTUALIZATION EXAMPLE

Presenting Problems

Tessa is a 9-year-old African American girl who is being cared for by her mother and her aunt. She presents as a well-behaved but fearful and sad child. Her schoolwork consistently receives A's and B's. However, her teachers complain that Tessa is slow to complete her assignments and frequently requires considerable reassurance. She often cries in class during new assignments or during group projects. At lunch and recess, she wanders around the playground, sits by herself, or elects to stay in the classroom to read with the teacher rather than play with her classmates. More specifically, the physiological components of Tessa's problems include stomachaches, sweating, and headaches. Her mood symptoms are marked by fear, anxiety, and sadness. Behaviorally, she cries frequently, is restless and fidgety, is slow to turn in work, and requests to see the nurse frequently. Interpersonally, she appears shy and withdrawn. Her cognitive components include automatic thoughts such as "I'm going to mess up and everyone will notice," "Everybody is waiting for me to mess up," "I'm not going to be OK at school without my mom," and "The other kids in class don't like me."

Test Data

Tessa completes the Children's Depression Inventory (CDI) and Revised Children's Manifest Anxiety Scale (RCMAS). On the CDI, Tessa obtains a raw score of 18, which suggests a moderate level of depression. On the RCMAS, her total score is 18, indicating moderate anxiety. She scores relatively high on subscales for worry and social concerns.

Cultural Context Variables

Tessa's mother's income is quite limited. They struggle to make ends meet but they live above the poverty line. Tessa, her mother, and her aunt all belong to the same Baptist church. The church offers some social support to them. They have a few relatives in the area who occasionally visit and babysit. The family lives in a low-rent area where rates are relatively moderate. Tessa attends a predominantly Caucasian school and she is one of a few African American children in her grade. Both Tessa and her mother did not report specific instances of Tessa experiencing prejudice or racism. Her mother did say, "I tell her she has to be twice as good, well-behaved, and smart to compete with her white friends." Tessa's mother describes her daughter's teachers as "friendly and cooperative" but she says she gets a feeling that school personnel are walking on egg shells. "I think they are afraid or uncomfortable about dealing with me. I don't know why. Maybe they just aren't used to people like me."

Mother gives Tessa lots of "survival instructions." She warns her about walking home from the bus stop and gives her specific instructions on how to walk from her house to a nearby grocery store. "I don't want anybody to mess with her. When I was her age I could defend myself but Tessa is different. She takes things personally."

History and Developmental Milestones

Tessa reached and completed all her developmental milestones within normal age limits. In the past she is described as a serious and anxious child, but her mood symptoms have exacerbated within the last several weeks. Her mother, who is diagnosed with major depressive disorder and takes Prozac, discloses that her own depression seems worse during the last few months.

Tessa has always been a good student. Her grades remain consistently good and she presents with no behavioral problems. As a toddler and preschooler, she attended daycare and preschool where she initially displayed some separation anxiety, but she subsequently adjusted to the school routine. Tessa regularly gets quite nervous the week before the first day of a new school year and seems worried on Monday mornings. She says she does not like waiting for the bus or riding on the bus. Sometimes she worries that her aunt will not pick her up at the bus stop. She recalls that her most embarrassing moment at school was when the other kids made fun of the gift she gave for a holiday grabbag ("It's so small and cheap!").

Tessa plays soccer and baseball, and takes flute lessons. In her free time, she enjoys reading and watching television. She has a few friends in her neighborhood, with whom she plays typical childhood games. Tessa likes to play with younger children and take care of them. She rarely fights or argues with friends. She gets invited to birthday parties for her school friends but elects not to go. Her invitations in the last year seem to have decreased.

Tessa's father left when she was 9 months old; she has not seen him since that time. Her mother and aunt get along well and generally agree on disciplinary practices. Tessa's mother claims that her sister thinks she is "babying" Tessa. Her mother reports that she is the "authority" in the house, but also discloses that she thinks she has been more lax in her discipline since she has been more depressed. Her primary disciplinary techniques are praise, hugging, time-out, and removing rewards and privileges. Mother says she does not believe in physical punishment because she was "whooped" as a child. She did not want to spank her daughter. Mother also reports she has not had much energy to do one-on-one activities with Tessa. She feels guilty about this and blames her tiring schedule and increasing depression for her low energy level.

Tessa does not use drugs or drink alcohol. She has no legal troubles. This is her first psychotherapy experience. Mother has seen a family practice physician for her medication but has never seen a therapist. Mother hopes Tessa will find "someone she can talk to and confide in" in therapy. Tessa is not quite sure what to make of coming to therapy.

Cognitive Variables

Tessa's automatic thoughts include beliefs such as "I'm going to mess up and everyone will notice," "Everybody is waiting for me to mess up,"

"I'm not going to be OK at school without Mom," "The other kids in class don't like me," "I have to be good so I don't tire Mom out," "The world has lots of awful dangers," "I don't think I can protect myself," "I'm not as smart or strong as most other kids," "Being frightened means something bad will happen," and "I don't think I fit in." Her characteristic cognitive distortions include all-or-none thinking, personalization, overgeneralization, emotional reasoning, and labeling. Since Tessa is only 9, it is likely that her schemata are not fully formed. However, she may be vulnerable to developing core beliefs such as "I'm vulnerable and fragile in a critical and harsh world where others are unresponsive and judgmental," "Being different makes me an outcast in a world where others are smarter and stronger," "I must be constantly alert to all the dangers so I can avoid them," and "Mistakes are catastrophic in a critical world where others are critical and I am weaker than they are."

Behavioral Antecedents and Consequences

Transitions from home to school, especially on Monday mornings, are clear triggers for or antecedents to Tessa's symptoms. Additionally, new assignments, group projects, critical feedback, and ambiguous situations such as recess stimulate her anxious and depressed feelings. Unresponsiveness by adult caretaking figures and other children (e.g., mother, aunt, teachers) also triggers beliefs such as "They don't care about me" or "They don't like me." Tessa's avoidance, withdrawal, and checking behavior on her assignments are not only emitted in these stimuli but are reinforced by relief from anxiety. Her checking is positively reinforced by her good grades and praise from Mom. Her reassurance seeking is also intermittently positively and negatively reinforced. At times, she feels comforted by authority figures; the simple act of seeking reassurance provides anxiety relief. Her quiet behavior is reinforced in the classroom. Tessa's somatic complaints also have functional value. They elicit caretaking from others, which Tessa finds satisfying. Tessa's eagerness to please is also positively reinforced by others' approval.

Provisional Formulation

Tessa is a young African American girl who is experiencing primarily anxious and depressive symptoms. Her cognitions are marked by themes of fear of negative evaluation and self-criticism. Behaviorally, she responds to such threats through hypervigilance, approval/reassurance seeking, and withdrawal from peers. Many of her psychological symptoms are translated into somatic symptoms. It is possible that

Tessa fears negative evaluation by others if she is more emotionally expressive.

Certainly, environmental factors feed into the initiation, maintenance, and exacerbation of her distress. Both Tessa and her mother are aware of the racial differences between her and her classmates. Tessa has likely internalized Mom's encouragement to "work twice as hard as her white friends." Therefore, she feels put on the spot to perform, compete, and fit in. These are a lot of strong feelings for a young child. Moreover, thoughts such as "Everybody is waiting for me to mess up" reflect her sense that she is on display. This propels her social anxiety. For a youngster who experiences such pressure in a context where people are walking on egg shells, reassurance is expected. Indeed, it is a way for Tessa to gage how she is doing.

Tessa sees herself as fragile in a critical and threatening world. In order not to be damaged, she withdraws and behaves extremely cautiously. Indeed, cautious behavior is adaptive in her neighborhood and at times with her classmates. However, because she is so cautious, her peers taunt and intimidate her. Mom also tends to be overprotective. The overprotection and peer teasing further reinforce her negative self-perceptions.

Anticipated Treatment Plan

1. Due to Tessa's high level of somatic complaints, relaxation training should be initiated.
2. Pleasant event scheduling should be attempted to increase her level of positive reinforcement.
3. Cognitive interventions aimed at ameliorating her fears of negative evaluation should begin with self-instructional approaches and progress to techniques involving more rational analysis.
4. Care should be directed toward Tessa's attributions around her awareness of the racial differences between her and her classmates. If she is making self-damaging attributions, cognitive techniques such as reattribution procedures should be employed.
5. Problem-solving strategies should be taught to Tessa throughout the treatment process.
6. Cognitive techniques aimed at Tessa's view of herself as fragile should also be initiated.
7. Tessa's mother should be included in child-centered parent training to develop a contingency management program for therapy homework completion. Additionally, therapy should focus on helping the mother decrease her overprotectiveness and increase

her consistency in responding to Tessa's needs. Care will need to be directed toward increasing consistency and communication between Tessa's major caretakers (i.e., mother and aunt).

8. Depending on Tessa's social skill level, social skills training in response to peers' teasing should be considered.

9. After Tessa has sufficiently acquired, practiced, and applied her skills, behavioral experiments should be collaboratively designed that will test Tessa's inaccurate predictions.

10. Ongoing collaboration with the teacher and other school personnel should be maintained.

Expected Obstacles

Tessa is an eager and motivated young client. Therefore, noncompliance is not expected to be an issue. However, Tessa does have a tendency to "overdo." Therefore, we should be alert to perfectionistic efforts at homework completion. Additionally, since Tessa is so eager to please and fears negative evaluation, we will have to watch out for signs that she is minimizing her symptoms or inhibiting dissatisfactions about the therapy. Finally, due to Tessa's strong written and oral expressive skills, we will have to be alert to the possibility that Tessa will initially provide intellectualized responses rather than emotionally present ones.

Working with Tessa's attributions regarding racial differences will be crucial. Helping Tessa to comfortably explore her thoughts and feelings about these issues without exacerbating her social anxieties will be difficult. Focusing on both the content and process issues in therapy (e.g., What is it like to talk about these thoughts and feelings?, What is the danger in talking about these thoughts and feelings?) is important.

Parental work will also present challenges. Mother's level of depression will need to be monitored. If indicated, individual therapy for mother may need to be recommended. In this instance, attention to the cost of care is critical. Regardless, the child-focused parental work will need to be sensitive to mother's depression. For instance, pleasant activity scheduling may be an arduous task when Mom is depressed. Due to her depressed mother, attention may be inordinately focused on Tessa's vulnerabilities. Finally, Mom may find it difficult to marshal the psychological energy to respond to Tessa and increase her communication with her sister.

Consulting with the school may also present some obstacles. Establishing a partnership with Tessa's teacher is a good idea. We likely would coach the teacher on ways to help reduce Tessa's reassurance seeking and avoidance. Increasing the teacher's sensitivity to Tessa's anxiety would be another proper strategy.

CONCLUSION

Case conceptualization brings together the processes and procedures outlined in the following chapters. Each case is unique; the clinical application of the general techniques described must appreciate this uniqueness. By emphasizing case conceptualization, you avoid a "one-size-fits-all" clinical mentality. When you get stuck with your cases, refer back to this chapter and allow yourself to reconceptualize, redesign, and ultimately refresh your therapeutic work.

3

❖

Collaborative Empiricism
and Guided Discovery

Each cognitive-behavioral technique is adapted to the individual child through empiricism and guided discovery. These concepts allow us to adjust our treatment to the dynamic needs of different children. In this chapter, we define collaborative empiricism and guided discovery. In addition, we discuss how various issues (e.g., age, motivation, ethnicity, stage of therapy) influence collaborative empiricism and guided discovery.

Critics often argue that cognitive therapists neglect the therapeutic relationship (Gluhoski, 1995; Wright & Davis, 1994). However, this argument is ill-founded and paints a caricature rather than a true picture of cognitive therapy. Indeed, the seminal cognitive therapy manual (A. T. Beck et al., 1979) explicitly states that therapists must be able to communicate in an empathic, concerned, warm, and genuine manner. Moreover, "slighting the therapeutic relationship" (p. 27) is decried as a common therapeutic pitfall. Collaborative empiricism and guided discovery go beyond mere rapport building to concretely construct productive therapy relationships that encourage therapeutic momentum.

A. T. Beck et al. (1979) aptly state that "the therapist applying cognitive therapy is continuously active and deliberately interacting with the patient" (p. 6). Cognitive therapy embraces the notion that the therapy relationship reflects a collaborative balance between therapist and clients. Therapists and children are true partners in the therapeutic journey. Of course, collaboration does not imply equality. We often talk to children about being teammates in their treatment and discuss the therapeutic relationship in terms of "teamwork." Some children and adolescents are initially surprised by this approach: "Imagine—an adult authority figure is giving me a chance to shape my treatment!" We have found that youngsters welcome this stance. Moreover, many youngsters come to realize that while a collaborative approach offers them opportunities for input, it also encourages responsibility. The following exchange illustrates a collaborative process.

THERAPIST: It would help me if you would write down a list of things you would like to work on when we talk together. How does that sound to you?

JAKE: Why do we need a list?

THERAPIST: A list can help us keep track of things so we don't forget something that might be important later on.

JAKE: I'm not sure about this list.

THERAPIST: Let's talk about it then. What troubles you about making this list?

This example illustrates the importance of collaborating even on the most ostensibly benign therapeutic tasks. Obviously, Jake had some objections to making the list. If the therapist did not check in with Jake, she might have steamrolled through the technique, flattening Jake in the process and triggering his avoidance. By addressing Jake's objections early and explicitly, the therapist communicates respect for him, honors his hesitancy, and directly involves him in the therapeutic process.

The "empiricism" in the term *collaborative empiricism* refers to the data-based approach of cognitive therapy. Data comes directly from the client and reflects cognitive therapy's phenomenological foundations (Alford & Beck, 1997; Pretzer & Beck, 1996). "The client's experience dictates how general principles will be applied to help current problems" (Padesky & Greenberger, 1995, p. 6). Children's beliefs are viewed as hypotheses to be tested. Thoughts are not a priori viewed as distorted or inaccurate (Alford & Beck, 1997). Rather, the accuracy and functional value of the thoughts are evaluated through an empirical process wherein children and therapists function like detectives sifting through various clues (Kendall et al., 1992).

Dattilio and Padesky (1990) aptly wrote that "emphasis is placed on the collaborative aspect of the approach, on the assumption that people learn to change their thinking more readily if the rationale for change comes from their own insights rather than from the therapist" (p. 5). Guided discovery helps youngsters build a database for rational analysis.

A proper guided discovery recipe has many different ingredients. Empathy, Socratic questioning, behavioral experiments, and homework may compose the guided discovery process. Like a recipe, the particular ingredients will vary from child to child depending upon what the therapy is designed to "cook up."

The guided discovery process is designed to cast doubt on the certainty of clients' beliefs (A. T. Beck et al., 1979; Padesky, 1988). Rather than coercing the child to think what he/she thinks, the therapist employs guided discovery to encourage children to create more adaptive/functional explanations for themselves. The simplicity and straightforwardness of this principle is deceiving. In fact, when we reflect back on our own training experiences, we both remember that promoting guided discovery was one of the most difficult lessons to learn. The therapist's urge to provide the child or adolescent with an answer or a new interpretation is an understandable one. Many times we want to say, "Let me tell you what to think." Guided discovery requires more patience and artful questioning on the part of the therapist, which permits children and adolescents to build new appraisals for themselves. In our experience, remaining faithful to guided discovery enables us to sensitively tune into youngsters' inner worlds.

Guided discovery and collaborative empiricism foster an atmosphere of curiosity shared by therapist and child (Padesky & Greenberger, 1995). The therapist is interested, inquisitive, and eager to learn more about the child's personal paradigms (A. T. Beck et al., 1979). By sticking to a curious stance, therapists model and promote flexible thinking, which leads to examining the problem from many angles. In order to see each corner of a child's experience, we often turn the problem on its ear to get a different perspective. For us, this is one of the most exciting aspects of cognitive therapy. Quite frankly, it keeps the work fresh. For example, a youngster was unwilling to show his parents some of the work he was doing in therapy. We initially thought he was ashamed of what he was thinking or feeling or was worried about his parents' reaction. When we asked him about sharing his homework, his response surprised us: "It's my special time. It's something I want to keep just to myself."

Consider the following example. A 14-year-old African American honor student has moved from a school with predominantly African American students to one with a predominantly Caucasian student body. Prior to the move, she experienced no symptoms and was functioning at an extremely high level (e.g., class president, star athlete). After several months at the new school, she develops various anxious and depressed symptoms. While there are some expected cognitions associated with her symptoms (e.g., "I'm not making the grade, I'm letting my family down. Nothing will work out."), these thoughts are not directly tied to the most pressing problem. This young woman perceives rejection from the Caucasian students due to her ethnicity, as well as rejection from the few other African Americans due to her scholastic ability. Through collaborative empiricism and guided discovery, the youngster finally admits her true thoughts: "I'm all alone. I can't fit in anywhere. The black kids think I'm acting white and the white kids want nothing to do with me. I think they're scared of me." Through collaborative empiricism and guided discovery, the core subjective experiences impinging on the youngster's humanity are identified and worked through.

CONTINUUM OF COLLABORATION
AND GUIDED DISCOVERY

Collaborative empiricism and guided discovery are not all-or-none constructs. Figure 3.1 represents the continuum of guided discovery and collaboration. Over the course of treatment, clinicians adjust the level of collaboration and guided discovery. In some instances therapists are highly

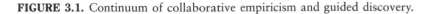

Low Collaboration Low Guided Discovery	Early in Treatment	Later in Treatment	High Collaboration High Guided Discovery
	High acuity	Low acuity	
	Younger children	Older children	
	Low motivation	High motivation	
	Passive, dependent children	Autonomous, active youngsters	
	Less reactant to control	Highly reactant to control	
	Client has more adherence to cultural prescriptions regarding obedience to authority	Client has less adherence to cultural prescriptions regarding obedience to authority	
	Questioning seen as unacceptable by client's culture	Questioning seen as acceptable by client's culture	
	Low tolerance for ambiguity	High tolerance for ambiguity	
	Low frustration tolerance	High frustration tolerance	
	High impulsivity	Low impulsivity	

FIGURE 3.1. Continuum of collaborative empiricism and guided discovery.

collaborative (e.g., with lower acuity, highly motivated, autonomous youngsters), whereas in other circumstances they may employ a lower level of collaboration (e.g., with higher acuity, lower motivation, more passive children). When therapists become frustrated, they often lapse into an authoritarian role rather than maintain an authoritative collaborative stance. In these cases, the therapeutic relationship grows more adversarial and debating and arguing moves the therapist away from an advocacy position. Of course, mindlessly agreeing with or refusing to challenge clients does not propel therapy forward. Both stances force therapists into increasingly narrow clinical options.

The *stage in therapy* is an important consideration for determining the level of collaboration and guided discovery. Early in treatment, we generally assume a more active role in the treatment process. Most children and adolescents do not yet know the rules, roles, responsibilities, and expectations of therapy. Families see us as experts and then naturally behave as more passive recipients of treatment. Accordingly, the socialization to treatment described in Chapter 5 requires therapists to assume relatively more directive roles. Later in therapy, after youngsters and their families know more about the structure of cognitive therapy, the therapist should promote greater collaboration. In these instances, the youngsters and their families are directing their own treatment.

The nature of guided discovery differs with each child. With some youngsters (e.g., older children, psychologically minded youngsters, youngsters well skilled in self-instruction), guided discovery is punctuated by self-initiated exploration and rational analysis. Take the case of Amy, a 14-year-old depressed girl who took to rational analysis like a duck to water. She readily saw connections between thoughts and feeling, easily grasped her automatic thoughts, and was quickly able to construct counterthoughts. However, other clients (e.g., younger children, impulsive clients, children with low tolerance for ambiguity) need more self-instructional/self-control methods. Elise was an 8-year-old emotional juggernaut who found stopping and thinking to be a foreign idea. Her credo, like the Nike slogan, was "Just do it." She needed structure badly. Additionally, Elise had trouble catching her thoughts and feelings. Therefore, in her case we began with more self-instructional tools.

The *nature of the presenting problems* also dictates the level of collaboration and guided discovery. In highly acute crisis situations such as possible suicide attempt, intent to harm someone else, and ongoing child abuse, therapists literally have to take charge of the situation. Ideally, suicidal youngsters will work with the therapist to reduce their distress. However, with severely acute hopeless and suicidal youngsters, unilaterally breaking confidentiality or involuntarily hospitalizing a youngster is sometimes the best option (e.g., "I'm concerned about your safety. Since you cannot commit to staying safe and taking care of yourself, I'm going to have to help you stay in control and out of danger."). Highly acute crisis situations do not generally lend themselves to high levels of collaboration.

Developmental capacity also influences the degree of collaboration and guided discovery. Younger children have shorter attention spans, have less tolerance for ambiguity, and are more concrete in their reasoning processes. Moreover, in general, younger children are more impulsive and less self-reflective than older adolescents. Consequently, we rely more on the collaborative end of the continuum with older children.

In our experience, titrating the level of collaboration and guided discovery is difficult. Errors in both overestimating and underestimating children's capacities are commonplace. The following exchange reflects too much emphasis on guided discovery with Sonya, a 9-year-old child.

SONIA: I get upset when my dad makes these faces when I tell him about school.

THERAPIST: What do these faces mean to you?

SONIA: I don't know.

THERAPIST: What goes through your mind about these faces?

SONIA: He doesn't like me.

THERAPIST: What convinces you about that?

SONIA: His face.

THERAPIST: What about his face?

SONIA: The frown.

THERAPIST: What does the frown mean?

SONIA: I don't know.

In this example, the therapist is unwittingly taxing the child's developmental capacity. The therapist's questions are too abstract and strain Sonya's resources. More specific, concrete questions would have been more useful here.

Age also influences the level of collaboration and guided discovery that can be expected. In general, most adolescents will obviously have a greater capacity for collaboration and rational analysis than first graders. Once younger children become more familiar with treatment processes and direction, the therapist may increase the level of collaboration.

The child's *motivation* also shapes collaborative empiricism and guided discovery. Highly avoidant and unmotivated youngsters will generally react strongly when they think they are being controlled by others. Prescriptive and overly directive approaches with recalcitrant youngsters may meet with understandable obstacles. When you approach a recalcitrant child too forcefully, she's likely to withdraw. Yet, when you find a way to invite her into the collaborative adventure, she may become more invested. The following transcript illustrates a potentially useful stance with an ostensibly unmotivated youngster named Claudia.

CLAUDIA: I'm just telling you, I'm not talking.

THERAPIST: I see. Tell me what is making you not want to talk.

CLAUDIA: (*Sullen stare and silence.*)

THERAPIST: Well, this could be a very long 50 minutes.

CLAUDIA: (*Wry smile.*)

THERAPIST: You really seem more interested in fighting with me than in working with me. I'm trying to figure out a way we might work together. How does that sound?

CLAUDIA: (*Stares.*)

THERAPIST: (*Pauses for several moments.*) Well, I'm kind of stuck about what to do. Should we stop now?

CLAUDIA: (*Smiles and shrugs her shoulders.*)

THERAPIST: (*Smiles.*) I'll take that as an "I'm not sure" or "I don't care."

CLAUDIA: (*Shrugs again.*)

THERAPIST: (*Pauses.*) I think we need to develop this a bit more.

CLAUDIA: (*Sighs and rolls her eyes.*)

THERAPIST: I'll take that to mean this is kind of pissing you off. Boy, this is hard. You're really making me work. How am I doing so far?

CLAUDIA: (*Shrugs.*)

THERAPIST: We need another cue. Would you be willing to simply tell me "Yes" or "No"?

CLAUDIA: (*Shrugs.*)

THERAPIST: OK, you're not sure. What if you give me some signal? Like if you thought "Yes," you could nod your head like this and if you thought "No," you could shake your head sideways. Are you willing to do this?

CLAUDIA: (*Shrugs and stares.*)

THERAPIST: Not sure, I guess. Should we add another session per week?

CLAUDIA: (*Shakes head vigorously from side to side.*)

THERAPIST: Well, that's clear. What signal should we use if you want me to stop talking?

CLAUDIA: (*Pauses, smiles, raises middle finger skyward.*)

THERAPIST: I'll remember that one. OK. So we have an "I don't care," a "No," a "Yes," and a "I'm pissing you off" signal. What more do we need?

Eventually, the youngster began to use the hand signals regularly and then to actually verbalize her thoughts and feelings. This exchange illustrates the laborious yet ultimately productive way collaboration facilitates greater motivation. Clearly, at this stage, the therapist has assumed more responsibility for the direction of the session. By enlisting the child's cooperation, he moved away from such a direct approach as the child's investment in therapy increased. The therapist did not berate or blame Claudia for her avoidance. Rather, he maintained a curious attitude and developed a problem-solving strategy that respected the girl's avoidance yet gently nudged her toward greater expressiveness.

Individual children's *interpersonal styles* impact collaborative empiricism and guided discovery. Some children behave more passively than others and characteristically rely on others for direction and support. Fifteen-year-old Oscar was shy, quiet, and fearful of appearing too demanding or controlling. He looked to the therapist for direction and constantly scanned for signs on how he was doing. Other children are more self-directed and may act more autonomously. Twelve-year-old Ricky lived to "be in charge" and spent much energy staking out his territory. Therapist responsiveness to these tendencies individualizes treatment and necessarily modifies collaborative empiricism and guided discovery. For instance, collaboration with a more passive youngster will be arduous at first. You will need to establish collaboration as a goal and introduce graduated steps for the child. You will need to work with this child's shyness, reticence, and withdrawal, gently shaping the collaborative stance accordingly. The following transcript illustrates the way you might work with a child who is unaccustomed to collaboration.

THERAPIST: What would you like to talk and play about today?

MIA: I don't know. You decide.

THERAPIST: Deciding what to play about can seem a little risky. What makes you want me to take the lead?

MIA: You know what to do.

THERAPIST: I see. Do you think you might know what are the important things going on inside you?

MIA: Yes.

THERAPIST: How would it be if we worked together like a team to figure out things to help you?

MIA: That would be good, I guess.

THERAPIST: The thing we could do as teammates would be that if you saw me going off track you could tell me . . .

MIA: And if I went off track you could tell me.

THERAPIST: Exactly.

This transcript amplifies several pivotal points. First, the therapist takes a gentle approach to nudge the initially reluctant child toward increased collaboration. Second, through the therapist's systematic questioning, the child comes to a new perspective on the therapy process. Mia shifted from a position emphasizing total reliance on the therapist for direction to a position where the two partners formed a team. Third, the therapist worked diligently to empower the child throughout the process.

Other children may be especially sensitive to control issues. These children may balk at the idea of anyone providing direction for them. Adolescents will often react strongly to perceived and real threats to their autonomy. Not surprisingly, collaboration is essential in reducing youngsters' antagonism and recalcitrance. Often, the collaboration and guided discovery process involves "going with" youngsters' avoidance rather than fighting it. The following exchange illustrates the process with 15-year-old Edgar.

EDGAR: This is boring. I hate doing these stupid games and worksheets.

THERAPIST: What about these things are boring?

EDGAR: Everything. I hate coming here. You ask too many stupid questions.

THERAPIST: I can see you are angry at me and many of the things we do in here.

EDGAR: I'm not angry, I'm just bored.

THERAPIST: I see. You sure sounded angry to me. What is it about these worksheets that make you feel so bad?

EDGAR: These worksheets make me sick.

THERAPIST: How easy is it for you to talk about your feelings?

EDGAR: Very hard. I don't like this stuff at all. It makes me feel bad to talk about my feelings.

THERAPIST: I think I understand now. These worksheets make you feel bad because they make you think about your troubles.

Initially, Edgar is unexpressive and disengaged. He lashed out and blamed therapy. The therapist empathized with his discomfort and aligned with his avoidance. As the therapist collaboratively joined with him in his struggle to express and tolerate the negative feelings associated with his schoolwork, Edgar's recalcitrance lessened. Through the guided discovery process, Edgar learned to put words to his thoughts and feelings.

Cultural factors set broad parameters for collaborative empiricism and guided discovery. For example, Rotheram and Phinney (1986) as cited by Canino and Spurlock (2000) outlined interdependence versus dependence, active achievement versus passive acceptance, authoritarianism versus equalitarianism, and expressive/personal versus restrained/formal/impersonal communication as salient dimensions relevant to child psychotherapy. The way children and their families enter the collaborative venture is mediated by their cultural context. For instance, some families may view therapists as ultimate authorities and their cultural background may dictate deference. These families are simply interacting in a culturally determined manner. In these instances, therapists must adjust their expectations for collaboration so that they are culturally responsive.

Families also have culturally prescribed communication styles. Some may be more restrained and formal, for example, and may prefer to call the therapist "Mr.," "Ms.," or "Dr.," and in turn expect the same courtesy from the therapist. If the therapist unwittingly calls the parent by his first name, he/she may damage the collaborative relationship. The best approach is to simply respectfully ask the client how he/she would like to be addressed. Moreover, the therapist can ask parents, "What are you comfortable calling me?"

Minority culture clients may view language differently from individuals from the dominant culture (Johnson, 1993). For example, some types of questions that would seem normal to someone from the mainstream culture may be seen as rude to someone from the Native American and Asian American cultures (Johnson, 1993; Sommers-Flannagan & Sommers-Flannagan, 1995). Thus, the Socratic questioning component may need to be adapted to fit the needs of these clients. Questions may need to be posed in a less invasive, more indirect way in some circumstances. Additionally, in some cultures silence and lack of eye contact may be viewed as a sign of respect rather than as a signal of avoidance or resistance. Language will also influence collaboration.

CONCLUSION

Collaborative empiricism and guided discovery honor the unique characteristics each individual child brings to therapy. If learning to do cognitive
therapy with children can be equated to a children's coloring book, the
techniques represent the outline of the drawing. Collaborative empiricism
and guided discovery represent the color each therapist adds to the standard outline. Like a super box of crayons, there are many shades of collaborative empiricism and guided discovery.

In this chapter, we presented a continuum of collaboration and
guided discovery. In your work with children, you will need to decide
where on the continuum to begin and how to gage the level of collaboration in each phase of treatment. The child's acuity and the severity of his/
her problems, the child's developmental capacities, the child's cultural
context, and the child's personal style will guide your decision making.
Collaborative empiricism and guided discovery are embedded within
every clinical action and decision. The session structure, problem identification, introduction to the treatment model, identifying feelings
and thoughts, traditional cognitive-behavioral interventions, and creative
modifications of techniques—all require an understanding of collaborative empiricism and guided discovery. In short, now that you know about
collaborative empiricism and guided discovery, you are ready to dive in
with specific processes and techniques. Remember, you can always return
to this chapter when the therapy seems offtrack and you want to refresh
your interventions.

4

❖

Session Structure

Can you juggle? Juggling is an apt metaphor for what we need to do when we adopt cognitive therapy's trademark session structure. The session structure includes six central components: mood check-in, homework review, agenda setting, session content, homework assignment, and eliciting client feedback. Like the balls jugglers toss and catch in their amazing balancing display, these clinical components must be kept in motion during therapy. Each separate component must be mindfully considered so that therapeutic momentum is maintained. You want to be careful not to drop a ball!

As a cognitive therapist, you will always have these six balls in your hands. However, the way you juggle the components will vary from child to child. Sometimes you will be able to juggle faster than at other times. In other instances, you will vary the pattern of your juggling. As you become more comfortable with each component and your capacity to juggle them, you will develop more flexibility and creativity in your session structure. In this chapter, we will explain session structure, discuss why it is important, and offer you specific ways to implement the session structure with children and adolescents.

What do we mean by "session structure"? The *session structure* is a general template for conducting cognitive psychotherapy. The components are the "things you do" in session. While session structure involves a logical sequential order of steps, it is far from a lockstep process. When applied flexibly, the session structure evolves into an individually tailored clinical approach.

The six distinctive components of cognitive therapy session structure are interrelated and form a coherent treatment approach. Sessions begin with a mood check-in, which is followed by homework review. The therapist and client then collaboratively set the agenda. Based on this agenda setting, the session content emerges. Homework assignments evolve gracefully from session content. Finally, the client's perceptions of the session are elicited in the feedback phase.

Why is this session structure so important? In our minds, session structure provides direction to, focus for, and substance in therapy. The session structure helps children and their therapists sharpen the focus on the issues that bring youngsters to therapy and provides for an organized flow of information. For instance, due to no fault of their own, many clients begin therapy by aimlessly rambling on about multiple events or circumstances in their lives. They simply do not know how to organize and manage their inner experiences. The session structure teaches them a way to clarify their often chaotic and confusing experiences. Put simply, session structure is another means to promote self-control and self-regulation.

Session structure often provides youngsters with a sense of predictability. Consequently, they may feel "safer" in treatment. For instance, many clients feel more at ease knowing what to expect from therapy (J. S. Beck, 1995). Session structure provides a "containment" function for children, supplying them with an organized format for the expression and modulation of their distressing thoughts and feelings. Youngsters are frequently told what to do, and life may seem very unpredictable to them. Increasing the child's sense of control and decreasing their sense of unpredictability can lead to their greater investment and participation in treatment.

For instance, an 8-year-old boy with behavior problems is brought into therapy by his parents. Due to his acting-out behaviors, the majority of his interactions with adults result in scolding, nagging, criticism, and punishment. His teachers and parents frequently correct his behavior and tell him what to do ("Stop running!"; "Clean your room."). Decisions, even small ones, are rarely left up to the boy himself. Although you would want to work with the parents on these issues, your session structure can also help the child perceive that he has some real control over his life, his feelings, and his treatment. By collaboratively participating in agenda setting, homework assignments, and providing feedback, the boy is empowered to make relevant decisions, and even to become more comfortable disclosing and examining his thoughts and feelings. The predictability and perceived control of the cognitive therapy session may also lead to less limit testing. The structure increases the trust the child has in the therapist, promotes rapport building, and thus facilitates the therapeutic relationship and specific change processes.

MOOD OR SYMPTOM CHECK-IN

The first ball you put in motion is the mood or symptom check-in (J. S. Beck, 1995). The check-in serves several purposes. First, it provides therapists with baseline information about children's emotions and current symptoms and gives them a chance to take a youth's "psychological temperature." Second, the mood check-in compels youngsters to reflect on their own mood states and behaviors, requiring them to identify feelings and rate the feelings on a scale (e.g., Feeling: Sad; Rating: 8). The check-in also includes recapping the last session or comparing the youth's current mood with his/her mood ratings from previous sessions. The child's self-report and parents' observations can both be considered to identify changes in the child's symptoms. However, we do not recommend relying solely on the parents' report because overall children may be better reporters of their own mood states (Achenbach, McConaughy, & Howell, 1987).

How you elicit youngsters' ratings of their mood and symptoms differs with each child. You might encourage youngsters to verbally report their moods via a rating scale such as a point or percentage scale. With others, you may ask the child a series of questions, such as "How will we know how strong that feeling is?" or "What would you like to use to rate how strong the feeling is?" Most children need guidance with feeling identification. You can help them along by stating, "We could rate it on a scale of 1 to 10. What should be the strongest?"

Mood Check-In with Children

Depending on children's verbal fluency and expressiveness, inventive means of reporting their feelings may be used. Many of the children we have worked with find it easier to draw a face showing how they feel as illustrated in Chapter 6. The children then keep the drawings from week to week, which allows them to track their mood changes. We have found that children become quite invested in this simple self-monitoring task. These methods should be coupled with the therapist modeling skills in emotional expression.

The following dialogue shows how to use a verbal report during a mood check-in to gather information about a child's mood state.

THERAPIST: I am wondering how you have been feeling since we met last week. Why don't you draw a feeling face to show your mood?

SERENA: OK (*draws feeling face*).

THERAPIST: I see the feeling face you drew has a frown and tears on her face. Is that feeling mad, sad, glad, or scared?

SERENA: Sad.

THERAPIST: So you are feeling sad. What feeling face did you draw last week?

SERENA: That one was sad too (*takes out old feeling face*).

THERAPIST: And how did we know how strong the feeling was?

SERENA: By how big it is. Last week I was very sad so it was this big (*draws a circle that covers the entire page*).

THERAPIST: And this week?

SERENA: I am a little less sad so it is only this big (*draws a circle that covers three-quarters of the page*).

THERAPIST: Remember we talked about how the same feelings can be strong, weak, or in between, like the circles? What makes it less sad today?

SERENA: Well, my tummy didn't hurt so much this week and I didn't cry at school.

THERAPIST: So you have noticed several changes. What do you think it means that you have changed?

The mood check-in provides valuable information on Serena's symptoms in the past week. Skills in feeling identification and their connection to physiological and behavioral symptoms are also reinforced in the exchange (e.g., "Well, my tummy didn't hurt so much this week and I didn't cry at school."). By comparing the intensity of the child's feelings from week to week, the therapist can track change or lack of change. Consequently, the therapist can identify antecedents to feeling states, situational or environmental influences, and accompanying cognitions.

By tuning into their own emotions children begin to distinguish between different mood states. For example, many children begin therapy being able to say no more than that they are either feeling "good" or "bad." Over time, the mood check-in gives them an opportunity to learn to express different shades of their feelings and to develop a broader emotional vocabulary, such that they learn to say that they are feeling "lonely," "sad," "embarrassed," or "mad." The mood check-in also promotes monitoring feeling intensities. Various scales, such as a 10- or 100-point scale, may be used. Further, a thermometer or traffic signal could be used for scaling. By learning to distinguish between various feeling states and to scale their intensity, children learn to "fine-tune" their emotional expression.

Mood check-ins allow you to gage symptom relief. Session content and subsequent treatment foci should be guided by changes in moods and symptoms. For example, imagine that your client, Isaac, has been experiencing a steady decrease of depressive symptoms and an increase in positive mood. Through the mood check-in, you sense Isaac's mood has suddenly worsened. The following transcript illustrates the way you might use the mood check-in to monitor Isaac's progress.

THERAPIST: How was your week?

ISAAC: I feel worse today. Actually, more depressed than last week.

THERAPIST: Last week you said you felt about a 5 for depression.

ISAAC: Yeah, and I felt OK until yesterday. The past 2 days, it was more like an 8.

THERAPIST: So you noticed a change yesterday. When exactly did that change occur?

ISAAC: Well, I guess it was around lunchtime. I overheard some boys talking about going to the park on Saturday. I got upset because I know no one will invite me to go with them.

THERAPIST: So the situation was that some boys were talking about plans for Saturday. You had the thought, "No one will invite me to go with them," and you noticed your depressive feelings increased. How did your body feel?

ISAAC: Really tired.

The therapist's questions help Isaac to focus on identifying the situation that led to his mood shift. Through this process, the cognitive model is reinforced by the therapist, who helps Isaac draw connections between the various components of the cognitive model (physiology, mood, behavior, cognition, and interpersonal). Mood states are identified and cognitions, behaviors, and physiological reactions that accompany the emotions are discussed. Work on identifying cognitive distortions, connections between cognitions and mood states, and problem solving can begin.

Using self-report measures, such as the CDI (Kovacs, 1992), the RCMAS (Reynolds & Richmond, 1985), and the MASC (March, 1997) to monitor youngster's emotional functioning is a common clinical practice for us. For a variety of reasons, many children find endorsing items on a self-report scale easier than expressing these feelings verbally. First, the items are supplied for them on a self-report measure. Thus, they do not have to access these experiences themselves. Second, checking or circling items on a list is a far simpler task than translating their inner experiences into words. Third, filling out a checklist offers children somewhat greater psychological distance from their emotional experiences than directly sharing these feelings with an adult authority figure. Thus, doing so serves as a graduated task for identifying and discussing feelings. Further, the self-report instruments provide a more objective measure for tracking progress in symptom reduction over the course of treatment.

Mood Check-In with Adolescents

Generally, adolescents are better equipped to identify their feelings than younger children. But some adolescents may not be so adept at the process. Therefore, when completing the mood check-in, you must not assume that your adolescent clients have a clear understanding of their different mood states. Depending on the adolescent's gender, cultural background, family interactions, and temperament, values and expectations regarding the discussion of feelings may vary greatly. The following transcript illustrates the mood check-in with a 15-year-old girl.

THERAPIST: How have you been feeling the past week?

TINA: (*Shrugs shoulders.*) Not so great.

THERAPIST: Can you describe that "not-so-great" feeling a little more?

TINA: I just feel bad.

THERAPIST: Sounds like you have had a hard week. When you were feeling bad, was it more mad, sad, or scared?

TINA: It was sad—really sad.

THERAPIST: What made you know it was sad rather than mad or scared?

TINA: Well, I cried a lot and everything went wrong.

THERAPIST: If you were to rate your sadness for the week, how sad did you feel?

TINA: Mostly it was an 8 out of 10.

This transcript illustrates how the therapist helped Tina distinguish between different negative affective states ("What made you know it was sad rather than mad or scared?"). Some adolescents are very skilled at identifying their feelings, but others require some guidance. It is your job as a therapist to guide the adolescent through the task of mood identification without being overly directive. The therapist in the above transcript provided Tina with options to choose from and allowed her to describe her feelings (e.g., "Can you describe that 'not-so-great' feeling a little more? . . . Was it more mad, sad, or scared?"). Once she identifies her feeling, Tina is able to rate it using her own scale to communicate the severity of her sadness.

Many youngsters group all negative affect under one "bad" label. Distinguishing between different negative affective states is helpful to set the stage for later identifying accompanying cognitions. Affective responses become more salient and are described, identified, and evaluated for intensity. If you work with an adolescent who has frequent difficulty identifying feelings, you may want to put that topic on the agenda and spend more time building his/her skills in identification of feelings.

HOMEWORK REVIEW

The second ball to toss in each session is homework review. You examine whether the child has completed the assignment, the content of the assignment, and the youngster's reaction to the assignment. Children's responses and reactions to the process and content of therapeutic assignments provide a meaningful glimpse into their inner worlds. Reviewing homework underscores the importance of the assignments and their role in the treatment process on two levels. Homework assignments allow the child to practice skills important for decreasing symptoms and improving mood. In addition, the process of reviewing homework conveys your interest in the child's feelings, thoughts, and reactions regarding the homework.

Reviewing homework assignments communicates the therapeutic message that the homework is central to treatment and reinforces the client's efforts (A. T. Beck et al., 1979; J. S. Beck, 1995; Burns, 1989). By discussing the specifics of previously assigned homework, and by processing the children's experience of completing the assignment, therapists emphasize the value of the work. Overall, incorporating homework tasks into treatment, spending time each week discussing them, and integrating the previously learned skills into other sessions demonstrates that the tasks are valued. The following transcript shows how to review homework.

THERAPIST: I see you brought your activity schedule back this week.

NICK: Yeah. I made plans to see a movie with a friend and I played basketball once this week like we talked about.

THERAPIST: What was it like completing your homework over the week?

NICK: It was kind of hard at first. I really didn't feel like doing it. But then I decided I would try and see if it helped me feel better.

THERAPIST: What went through your mind about doing the homework?

NICK: I thought that I was too tired and it would never work.

THERAPIST: What made you decide to do it anyway?

NICK: Well, I thought that we had talked about that, and I should try the experiment to see if it worked or not.

THERAPIST: What did you notice about how you felt before doing the activities?

NICK: Both times I rated my sadness as a 7. I did not feel like doing anything.

THERAPIST: And right after the activity?

NICK: After the movie, it was a 3. I really had a good time, and the movie was really funny. After basketball, I felt like a 5. It was not as much fun as the movie, but it still seemed to help.

THERAPIST: What do you make of the changes in your mood?

NICK: My feelings changed when I did stuff, so maybe the experiment worked.

In this exchange, the therapist and Nick not only reviewed the content of the homework but also discussed the process of completing the assignment. First, attending to Nick's feelings and thoughts about completing the assignment (e.g., "I thought that I was too tired and it would never work.") was revealing. Second, the therapist tested Nick's beliefs about whether his feelings would change with activity. Third, the therapist gently used Socratic questions to guide the dialogue.

Homework Review with Children

We are challenged by homework review with young children. Due to their developmental level, younger children use more concrete thought processes. Homework review translates the often abstract therapeutic principles into concrete practices for young children. Not surprisingly, younger children have shorter attention spans than older children. Therefore, we try to review homework in a playful manner. Finally, homework review supplies more opportunities for skills practice. Greater practice increases skill acquisition and recall. The following brief exchange shows you how to review a homework assignment with a young child.

THERAPIST: I see you did your feeling faces this week. Nice job bringing your work back to session. What feeling face would you like to share first?

DOUG: Mad.

THERAPIST: Oh, let's see that mad face. Make a mad face with your face now.

DOUG: (*Makes a mad face and laughs.*)

THERAPIST: Wow, what a mad face! How can you tell when your face looks mad?

This example demonstrates how you can engage children in the review rather than simply checking the completion of the assignment. The therapist was very playful and interactive (e.g., "Wow, what a mad face!"). Additionally, Doug's homework completion was reinforced (e.g., "Nice job bringing your work back to session."). The fun and playful manner likely made the task more memorable for Doug.

Particularly for children who have trouble in school or with completing schoolwork, the term "homework" may carry a negative connotation. Other creative titles may be used, such as "weekly projects" or "helping sheets." Generating a new name for the tasks may avoid a negative association between therapeutic assignments and schoolwork. Kendall and colleagues (1992) cleverly refer to homework as "Show That I Can" (STIC) exercises. Thus, rather than saying "This is a homework assignment" to children, you may encourage children to "show that they can" by completing various tasks. Further, you can discuss with the child the difference between school homework and therapy homework. Therapy homework does not have right or wrong answers. It is a chance for children to identify thoughts and feelings, and to do things to help themselves feel better.

Homework Review with Adolescents

Adolescents enjoy testing the limits of their autonomy. Their noncompliance, avoidance, and reactance to homework may reflect their natural rebelliousness and drive for independence. At the same time, adolescents are very experimental beings. We find that by offering techniques as experimental hypotheses rather than as requirements, we avoid taking on the role of an ultimate authority telling the adolescent youth what to do. Rather, adolescents are left to learn through experience what interventions work best for themselves. Behavioral experiments can be used to test the effectiveness of interventions. You do not have to take a position contrary to the adolescent; rather, you can collaborate with the teen on determining whether the homework is worthwhile. The following example depicts an approach to homework review.

THERAPIST: I see you brought your homework back this week?

MARCUS: Yeah, I got all three thought records done.

THERAPIST: Nice job remembering to complete the thought records. What was it like doing this assignment?

MARCUS: I like this one better than that one from last week where I just wrote down how I felt. This one seemed to help more because I could figure out why I felt bad by paying attention to what was going through my mind when I felt bad.

THERAPIST: So, do you think it would be worth it to use this again?

MARCUS: Yeah, even though I hate having to write stuff down, it really seemed to help.

The therapist included Marcus in the evaluation of the effectiveness of the assignment (e.g., "What was it like doing the assignment?") rather than dictating future assignments to him. Thus, Marcus becomes involved in objectively comparing different assignments and choosing what works best for him (e.g., "This one seemed to help more because I could figure out why I felt bad by paying attention to what was going through my mind when I felt bad."). Finally, the therapist includes Marcus in the decision to continue to use the homework (e.g., "So, do you think it would be worth it to use this again?").

AGENDA SETTING

Agenda setting, a third major component of session structure, sets the stage for and adds direction to therapeutic work (Freeman & Dattilio, 1992; Friedberg, 1995). Together with eliciting feedback, agenda setting is considered central to therapeutic success (Burns, 1989). *Agenda setting* itself involves identifying items or topics that will be addressed during the session. The process entails listing items and allocating approximate session time to be spent on each item. In this way, important items are prioritized. Specific agenda items may vary depending on the stage of therapy, the client's progress, his/her most pressing problems, the severity of his/her symptoms, and items carried over from the previous session (A. T. Beck et al., 1979). Collaboration between the therapist and the youngster is key in establishing the agenda. If the therapist and the child are not working collaboratively on the agenda, progress is less likely to occur.

Agenda setting is an unfamiliar task for children and adolescents. Therefore, explaining the process to youngsters is a useful therapeutic strategy (J. S. Beck, 1995). Typically, we engage in a Socratic dialogue with the child to discuss the advantages and disadvantages associated with agenda setting. Then we expand on ideas by explaining the rationale behind agenda setting. Further, we model the agenda-setting process for the youngster by concisely stating agenda items. For instance, an adolescent may respond to the therapist's inquiry regarding additional agenda items with a description of a problem that occurred since the last session.

THERAPIST: What would you like to add to the agenda to make sure we discuss today?

ELIZABETH: I got in a huge fight with Mom. She wouldn't let me go out with my friends. She is such a jerk—everyone else got to go. I got so mad! Then she grounded me for no reason because she said I was talking back to her.

THERAPIST: So, you'd like to discuss the fight with your mother?

ELIZABETH: Yeah, she is so unreasonable. She was yelling at me first and then I got grounded.

THERAPIST: I can tell you are really upset and would really like to talk about what happened. Is this something you would like to put first on our agenda?

ELIZABETH: Sure.

THERAPIST: OK. Why don't you write that down as the first agenda item?

This example demonstrates how you can grasp the opportunity to teach and model for the youth how to turn a lengthy description into an agenda item. Further, writing down agenda items can help keep the session focused. It also provides a record for reviewing content after the session. Often youngsters will change topics when they become emotionally aroused in an attempt to avoid the arousal and decrease distress. Through reliance on agenda setting, you can gently return the youngster to the avoided topic.

We recommend that you use children's *difficulties* in setting agendas as *agenda items*. For instance, the therapist can meaningfully work through children's difficulties in agenda setting. The following key questions may guide your processing of children's difficulties in setting an agenda:

- What are the pros and cons of setting an agenda?
- What do you gain by setting an agenda?
- What do you gain by not setting an agenda?
- What do you lose by setting an agenda?
- What do you lose by not setting an agenda?

- What does it mean to you to set an agenda?
- What is the danger in setting an agenda?

Agenda Setting with Children

Children are accustomed to parents and teachers imposing goals on them. Agenda setting allows children to bring their own issues to the table. We rarely use the term "agenda setting" with young children. Rather, we typically ask them, "What is it you want to make sure we talk about today?" We find including one to three items on the agenda is a realistic goal for young children. If the child has difficulty keeping items concise, you may have the child name what he/she wants to talk about as if he/she were naming a movie, book, or television show. The following transcript illustrates the process.

THERAPIST: What would you like to put on our list to talk about today?

MILO: I am mad at my brother. He's a big goof and always gets me in trouble. Last night he took away my game and then I tried to get it back. He told Mom on me and I didn't get to play the whole night.

THERAPIST: Wow, I can tell you are mad. When you were saying that your voice got louder and your eyes opened real wide. OK, why don't we put that on our list to talk about today? What short title can we use to write that on our list?

MILO: I think we should call it "No fair" cause it wasn't fair that I got in trouble.

This exchange illustrates how the therapist elicited a topic for the agenda from the child ("What would you like to put on our list to talk about today?"). While still honoring the client's report, the therapist guided Milo to concisely identify the problem ("What short title can we use to write that on our list?"). Additionally, the therapist conveyed empathy and respect for Milo's experience. Thus, the child's concerns were addressed, he felt understood, and the agenda setting propelled the therapeutic momentum.

Agenda Setting with Adolescents

Adolescent clients are particularly sensitive to being controlled or coerced. However, by enlisting the adolescent in the process of setting the agenda, the therapist has an opportunity to help the teen feel he/she has an active role in the treatment. Agenda setting provides adolescents with a greater sense of control, which in turn may foster their greater investment in the therapy. For instance, you can ask, "We have already talked about why your parents have brought you in, but I am interested in hearing what things you would like to work on. What would you like help with improving or changing?" The adolescent may identify a variety of issues—including wanting to terminate treatment. You and the adolescent can then work on identifying clearly defined subgoals, such as reduced fighting with siblings, so his/her parents will not be so upset. In this way, you are working together on a common agenda item (e.g., ending treatment).

Agenda setting is also difficult for adolescents because they often have so many topics they want to talk about, they can't decide where to begin. We find a question such as "If we could only talk about one thing today, what would you want it to be?" to be helpful. Teaching adolescents to identify areas they most want to work on also facilitates increased satisfaction with treatment (e.g., "What are the most important things you want to talk about? What makes this important?"). Adolescents are more likely to be motivated when they are working on goals they themselves have identified.

Agenda setting may also be hard for adolescents who resist structure and enjoy testing limits. When the adolescent is testing the therapist's limits, maintaining a consistent session structure is very important. If the adolescent sees that you are not consistent in maintaining the session structure, the youth may begin to doubt your commitment to other areas of treatment. Consistency serves to contain youngsters and contrasts with the chaos that may characterize other aspects of their lives. Establishing firm boundaries and setting limits sends the message that you will follow through and encourages trust.

THERAPIST: What would you like to put on the agenda to talk about today?

MELISSA: You asked me that last time. This time you decide.

THERAPIST: Well, I am most interested in talking about the things that are important to you.

MELISSA: So, you're the expert. You tell me what is important to talk about.

THERAPIST: Actually, Melissa, you're the expert on you. It's your choice whether we talk about the things that are important to you and bothering you. If you choose for us to do so, then together maybe we can figure out ways to help make things easier for you.

MELISSA: Yeah, right! How are we going to do that?

THERAPIST: Well, first we need to figure out what are the things that you want the most help with today.

MELISSA: My biggest problem this week is that my parents are always telling me what to do.

THERAPIST: OK. Why don't you put that down on our agenda. What other problems should we talk about today and try to solve?

Melissa may have perceived a loss of control in her life, and attempted to regain control by refusing to collaborate with the therapist in agenda setting. Adolescents are often torn between wanting to assert independence and feeling unsure of how to handle that independence. Here, for instance, Melissa may not have been aware of how to best choose items for the agenda. At the same time, anxiety may have prevented her from admitting her uncertainty, and thus led to an oppositional stance. By reminding Melissa of the purpose of agenda setting and guiding her through the process, the therapist aided in the agenda setting while maintaining the focus on issues important to Melissa. Additionally, the therapist allowed Melissa to remain in control, so as not to challenge her independence (e.g., "It's your choice whether we talk about the things that are important to you and bothering you.").

SESSION CONTENT

Specific agenda items are addressed during the content section of the session. Therapeutic content is processed using a variety of techniques such as empathy, Socratic questioning, problem solving, and behavioral experimentation. The goals of the session content include maintaining and building rapport, reinforcing the cognitive model, problem solving, addressing therapy goals, identifying automatic thoughts, and providing symptom relief (J. S. Beck, 1995). During this portion of the session, the clinician may use questions to aid the client in attending to a particular area, generate problem-solving methods, assess client's functioning and coping, and elicit specific thoughts and feelings (A. T. Beck et al., 1979).

Balancing content, process, and structure is yet another critical element in doing cognitive therapy with children (Friedberg, 1995). *Therapeutic structure* encompasses the tasks embedded in therapy such as thought diaries, games, homework assignments, and so on. Therapeutic content is produced by the structure. *Therapeutic content* consists of the thoughts, feelings, and behaviors elicited by the various therapeutic procedures. For instance, a thought diary (or thought record) is a form of therapeutic structure, whereas the thoughts, feelings, and events recorded in the thought diary are therapeutic content (Some therapists prefer the term "thought diary," others the term "thought record." We will be using both terms throughout the book.) *Therapeutic process* denotes the way the child goes about completing tasks, responding to questions, and/or solving problems in therapy. You will find that some children will dutifully complete a thought record and answer with emotionally honest responses. Others will platitudinously finish one with emotionally insignificant material. Still others will simply refuse to do the task. Each response reflects an individual psychological process. Accordingly, while the task structure remains the same, content and process vary with each individual child. Attending to and negotiating structure, content, and process issues in therapy with children is a way the therapist honors each particular child.

Session Content with Children

Your word choice and sentence length can significantly impact young children's understanding (e.g., "Your anger is really heating up."). Thus, developmentally appropriate language, including short, simple words and sentences, should be chosen when communicating with children. Young children also have difficulty attending to multiple tasks at one time. Thus, skills and instructions should be given individually, with opportunities to check for understanding and practice in between.

Session content is also influenced by the child's motivational level. Less motivated youth are more reluctant to engage in the session activities. By making tasks more attractive and encouraging collaboration, the therapist can increase motivation. You can apply skills with creative presentations to capture children's interest. One way of enhancing a child's responsiveness is by remaining animated and engaged as a therapist. Use props, stories, colorful drawings, and hands-on activities to increase the appeal of therapeutic tasks. The following transcript shows how a therapist might ignite a child's motivation.

JENNIFER: I don't want to talk today. All we ever do is talk and fill out worksheets! This is so boring. I'm not doing anything today!

THERAPIST: I planned a game for us to play today. I even got some new prizes to pick from if you won the game.

JENNIFER: It's probably a trick and probably boring.

THERAPIST: I don't know if it will be boring for you, but there is only one way to find out. Would you like to learn the game and try to win a prize?

JENNIFER: What are we going to do?

THERAPIST: See these cards? They are blank on one side and have questions on the other side. They ask about things you like and don't like, your feelings, and other questions. We are going to spread them all over the floor with the questions facing down so we can't see them.

JENNIFER: Can I help spread them out?

THERAPIST: Now you toss this token and try to hit a card. If it lands on a card, pick it up and read the question. If you answer the question, you earn a chip. If you miss the card and the token lands on the floor, then it is my turn. Ready?

Jennifer was initially unmotivated to participate in the session. She likely would not have responded to activities or skill building that involved a lot of discussion or writing. However, the therapist offered a creative twist on identifying thoughts and feelings by presenting the skill through an interactive game. The therapist hooked Jennifer's interest without demanding that she participate or guaranteeing that she would enjoy the game ("I don't know if it will be boring for you, but there is only one way to find out. Would you like to learn the game and try to win a prize?"). Later, if Jennifer enjoys any aspect of the game, the therapist should seize the opportunity to illustrate how "guesses" can sometimes be wrong ("It's probably a trick and probably boring.").

Session Content with Adolescents

Creativity and flexibility enable therapists to effectively negotiate session content with adolescents. Incorporating adolescents' interests into the session content often clicks for teens. For example, if an adolescent enjoys writing, he/she may warm to the idea of keeping a journal to record emotions. Giving the adolescent some sense of control or choice in the treatment is particularly important. By helping the adolescent recognize the control and choices available, the therapist increases his/her empowerment and motivation.

THERAPIST: You said that the agenda item you wanted to talk about first was a problem you are having with your sister.

KELSEY: Yes. She is 2 years younger than me, but she is always trying to hang around when my friends are over and it is so annoying. She is just a kid, and we are trying to talk about personal things. I can't get her to leave us alone. I've tried everything, and there is nothing else to do.

THERAPIST: Sometimes it's helpful to make a list of all the possible things that you could do, and then to decide which ideas are worth trying.

KELSEY: You mean write them down?

THERAPIST: How might that be helpful?

KELSEY: Well, I guess if I wrote them down then when she starts bugging me I could find something on the list to try. I know—I will write it in my notebook so I always have it with me.

THERAPIST: So, what things have you already tried to solve this problem?

In this example, the session content begins with the problem that Kelsey identified as most important to her this session. The therapist uses Kelsey's problem to help teach problem-solving strategies, thus keeping the content meaningful and therefore more salient for her. Further, the task is individualized to Kelsey's problem so that the skill is applied to a meaningful situation for Kelsey. Finally, Kelsey individualizes the task herself by opting to record her responses in her personal notebook.

While discussing session content, you may invite the adolescent to take notes, practice skills, and write down homework assignments to aid in the generalization of the skills (J. S. Beck, 1995). You may have the adolescent record such information in a notebook with the youth's favorite sports team or actor on the cover. Subsequently, the adolescent's interest in the activity and compliance with the task will increase because the notebook will not be stigmatizing. In addition, special pens could be earned and used to complete assignments.

HOMEWORK ASSIGNMENT

The essentials of assigning homework are fully described in Chapter 10. What is important to note here is that homework occupies a central place in every session and it follows from the session content. You want to make the assignment meaningful and increase a child's motivation for continuing therapy. The following brief example shows how to assign homework with an unmotivated teen.

JOEY: I don't want to do the stupid homework!

THERAPIST: I'm confused. You said a minute ago that you wanted help learning how not to worry so much. Now you're saying you don't want to try what we have been talking about?

JOEY: This will never work. These worksheets are dumb and I don't want to do them.

THERAPIST: This assignment may or may not help you worry less—I don't know. Why don't we do an experiment and see how filling out the worksheet and practicing the skill affects your worried thoughts and feelings.

JOEY: No way! I don't want to do this stupid worksheet at all.

THERAPIST: What might happen if you do try to do it?

JOEY: I already told you, it won't work. Then I'll have done the stupid work for no reason. That will just prove I am hopeless.

THERAPIST: What do you think we would do if we find out this doesn't help with your worried feelings?

JOEY: Nothing.

THERAPIST: Do you remember when I told you the assignments were like experiments?

JOEY: (*Nods.*)

THERAPIST: Well, if this experiment shows us that this skill doesn't help you worry less, what do you think our next plan will be?

JOEY: Try another experiment?

THERAPIST: That's right! We will keep trying new things until we find a way to help you worry less. It will take some work on your part, so are you willing to give it a try?

JOEY: I guess it can't hurt.

Joey initially refused to complete a homework assignment ("I don't want to do the stupid homework!") Rather than arguing with Joey, the therapist took the time to process his resistance and reveal cognitive distortions, thus leading to more successful homework assignment and completion. Joey's resistance stemmed from his worries and beliefs that failure in the homework would mean that he was hopeless. The therapist used Socratic questioning to develop a plan with Joey if the homework did not help ("Well, if this experiment shows us that this skill doesn't help you worry less, what do you think our next plan will be?").

ELICITING FEEDBACK

The final component of the session structure, eliciting feedback, represents a significant relationship-building and therapeutic strategy in cognitive therapy with children. At a minimum, you should elicit feedback toward the end of each session. You may also ask for feedback at the beginning and throughout the session (A. T. Beck et al., 1979; J. S. Beck, 1995). The child is asked what was helpful, unhelpful, or annoying about the session and the therapist. Early in the session, you might ask questions such as the following:

- "What went through your mind about last week's session?"
- "What thoughts and feelings about last week's session would you like to share with me?"
- "What things about last session were left over?"
- "What was last week's session like for you?"
- "What things about last session did you enjoy?"
- "What things did you not enjoy?"

Eliciting feedback also occurs at the end of each session. You should allocate about 10–12 minutes for feedback at the end of the session. You might ask questions such as the following:

- "What was helpful about today's work together?"
- "What was not helpful about today's work together?"
- "What was fun?"
- "What was not fun?"
- "What did I do today that bugged you?"
- "What did we do today that didn't seem right for you?"

By eliciting feedback, client misperceptions, dissatisfactions, or distortions regarding treatment, the therapist, or the relationship are prevented from continuing for weeks and stifling progress.

Not surprisingly, some children are reluctant to give feedback. Some children fear disappointing or upsetting the therapist. Others may be overly obedient and compliant. Some children may be influenced by cultural constraints that inhibit giving feedback. Still others may be passive and withholding. Regardless of the individual beliefs and motivations behind their reluctance to give feedback, you should explore the difficulty with them.

Feedback is elicited in various ways, but we suggest a straightforward approach: directly ask the youngster to reflect on the therapeutic process. However, giving adults in authority feedback is an unfamiliar and unsettling task for most children. If the child is uncomfortable, the therapist and youth must work together to problem solve the difficulty. The following dialogue shows how to process feedback with a youngster.

THERAPIST: What was helpful about today's work together?

JAMES: I guess it was good to just be able to talk to someone about what is going on and not have them tell me what to do.

THERAPIST: So you found it helpful to be able to express your thoughts and feelings today?

JAMES: Yeah.

THERAPIST: Well, I'm really glad you shared your feelings and thoughts. That took a lot of courage. What was unhelpful or annoying about today's session?

JAMES: I can't think of anything. Everything was great.

THERAPIST: Do you think you could tell me if there was something?

JAMES: (*Hesitates.*) I don't know. Maybe.

THERAPIST: If I did do something that really bugged you and you told me, what might happen?

JAMES: You might get mad at me and would not like me anymore.

What does this dialogue teach us? First, the therapist seized the opportunity to reinforce James's efforts in the session ("I'm really glad you shared your thoughts and feelings. That took a lot of courage."). Next, the therapist uncovered the youth's automatic thoughts embedded in his reluctance to provide negative feedback ("If I did do something that really bugged you and you told me, what might happen?"). By identifying the automatic thought, the therapist and adolescent can now work collaboratively to test the thought for accuracy.

Feedback also helps the therapist correct misperceptions and therefore solidify the therapeutic alliance (J. S. Beck, 1995). Such corrections are important because therapists are often misinterpreted by clients (A. T. Beck et al., 1979). Further, if feedback is consistently elicited and respectfully considered, honest reactions by the child are reinforced. Unexpressed dissatisfactions, which can sabotage therapy, may be avoided.

Eliciting feedback can be challenging for therapists. Initially, I (JMM) struggled with this component of the session structure for several reasons. First, at times when I doubted my own skills, I feared negative feedback would only validate my fears that I was doing something wrong. Second, I felt unsure of what to do with the feedback I might receive. What if it was something I could not change? How should I react to the feedback, be it negative or positive? How do I balance validating the child's perception and experience, while challenging any cognitive distortions embedded in his/her feedback? To face these fears, I thought I needed to do what I tell the children to do: gather data and test my fears! I listed the most challenging responses I could think of that a client might give to eliciting feedback and various ways to handle them. I soon realized that I could easily incorporate the child's feedback into the session.

Further, some feedback would clearly add to the conceptualization. Then I began asking children for feedback. I found myself feeling more prepared to elicit and process feedback with the clients. Consequently, I elicited some very meaningful beliefs and reactions from the children that may have otherwise gone undetected. Therefore, some problems were quickly identified and resolved through eliciting feedback.

Eliciting Feedback from Children

Youngsters may be uncertain about how you will react to feedback. Thus, it is important for you to simplify the process for the child. When a child does not provide you with negative feedback, you ask the child, "If there was something that bugged you, what would it be like to tell me? How do you guess I would react?" To promote greater comfort with giving feedback, therapists may demonstrate that they make mistakes and do not respond negatively to errors. For instance, in running a group I (JMM) forgot to bring a three-hole punch two sessions in a row. We needed the hole punch for the children to punch their worksheets and put them in their personal notebooks. The second time I forgot I commented, "That's the second time I forgot the hole punch! Oh well! I wonder what I could do next time to help myself remember?" The children in the group generated several ideas (e.g., put it with the other materials for group, write myself a note, ask my cofacilitator to remind me). I then turned the situation toward them to help them generalize their problem-solving strategies to their own lives: "What kinds of things do you sometimes forget? Would those ideas help any of you remember things in your own lives?" Doing so not only demonstrated an adaptive way for me to handle a mistake, and ways they too could use to deal with errors, it also provided them with a model that I was comfortable acknowledging errors and did not react negatively to such errors.

Various beliefs contribute to children's reluctance to give feedback. Young children may believe giving feedback is disrespectful. They may fear that they will be rejected or reprimanded for giving feedback to an authority figure. Other children may believe they will hurt the therapist's feelings if they share negative feedback. A brief example illustrates how a therapist may address a child's reluctance and identify the beliefs linked to the youth's hesitancy to provide feedback.

THERAPIST: What did you like about our work today?

KIMBERLY: I liked the puppet. The turtle puppet is my favorite!

THERAPIST: The puppets are fun! What didn't you like about our work today?

KIMBERLY: I liked everything.

THERAPIST: What kind of bugged you about today?

KIMBERLY: Nothing—I liked it all.

THERAPIST: If there was something that bugged you would you be able to tell me?

KIMBERLY: Umm. Yeah.

THERAPIST: You don't sound very sure. What might be hard about telling me that something bugged you?

KIMBERLY: You might feel bad.

THERAPIST: And then what might happen?

KIMBERLY: You wouldn't like me anymore.

What can we learn from this example? First, the therapist identified parts of the session Kimberly found satisfying. Second, the therapist probed Kimberly's reluctance to give feedback and identified the beliefs that buttressed that reluctance. Third, by uncovering these hidden fears, the therapist laid the foundation for testing her negative expectations.

Eliciting Feedback from Adolescents

Like younger children, adolescents also fear the consequences of giving negative feedback. They may fear getting in trouble or being rejected. To help alleviate these concerns, the therapist can ask, "If you did tell me that I had done something that had annoyed or bugged you, how do you predict I would react? What might I say or do?" Approaching the feedback in this manner may serve to uncover beliefs that are interfering with the adolescent providing feedback. For example, teens may predict rejection, fear they will offend the therapist, and/or believe they will be punished for saying something negative. At the same time, adolescents are often more able to verbalize the cause of their hesitancy to give feedback, and therefore the source of their discomfort may be more easily discovered through discussion with the teen.

On the other hand, some adolescents may seize feedback as an opportunity to psychologically bash you! For instance, an adolescent may respond to the therapist eliciting feedback with a comment like, "Everything stunk. You are the worst therapist ever." In these cases, it is particularly important to consider the case formulation. For instance, the response to feedback might reflect a crucial testing of the therapist to determine if he/she can handle the adolescent's problems. Additionally, the adolescent may be resistant to treatment in the first place due to being mandated to attend by parents or teachers. Thus, uncovering the functional value of the therapist bashing is important. Doing so will provide insight into inaccurate thoughts or beliefs that may need to be addressed in session. Further, the adolescent's feedback could be discussed, and problem solving could be done to make specific changes in the treatment if appropriate.

CONCLUSION

Skillfully juggling and keeping each of the six balls in the air clearly facilitates effective and efficient interventions. Each component of the session serves an integral part of the session. While each component of the session is important, the juggling process of implementing the session structure also propels skill building. Being flexible in the application of session structure allows you to effectively adapt sessions to meet the needs of various clients while still maintaining the basic components of the session. Further, collaboration with youngsters is maximized in a manner that facilitates client participation in treatment.

Juggling six balls at one time can seem overwhelming at first. Like juggling, the more you practice session structure, the easier it will become. With practice, you will find you will be able to juggle faster when needed or change the pattern of your juggling to fit the needs of individual clients. In this chapter, you have learned the link between session structure and cognitive therapy with children and adolescents, including suggestions for implementing each component of the cognitive therapy session. It is within this context that you will now apply some of the interventions and techniques described in subsequent chapters.

5

❖

Introducing the Treatment Model
and Identifying Problems

Educating clients and parents about the treatment model is a critical step in demystifying therapy and fostering a collaborative stance (A. T. Beck et al., 1979). We need to describe treatment in simple, understandable, and developmentally sensitive ways. This chapter describes several methods for introducing treatment to children, adolescents, and their parents.

Children, parents, and therapists need a degree of consensus regarding the problems to address in therapy. This first step can present challenges. Generally, parents, teachers, or other adults are first to identify and define the youngster's problems for him/her. You need to solicit input from the youngster in order to establish genuine agreement on the problem. Proceeding with treatment before problems are collaboratively defined will likely lead to therapeutic roadblocks. For instance, if a child does not agree with the therapist about his/her problem, he/she may not be motivated in treatment. This chapter also offers several recommendations for identifying problems with children and adolescents.

INTRODUCING THE TREATMENT MODEL TO CHILDREN

How do you introduce therapy to children of elementary school age in an engaging and understandable manner? Obviously, children need to be given simple concrete information. If they sense you are lecturing them, they won't hear you. While this may seem like a clinical "no-brainer," it is hard to accomplish in clinical practice. We have developed some strategies, stories, games, and metaphors to help minimize this problem.

For young children, we use a story- or picture-book format to illustrate the connection between events, thoughts, and feelings. The therapist asks questions to guide the telling of the story. The child provides answers to the therapist's prompts. Often the child will be asked to draw a picture. The process begins with the therapist drawing a picture of a child holding a balloon (Figure 5.1). We recommend you match the gender of the child in the drawing to that of the client. The drawing also includes a thought cloud. In the original drawing, the child is expressionless and the thought cloud is empty. You then proceed with the first prompt. The following exchange illustrates the process.

THERAPIST: I'm going to tell you a story about this girl, but first I will need your help. Hillary, are you willing to help me?

HILLARY: Yes.

THERAPIST: OK then. What should we name this girl?

HILLARY: Let's call her Lina.

THERAPIST: OK. This girl named Lina loved balloons. She thought that if

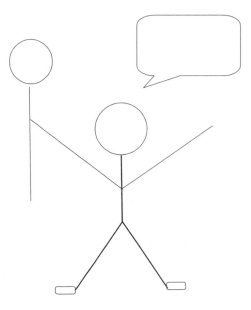

FIGURE 5.1. Therapist's picture of a girl holding a balloon.

she just had a balloon she would be the luckiest girl in the world. So one day her mom bought her a balloon. Here it is in the drawing. Lina got the balloon. How do you suppose she felt?

HILLARY: Really happy.

THERAPIST: She felt really happy. We need to find a place where we could know how happy Lina felt. Can you find a place on this drawing to show how happy Lina felt?

HILLARY: (*Nods.*) Yes. Right here. (*Points to drawing's face.*)

THERAPIST: We don't have any expression on Lina's face. What type of face should we put there?

HILLARY: A happy face.

THERAPIST: You draw a happy face on her.

HILLARY: (*Draws the face.*)

THERAPIST: She's feeling happy. Oh, look over her head. Do you see what that is?

HILLARY: (*Nods yes.*)

THERAPIST: That is a thought bubble. Do you know what goes in there?

HILLARY: The things she thinks about.

THERAPIST: That's right. So let's see if together we can come up with what Lina is thinking right now. She's feeling happy because she wanted a balloon and she got one. Now, what do you suppose is going through her mind?

HILLARY: I'm happy, I have a balloon.

THERAPIST: So when Lina feels happy because she has a balloon, what might that mean about her?

HILLARY: She's really lucky.

THERAPIST: Let's put that in the bubble. Let's see what we have so far. Lina is a girl who really loves balloons. Her mom gave her a balloon, she feels happy, and she thinks she is lucky. Does that make sense?

HILLARY: Uh huh.

Figure 5.2 shows the completed drawings. The transcript illustrates several important points. First, the therapist worked hard at involving Hillary in all parts of the story. Second, the therapist broke down the situational, cognitive, and emotional components of the story into simple and concrete terms. Third, the drawings and words represent cues about the

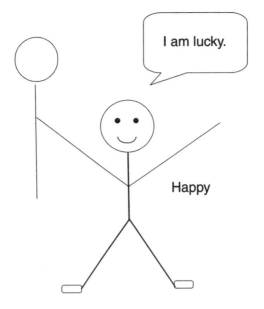

FIGURE 5.2. Drawing completed in first phase.

nature of therapy. Finally, the therapist summarized the story, connecting its situational, cognitive, and emotional components.

In the second phase of the story the therapist changes the situation. The therapist draws a picture similar to the one depicted in Figures 5.1 and 5.2. In this exercise the child learns that thoughts and feelings change in different situations.

THERAPIST: Hillary, do you want to know what happens next?

HILLARY: Uh huh.

THERAPIST: OK. Well, Lina is walking along holding her balloon and all of a sudden a car drives by and a pebble flies up and pops the balloon. So Lina's balloon is now gone. Will Lina still have a happy face?

HILLARY: No.

THERAPIST: That's right. Things have changed. What type of face will she have now?

HILLARY: A sad face.

THERAPIST: Can you draw a sad face on this picture? So her balloon popped and Lina is feeling sad. Will the same thing be in her thought bubble?

HILLARY: No.

THERAPIST: It wouldn't make sense that she would think she was lucky if her balloon popped and she felt sad. Her thoughts and feelings wouldn't match what happened. So we have to figure out what is going through her mind now. What do you suppose is in her thought bubble?

HILLARY: I lost my balloon.

THERAPIST: And when she lost her balloon and felt really sad, what did she say to herself?

HILLARY: I'll never get another one.

THERAPIST: That thought would sure go along with her sad feeling. Let's write it in the bubble. Let's see what we have so far. The balloon popped, Lina felt sad, and now she thinks "I'll never get another balloon." I would like to look at our two drawings and stories. What things changed in the second story?

HILLARY: Everything.

THERAPIST: What do you mean?

HILLARY: The balloon popped, she felt sad, and she thought she wouldn't get another balloon.

THERAPIST: That's right. The things around her changed, her feelings changed, and her thoughts changed. What were the things around her that changed?

HILLARY: The balloon popped.

THERAPIST: Can you tell me which are her feelings and which are her thoughts?

HILLARY: I'm not sure.

THERAPIST: Are you most in charge of the things that happen to you or of your thoughts and feelings?

HILLARY: My thoughts and feelings.

THERAPIST: These are the things you and I are going to talk and play about together. I am going to help you learn new ways to think about things and things to do when you feel badly. How does that sound?

Figure 5.3 shows the drawing completed in the second phase of this example. What has the therapist accomplished with this exchange? First,

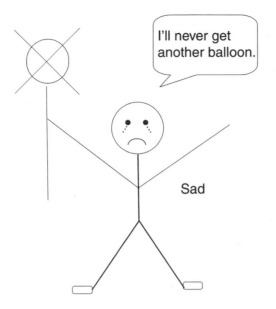

FIGURE 5.3. Therapist's drawing in second phase.

the therapist explicitly reviewed the event, feeling, and thought to help Hillary discuss the differences between the three elements. Second, the therapist also helped Hillary see the connection between events, feelings, and thoughts. Further, the therapist gently questioned Hillary to allow her to come up with an emotionally meaningful thought in the situation. This questioning process prepares Hillary for the Socratic-questioning and thought-testing procedures that come later in therapy. The therapist then asked her which of these factors she had the most control over. After Hillary responded with thoughts and feelings, the therapist followed with a concluding paragraph emphasizing that they will work on developing new cognitive and behavioral coping skills.

Another approach to teach about thoughts, feelings, behaviors, and situations is called Diamond Connections (Friedberg, Friedberg, & Friedberg, 2001). Diamond Connections uses a baseball diamond metaphor to illustrate the cognitive model. Each component (cognitive, behavioral, emotional, and physiological) of the model is symbolized by a base in the diamond. Children work their way through the worksheet base by base. They begin by identifying feelings and move on to recording bodily sensations, behaviors, and thoughts associated with sad or anxious feelings. After completing the exercise, the therapist explains that he/she will "cover all the bases" in his/her work with the child.

In our clinical experience, children seem to readily grasp the model presented in the Diamond Connections worksheet. The baseball diamond is familiar to most children and they quickly recognize that a diamond is not complete without all four bases. Therefore, the interactive relationship between components is easily communicated. The baseball metaphor lends itself to several experiential applications. Children can make bases out of cardboard and write "Thoughts," "Feelings," "Actions," and "Body" on them. They can then stand on each base while they share the appropriate symptoms. Therapists might toss a Nerf ball to them as they reach each base to add to the fun!

Therapists should note that as constructed the Diamond Connections worksheet addresses only sad and anxious feelings. However, therapists working with children experiencing other emotions could easily adapt the worksheet for their own purposes. This adaptation might simply involve adding a different emotion to the worksheet exercise or replacing worried or sad feeling words with the specific feelings children are experiencing.

INTRODUCING THE TREATMENT MODEL
TO ADOLESCENTS

Older adolescents are generally presented with the treatment model in the same manner as adults (J. S. Beck, 1995; Padesky & Greenberger, 1995). Typically, the cognitive model is presented after the assessment process is nearly or totally completed. The following transcript illustrates the way a therapist introduces the cognitive model to a depressed teenager.

THERAPIST: OK, Kendall. You have told me many things about yourself and the people around you. May I take this chance to tell you about how I work with young people like you?

KENDALL: All right.

THERAPIST: It always helps me to draw or write things down. I bet you noticed me writing lists while you were sharing things about yourself. As you can see (*shows model diagram*), there are four things about you that change when you feel depressed. All these things take place within your environment. The symptoms or signals of depression occur in these circumstances. How does this sound so far?

KENDALL: I'm not sure. What does "environment" mean?

THERAPIST: What were some of the things that happened which seemed to trigger your depressed feelings?

KENDALL: Well, I broke up with my boyfriend and my father left.

THERAPIST: That really hurts. Your dad and your boyfriend left you. These are all the things that are happening around you. (*Writes on paper.*)

KENDALL: (*Tears up.*) That's a lot of shit for one person.

THERAPIST: It sure is. You feel really sad, angry, and worried (*points to the feeling item on the model diagram*).

KENDALL: Yes. I get these stomachaches and awful headaches now.

THERAPIST: That's how they are connected.

KENDALL: I feel so shitty.

THERAPIST: So shitty that the things that were fun for you are no longer fun. You tend to keep to yourself and stay in your room.

KENDALL: That's where I feel safe.

THERAPIST: And if you look here (*points to the cognitive sphere*), on top of this you blame yourself and see most of your experiences as terribly unpleasant. You are kind of left with a pessimistic view of things.

KENDALL: Wouldn't you be?

THERAPIST: It certainly seems reasonable that if you see yourself as deserving of all the bad things that have happened and you expect more negative things in the future, you would be depressed and pessimistic. Now what we have to check out is whether the things you say to yourself about the terrible things that happened to you are accurate. Does that make sense?

KENDALL: I guess.

THERAPIST: Well, let me explain this model just a little bit more. (*Points.*) You see these lines? They connect each of these circles together. So if you make a change in one you can make a change in the remaining three. Which of these (*points*) are the ones you think you have most control over?

KENDALL: The thought and action ones.

THERAPIST: Exactly. What makes you think you have most control over these?

This exchange illustrates several critical points. Kendall's unique problems were explicitly addressed as part of the description, allowing her to personally relate to this approach. Additionally, the cognitive and behavioral focus of treatment was simply presented to Kendall ("Which of these are the ones you think you have most control over?").

Another method is a variation of a classic cognitive therapy procedure. The therapist first draws the situation, feeling, and thought columns on thought records or diaries, and then offers the following situation: Suppose you are at home and the telephone rings. Waiting for a telephone call is a prototypical event for many teenagers; often the telephone has a central role in their lives. After the situation is recorded, the therapist asks the youngster to report all the feelings he/she might have in response to the phone ringing (e.g., excited, angry, sad, nervous, calm). After the feelings are expressed, the therapist asks who it might be on the phone and records these explanations in the thought column. You should work diligently to compel the teen to explore all the possibilities about who it might be (e.g., boyfriend/girlfriend, mother/father, sibling, teacher, salesperson, friend of mother/father, friend of sibling). Figure 5.4 shows an example of the completed three-column table.

When the three columns are completed, the therapist works with the youngster to connect the thoughts and feelings (e.g., "If it was your teacher on the phone, which feeling would you have?"). At this point, the therapist explains that each thought uniquely shapes a feeling. The therapist draws lines to link different thoughts with different feelings. Moreover, the therapist calls attention to the finding that there are often multiple explanations for and feelings about the same single event. The therapist might elect to use Socratic questioning to explain the material (e.g., "How many feelings did we list?", "How many thoughts did we list?", "How many situations?", "What does this mean about a situation absolutely determining how you feel?").

The next step involves teaching the adolescent that not all explanations are functional or accurate. For example, the therapist might ask, "What if you thought it was your teacher calling to make a poor report

SITUATION	FEELING	THOUGHT
Phone rings at home	Excited Happy	It's my boyfriend/girlfriend.
	Sad	It's the doctor with bad news about my grandmother.
	Angry	It's my sister's stupid friend. It's a salesperson.
	Worried	It's my teacher. It's the police.
	Calm	It's my friend from school asking me a question.

FIGURE 5.4. Example of a thought record for introducing the model.

about you, but it was really a salesperson?" In this case, the youngster would become needlessly distressed. Subsequently, the youngster might be asked, "What if you thought it was a salesperson, but it was your teacher?" In this circumstance, the child is caught unaware. Thus, you conclude by explaining that in cognitive therapy we teach young people how to ask themselves better questions about the situations that occur in their lives so they do not become needlessly distressed or feel caught unprepared.

The last phase of this exercise provides the foundation for hypothesis formation, thought testing, and behavioral experimentation. In this phase, the therapist teaches the youngster that in order to know which thought is accurate he/she has to test them out and collect data (e.g., pick up the phone, ask who is calling, etc.). The therapist asks the youngster, "How will you know whether your guess about the caller is correct?" and "What do you have to do to find out?" Finally, the therapist concludes by connecting this metaphor to the concrete and specific tasks in cognitive therapy (e.g., "Together we will check out which of your conclusions are most accurate and useful for you in therapy. We will create different ways to find out which judgments best explain the things that happen to you.").

How do we decide which method to use? We tend to pick the telephone example for younger adolescents who need more concrete, specific examples. Further, the telephone method is preferable when the teenager is less motivated and less invested in treatment. Finally, the telephone method is well suited to group treatment.

IDENTIFYING PROBLEMS WITH CHILDREN AND ADOLESCENTS

Identifying problems with children and adolescents is a challenging process for even the most experienced therapists, but it is a crucial first step in treatment for several reasons. First, children may not know why they are coming to therapy and/or may be resentful about seeing a therapist. Second, in order to effectively address problems and compose a collaborative treatment approach, therapists, youngsters, and parents must form a consensus on the problem.

Considerable ingenuity is often required to engage youngsters in the problem-identification process. Some children may find the task boring and dull. Others may view it as painful. In fact, many therapists may see it that way too. However, the process does not have to be painfully dull! Therapists must make efforts to avoid making problem identification seem like a child's confession. If a child perceives criticism and believes the therapist is blaming him/her, he/she is likely to feel ashamed and resentful. Therefore, you must create an inviting way for the youngster to identify problems, a way that is empowering rather than belittling to the youngster. Accordingly, in this section, we suggest several methods for identifying problems with elementary school children and adolescents.

Identifying Problems with Children

Younger children may be especially clueless about why they are coming to therapy. They may think that they will be receiving a shot or medicine from the therapist. Other youngsters may view the therapist as a kind of principal or headmaster/headmistress who will penalize them now that they have gotten themselves into trouble. Correcting these mistaken assumptions is the first task of introducing therapy to a child and identifying target problems.

The "Dear Doctor" or "Dear Therapist" letter offers a way youngsters can tell you about themselves by doing something familiar to them, namely, writing a letter and identifying their problems (Padesky, 1988). Writing a letter serves as an initial step toward more direct self-disclosure by providing the child with a comfortable sense of distance from the therapist.

You could present the task in the following manner:

> "I want to get to know you a little bit better. One way I can learn more about you is if you tell me more about yourself. Have you ever written a letter to anyone before? Well, that's what I want you to do next week. I want you to write me a letter telling me whatever you want about yourself. Tell me about the things you do; your family; your sad, angry, or worried feelings; the things you enjoy; the things that get you in trouble; your school; and your friends. I really want you to write down whatever it is that you want me to know about you. Write both the things that make you happy and the things that trouble you. How does this sound?"

You may choose to write down the instructions for the letter and give them to children so they have a guide to help them complete the task. Younger children could speak into a tape recorder or dictate a letter to their parents instead of writing it themselves. Drawing pictures of things that make them happy, scared, or sad is another alternative for younger children.

Children often think about problems in global, impressionistic, and vague terms. Your first job in these circumstances is to help the youngster break the problem down into discrete, manageable, and understandable components. The Mouse-Traps and Fix-It exercises (Friedberg et al., 2001) are examples of fun methods designed to help children specify their problems. Children are invited to list the cognitive, emotional, and behavioral traps that snare them. Youngsters may be more willing to identify "traps" than "problems." You could have children draw pictures of nets, traps, or holes they fall into. They could write their problems down in the pictures of the traps. If children do not want to draw, they could cut out pictures of traps.

Identifying Problems with Adolescents

Identifying problems with preteens and adolescents presents unique challenges. In some ways, these youngsters are quite able to profit from traditional methods for identifying problems. In other ways, due to their mistrust and suspicion of adults, these youngsters are often quite reluctant to say what's really on their minds. Therefore, we need to make deliberate efforts to collaborate with adolescents in the problem-identification process.

The most conventional way to identify problems with adolescents is the problem list (Padesky, 1988; Persons, 1989). In developing the problem list, we recommend that you operationalize the cognitive, emotional, physiological, behavioral, and interpersonal components of the problem. It is relatively commonplace for reluctant adolescents to distance themselves from the problem or to describe the problem in terms of what others are doing to them. For instance, when asked about his problems, a recalcitrant teen responded, "My mother is a nagging bitch." We encourage you to initially accept this external definition of the problem and consider it as an initial step toward more productive work rather than automatically dismissing it.

The following transcript illustrates how to construct a problem list with a recalcitrant 15-year-old boy.

THERAPIST: What should we work on together today, Anthony?

ANTHONY: My mother nags me. She's always on my case. She treats me like I'm 5 years old.

THERAPIST: OK. Let's put that down on this paper (*writes*). Your mother treats you like a baby and is always on your case. You don't like that, do you? Let's see what else seems to be a problem.

ANTHONY: They bitch at me for not doing my homework and for watching too much TV. My dad wants me to turn down my music all the time.

THERAPIST: You think they don't give you enough freedom. Your mom and dad tell you how much TV to watch and they supervise your homework. I bet that kind of gets on your nerves.

ANTHONY: It sucks.

THERAPIST: So that sounds like another problem for you. We will write this one down too (*writes*). Now what we need to do next is to figure out how you can get what you want.

ANTHONY: That sounds good.

THERAPIST: What do you suppose you need to do to help Mom see you as a 15-year-old?

ANTHONY: I dunno.

THERAPIST: Oh. You gotta help me and Mom out here. What do you do that makes her treat you like a little kid?

ANTHONY: Ask her!

THERAPIST: Well, I could, but then she would be taking charge of your plan. I thought you wanted to be more in charge of things. Kind of limit Mom's nagging. If we allow Mom and Dad to define your problems, I think we're back to them treating you like a kid. What do you think?

ANTHONY: I guess so.

THERAPIST: So what is it that you do that makes Mom and Dad treat you like a little kid?

ANTHONY: Well, I don't listen to them a lot. Sometimes I forget to do all my crappy homework.

THERAPIST: So if your parents thought you listened more and paid more attention to your schoolwork, they might get off your back more?

What can we learn from this exchange? First, the therapist briefly explained the purpose of identifying problems (i.e., to know and understand you). Second, the therapist began the process from Anthony's perspective and through guided discovery gradually molded the definition to accommodate his own contribution to the difficulties. Third, the therapist wrote down the problems on paper, which communicated to Anthony that he was listening and is taking the report seriously. Finally, the therapist demonstrated both patience and confidence throughout the example.

You may also elect to use the standardized measures discussed in Chapters 2 and 4 as a way to identify problems. For instance, the CDI, MASC, and/or RCMAS are used to monitor progress and check-in on the level of emotional functioning. You can use children's self-reports of symptoms as a way to jump-start the problem-identification process.

The following transcript shows how you can use the CDI as a way to help a 13-year-old girl identify problems.

THERAPIST: I am looking over the sheet where you checked how you feel about certain things. I noticed that you checked you cried a lot. Do you cry a lot?

WENDY: Yes.

THERAPIST: Tell me, what do you cry about?

WENDY: Many things, really. When my friends make fun of me, when my father gets angry with me. When I can't visit my father on weekends.

THERAPIST: May I write these things down on paper?

WENDY: Sure, if you want to.

THERAPIST: (*Writes.*) I want to because I want to make sure I don't miss anything. What you say is important. What else makes you cry?

WENDY: I mainly cry when I am alone. My mom says I shouldn't. I cry sometimes when I get a bad grade.

THERAPIST: I see. I also noticed that you checked you are not having much fun. Tell me about that one.

Here the therapist used the child's report of her symptoms as a springboard for problem identification. This is a relatively efficient method for problem identification since it comes from the children themselves. The transcript illustrates how the therapist can delve deeper into the child's report and gain broader information.

CONCLUSION

Therapy is a mystery to most children and their families. People normally approach unknown territory with great trepidation and considerable ambivalence. By explicitly introducing the treatment model you can demystify the therapy process and make families more comfortable. Simple drawings and stories are inviting ways to introduce treatment to children. You can match methods for teaching children about the cognitive model to the children's interests and developmental level. Dear Doctor Letters, problem lists, and standardized self-report measures are helpful ways to identify problems. Problem identification and introduction to treatment propels therapeutic momentum and leads the way to pivotal therapeutic processes such as self-monitoring, self-instruction, rational analysis, and performance-based treatment options.

6

❖

Identifying and Connecting
Feelings and Thoughts

Identifying feelings and thoughts is a key self-monitoring task in cognitive therapy. This chapter begins with recommendations for helping children and adolescents identify their feelings. The second part describes the challenges involved in identifying and reporting cognitions. Next, the content specificity hypothesis, which states that different emotions are characterized by distinct cognitions, is explained and its clinical implications are explicated. Finally, the steps involved in completing a thought diary/ thought record are outlined and methods for avoiding common pitfalls are suggested.

IDENTIFYING FEELINGS WITH
CHILDREN AND ADOLESCENTS

Identification of feelings is a first step in cognitive therapy for several reasons. First, evaluating treatment outcome depends on children's ability to identify their own feelings. Unless children report their distressing emotions prior to any interventions, the therapist has no way to know whether his/her intervention effort resulted in any positive emotional changes. Second, distressing feelings are common cues for using thought-testing skills. Thus, recognizing when they feel badly prompts skill application. Third, the content-specificity hypothesis guides you in helping children reliably identify their feelings. Fourth, exposure exercises require children to identify and endure emotional expression.

Identifying and reporting feelings is difficult for many children. Therefore, designing ways to overcome these difficulties is incumbent upon therapists. Accordingly, the following section offers recommendations for helping children and adolescents identify their feelings.

Identifying Feelings with Children

Identifying feelings with young children often requires considerable creativity. Young children lack experience in articulating their emotional state. We recommend that you teach children how to report their mood states prior to beginning cognitive interventions.

Adopting a simple classification system for emotions is a good initial strategy. Young children will be overwhelmed by a complex system that requires them to make fine discriminations. For instance, understanding the fine distinctions among feelings such as annoyance, irritation, frustration, and upset may be too challenging for young children. Accordingly, we use the traditional classification system consisting of mad, sad, glad, scared, and worried feelings.

One useful tool is a *Feeling Faces Chart*. The chart offers pictures that demonstrate various facial expressions and includes labels naming the appropriate emotion beneath each picture. While these charts are helpful for many children, they do have limitations. First, younger children may be overwhelmed by the number of feeling faces from which to choose. Second, the words used to describe the children's feelings tend to be more sophisticated than the average 9-year-old child might employ (e.g., "devastated"). Third, depending on the version of the Feeling Faces Chart used, the chart may be culturally insensitive.

Our solution has been to develop our own charts. Indeed, we encourage children to make their own charts. They draw blank faces, elect skin color and facial characteristics, and offer their own labels for the feelings. Figure 6.1 illustrates the Feeling Faces Chart. Often, this is a useful icebreaker for children. Children are invited to draw three or four faces and then write labels beneath them. Laminated charts allow for additional flexibility: Children can write on them with erasable water-based markers, erase, and redo their faces and labels as needed.

A procedure developed in the Preventing Anxiety and Depression in Youth program offers another variation of this task (Friedberg et al., 2001). In this alternative, children draw their feeling on a picture of a mouse character named "Pandy" and then label the feeling on the drawing. Drawing the feeling face on Pandy seems to allow the child to identify with the mouse while also providing sufficient distance to facilitate emotional expression.

Employing pictures from a magazine is a third variation. We give the

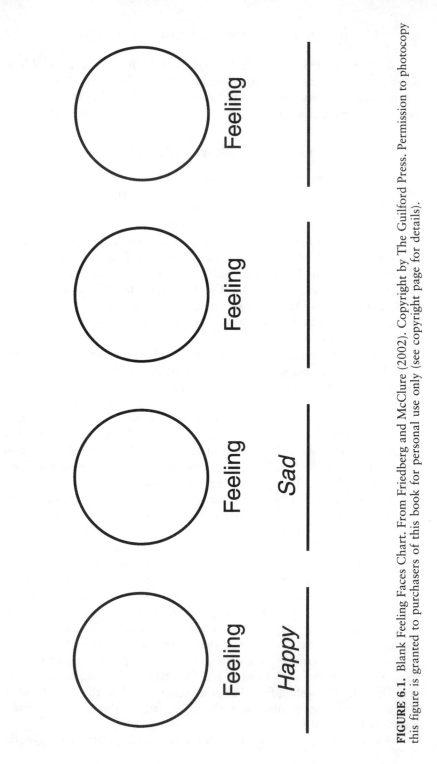

FIGURE 6.1. Blank Feeling Faces Chart. From Friedberg and McClure (2002). Copyright by The Guilford Press. Permission to photocopy this figure is granted to purchasers of this book for personal use only (see copyright page for details).

84

child old magazines and ask him/her to cut out pictures of people who are experiencing different feelings. The child pastes the pictures on cardboard or heavy construction paper and then writes the appropriate feeling word under each picture.

Creating an individualized Feeling Faces Chart has several advantages. First, by reviewing magazines, children are able to cut out pictures of people who are likely to be role models for them. Second, there is a potential for children to select pictures that most resemble themselves. In this way, the task becomes culturally responsive and can represent their real-life circumstances. Third, emotional expression becomes more normalized through this process. If children select pictures of people they admire showing various emotions, the act of identifying feelings becomes less threatening.

Reading *picture books* with young children is another way to explore emotional components. Obviously, you want to choose books with illustrations that are demonstrative and identifiable. In addition, you should try to provide books that are culturally sensitive. For instance, the *Amazing Grace* series (Hoffman, 1991) wonderfully portrays the struggles of a resourceful African American girl. Bill Cosby's (1997) *The Meanest Thing to Say* is also a nice choice. *Smoky Night* (Bunting, 1994) is an emotionally powerful depiction of the Los Angeles riots. *Mei-Mei Loves the Morning* (Tsubakiyama, 1999) and *Shibumi and the Kite-Maker* (Mayer, 1999) are expressive books with Asian American characters. Joy Berry (1995, 1996) has written specific emotionally focused books for children that include some children of color. Cartledge and Milburn (1996) provide a rich resource of recommendations for literature with culturally diverse children.

As you read through your chosen book together, you should pause and discuss its emotional components. You can then ask the child to identify the characters' feelings and talk about how they are similar or different from their own. The following transcript illustrates the process when reading *Alexander and the Terrible, Horrible, Very Bad Day* (Viorst, 1972).

THERAPIST: So, Alexander had a very bad day in this book. How do you feel when you have a very bad day?

JENAE: Bad.

THERAPIST: What does your face look like?

JENAE: (*Frowns.*)

THERAPIST: I see. A lot of things happened to Alexander during his bad day. What happens to make you feel sad?

JENAE: My friends are mean to me. My mom yells at me. My teacher gives me too much homework.

While reading books is a strategy that works for many children, some youngsters may not respond well to written material. In these instances, we recommend *movies, plays, television shows, and music* as ways to help children identify feelings. For instance, we showed clips from *The Wizard of Oz* to a child who was having difficulty identifying and labeling his feelings. We showed him the segment where Dorothy, the Cowardly Lion, the Tin Man, and the Scarecrow meet the all-powerful Oz. In this episode, each character displays different emotions in varying intensity. The child was then asked to notice each character's reaction; to note the character's facial expression, verbal comments, and behaviors; and consequently to identify the character's feelings. The therapist then asked the youngster if he had similar feelings. When the boy shared that indeed he had similar feelings as nearly every character, the therapist expanded the process by asking the youngster to show how his face looked when he was sad and inquiring what went through his mind when he felt low.

After children learn to identify and label their feelings, they are ready to rate their feeling intensity. Children see emotions categorically: they either have them or they don't. They are relatively unskilled in determining how much of the feeling they experience. Thus, therapists need to help youngsters understand that feelings vary in intensity. For example, 10-year-old Chester knows he is anxious but is unable to say when he feels more anxious and when he feels less anxious. For Chester, his anxiety is a backpack filled with rocks: he knows it is heavy but he is unable to measure its weight. In order for children to grasp this concept, we simplify the idea through more concrete exercises.

Building on the Feeling Faces exercise is a straightforward way to begin to scale the intensity of feelings. When children draw a feeling face, they are asked to rate how strongly they experience the emotion they have illustrated. Older children estimate their level of feeling on a simple 1–5 scale. Younger, less sophisticated children will likely require more assistance. In these instances, we add boxes to their Feeling Faces Charts. Figure 6.2 illustrates this practice.

When completing this worksheet, children draw their feeling face in the space provided and then add the feeling label (e.g., sad). Below the feeling label, five boxes representing varying levels of intensity are provided. The boxes range from an empty one to a moderately filled box to a completely filled box. Children are then asked to circle or point to the box that shows how much of the feeling they experienced. These boxes translate nicely into the more abstract 1–5 rating scale.

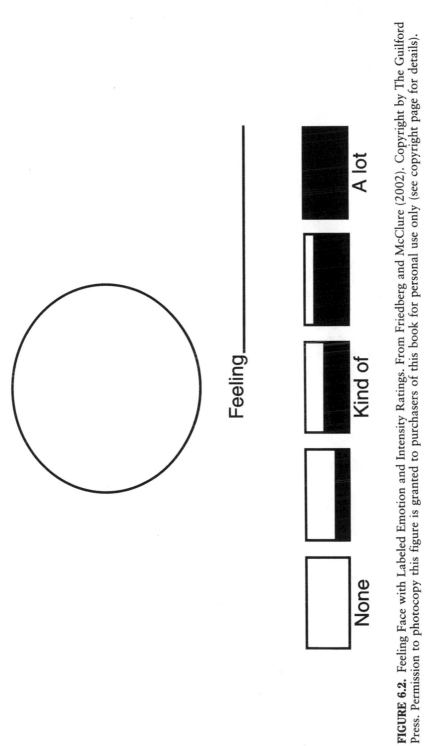

FIGURE 6.2. Feeling Face with Labeled Emotion and Intensity Ratings. From Friedberg and McClure (2002). Copyright by The Guilford Press. Permission to photocopy this figure is granted to purchasers of this book for personal use only (see copyright page for details).

The rating task can be made even more concrete. Hands-on experimentation helps teach children in a focused manner. Inviting the child to pour colored water into clear plastic cups is an engaging plan. The children are told to leave one cup empty, and to fill the other cups one-quarter full, half full, three-quarters full, and full. You can facilitate this process by premarking the different levels with a black marker on the cups. Instead of liquid, you could use beads, marbles, shells, or any fun object that could fill a cup. You then ask the youngster to point to the cup that shows how much they feel the feeling.

Feeling thermometers or Feeling Barometers are widely used tools for helping children identify emotional intensity (Castro-Blanco, 1999; Silverman & Kurtines, 1996). Most children know what a thermometer does. Moreover, it lends itself to useful metaphors. For instance, after a child has completed the Feeling Thermometer, the therapist might say, "Show me where your anger reaches the boiling point."

A *Feeling Traffic Signal* is another way to record emotional intensity (Friedberg et al., 2001). Like the Feeling Thermometer, the Traffic Signal exercise helps rate emotional intensity and provides a source for accessible metaphors. For instance, experiencing feelings at a high intensity may contribute to children's behavioral and cognitive paralysis. Indeed, they run into a red light and they are stopped cold in their tracks. Recognizing that these strong feelings may stop them in their tracks like a red light halts traffic may facilitate children's better understanding of the role emotions play in their lives.

Tying feelings to physical sensations is yet another way to help children identify their feelings. Children are often readily aware of their bodily/somatic sensations. Consequently, these physiological reactions represent viable anchor points for youngsters. Asking the child "How does your body feel when _____?" creates a foundation for emotional expression. You should tie a concrete behavioral referent to the question (e.g., "How does your body feel when you hear your mom and dad yelling at each other?"). Grounding the feeling in a physical sensation gives children a concrete referent for their feelings. The following transcript illustrates the process of connecting feelings to physical sensations.

THERAPIST: When your teacher gives you a spelling test, how does your body feel?

CARLY: All tight.

THERAPIST: What other changes in how your body feels do you notice?

CARLY: My stomach feels upset, my head is stuffy.

THERAPIST: If your stomach had a voice, how would she say she is feeling?

CARLY: Sick, like I'm going to throw up.

THERAPIST: How about your stuffy head? What would her voice say?

CARLY: I'm tired, I feel like I have the flu.

THERAPIST: So it sounds like spelling tests really make you feel sick. Can you draw a picture of your stomach and put a face on it?

CARLY: (*Draws the picture.*)

THERAPIST: What type of face does your stomach have?

CARLY: A worried one, I guess.

In this exchange, the therapist asked Carly specific questions that were connected to concrete referents (e.g., "When your teacher gives you a spelling test, how does your body feel?"). Additionally, the therapist helped the child express the feeling embedded within the physical sensation (e.g., "If your stomach had a voice, how would she say she was feeling?"). The therapist encouraged Carly to further specify her feelings in a concrete way by inviting her to draw a picture of her "sick stomach." In this example, Carly profited from some open-ended questions. Some children may need more guidance. In these instances, we give youngsters multiple choices ("Are you feeling mad, sad, scared, or worried?") Further, if the child does not respond verbally, we draw simple happy, sad, worried, and mad faces and ask him/her to point to the picture of his/her feeling.

Identifying Feelings with Adolescents

Given adolescents' emotional maturity, their ability to identify feelings is more developed than that of younger children. In cases where adolescents are more limited, you can rely on the techniques used for younger children. No matter what the youngster's age, you need to make sure your client is well skilled in identifying and reporting his/her feelings. This section offers several suggestions for helping adolescents identify their feelings.

Self-report inventories are handy methods for identifying adolescents' mood states. When completed by the adolescent, the CDI, MASC, or RCMAS provides a gross measure of mood states. These inventories are simple to complete and direct both the therapist's and the youngster's attention toward salient feeling states.

Switching Channels (Friedberg, Fidaleo, & Mason, 1992) offers several exercises designed to prompt emotional expression in adolescents. In a *story exercise*, teens are asked to write a story about a time they felt sad, angry, or depressed. The story can include the circumstances surrounding the feeling, the youth's physiological reaction, and cognitive and behavioral reactions. The teen provides a title for the story that also frequently reveals his/her emotional state.

The story exercise can clearly be modified by encouraging adolescents to *create a poem, song, or rap lyric* describing their feelings. Teens may find these creative outlets liberating and may consequently disclose more heartfelt emotions through a poem or rap. Moreover, songs and rap reflect these youngsters' social ecology. In short, it may be more permissible for a youth to express his/her feelings through a poem or a rap than to directly say them to another person.

Many teenagers suffer from a limited feeling vocabulary. For instance, they may refer to all negative emotional states by calling them "bad" or "upset." This restricted feeling vocabulary makes it difficult to distinguish between discrepant emotional categories (e.g., mad, sad, worried) as well as between varying intensities within the same feeling (e.g., annoyed, angry, furious). For example, when asked how he was feeling, Otto always had the same response: "bad." Moreover, youngsters may use idiographic labels to communicate their feelings (e.g., "Whatever"). Consider the example of Julian who repeatedly reports his feeling as "itchy." Thus, expanding a teen's feeling vocabulary provides the youth with a greater range of responses and incorporates personalized idioms. You can simply invite teens to list as many words as they can to describe their feelings.

Creating a *feeling poster or collage* is also a productive plan. In this exercise teens design a poster representing different feeling states from pictures cut out of popular magazines. A feeling collage is well suited to youngsters who have difficulty putting words to their feelings. The feeling collage is a graduated task. Youngsters begin the process with the collage assignment and then proceed to experiment with verbal expression.

Feeling charades, a therapeutic variation of the familiar party game, identify and express feelings (Frey & Fitzgerald, 2000). Youngsters select cards labeled with various emotions (e.g., angry, pissed-off, ashamed) and then act out the chosen emotion using only expressions and actions. Charades works especially well with groups and families. Participants divide into teams that earn points for correct identification of feelings. The game allows for practice in both expressing one's own emotions and recognizing feelings in others. Attention to nonverbal cues associated with emotional states is reinforced through this fun and interactive game. Similar to the feeling vocabulary list, this game is culturally responsive to different feeling labels and expressions. Individuals can create their own idiographic labels and demonstrate unique ways to manifest these feelings.

Deblinger (1997) offers an extremely creative *talk-show method* to facilitate a youth's emotional expressiveness. In her work with sexually abused youngsters, Deblinger inventively used the "call-in" format that characterizes many television and radio talk shows. Cognitive therapists might modify this strategy to help reticent teens express their feelings. Typically, the therapist pretends to be a talk show host and the teen acts like his/her guest. The therapist then pretends to take a call from a viewer at home who has specific questions about how the youngster felt in certain circumstances. The teen might find the "distance" from the "pretend caller" comfortable and demonstrate more willingness to express his/her emotions. Moreover, the fun and imaginative nature of the task might loosen the youngster's prohibitions against expressiveness.

IDENTIFYING THOUGHTS AND CONNECTING
THOUGHTS TO FEELINGS

The classic means to identify thoughts is the question "What is going through your mind right now?" This is best asked at the moment of a mood shift (J. S. Beck, 1995; Padesky, 1988). Remaining mindful of this practice makes cognitive therapy an "experiential here-and-now" type of approach. You should not ask the question in a overly stylized or stereotypical manner (A. T. Beck et al., 1979). Certainly, you can alter the question in a variety of ways. We encourage you to develop your own personal style. However, we strongly recommend that therapists stay away from questions such as "What are you thinking?" or "What thoughts are you having about _____?" These kind of questions may limit the youngster's responses by neglecting cognitive processes such as imagery. Rather, we invite therapists to embrace more open-ended queries such as:

"What popped into your mind?"
"What flew into your mind?"
"What zipped through your mind?"
"What breezed through your head?"
"What rushed through your mind?"
"What did you say to yourself?"
"What raced through your head?"

The most common device cognitive therapists use to connect thoughts and feelings is a *daily thought record* (DTR), also called a thought diary. There are several excellent DTR's in the literature on cognitive therapy with adults (A. T. Beck et al., 1979; J. S. Beck, 1995;

Greenberger & Padesky, 1995). In general, the DTR allows clients to chronicle their problematic situations, distressing thoughts and feelings, alternative responses, and the emotional outcome accompanying the counterresponse. The traditional DTR may be appropriate for older adolescents.

Identifying Thoughts with Children

Several child-friendly thought records have been created (Bernard & Joyce, 1984; Friedberg et al., 2001; Kendall, 1990; Seligman et al., 1995). Recent research has revealed that even young children understand that a thought bubble denotes cognitive content (Wellman et al., 1996).

Bernard and Joyce (1984) describe a particularly creative thought record for younger children called a *Thought Flower Garden*. In this procedure, children draw flowers whose blooms represent feelings and whose stems indicate thoughts; the soil denotes the precipitating event for their feelings and thoughts. Children color the blooms different colors to represent different feelings. In our experience, youngsters find this task fun and entertaining. The following transcript provides an example of how to use the *Thought Flower Garden* exercise with young children.

THERAPIST: Have you ever drawn a flower?

KENDRA: Yes, in my school.

THERAPIST: Go ahead and pick out some colors and I will show you how to draw a Thought Flower Garden.

KENDRA: (*Selects some crayons.*)

THERAPIST: OK. Let's draw the ground. What color should we make it?

KENDRA: Brown. I'll do it. (*Draws the ground.*)

THERAPIST: The flowers grow from the ground. The ground is like the things that happen to you when you feel bad. What happened this week that made you feel bad?

KENDRA: Mom and Nana got into a fight.

THERAPIST: OK. We'll put that in the soil here (*writes*). Now we have to figure out what thoughts and feelings grew from this. What went through your mind about the fight?

KENDRA: I'm a bad girl.

THERAPIST: That thought is the stem. You draw the stem. I'll write what went through your mind. Now, how did you feel when Mom and Nana argued and you believed you were a bad girl?

KENDRA: Sad.

THERAPIST: What color flower would this be?

KENDRA: Gray.

What does this example illustrate? First, the Thought Flower Garden did not demand much verbal expressiveness. Second, drawing was a nonthreatening task. Third, the garden metaphor allowed the therapist to present the psychoeducational material without lecturing the child. Fourth, Kendra identified her thoughts and feelings while coloring.

Simple *thought bubbles floating over a cartoon-like face or figure* is another useful way to identify thoughts (Padesky, 1986). In this type of thought record people or animal characters are expressing some emotion and children fill in the bubble (Kendall, 1990; Seligman et al., 1995). In Kendall's (1990) ingenious *Coping Cat* program, clever depictions of restful dogs and frazzled cats engage youngsters in the thought-identification task. Friedberg et al. (2001) use a mouse figure to identify the feeling, a traffic-signal icon to rate the feeling intensity, and a blank bubble to capture thoughts and feelings. Cartoon figures and drawings may make therapy seem less like work for children.

Older children may not require cartoon-like illustrations to grab their attention. With these youngsters, a blank face with a bubble above the head may suffice. Figure 6.3 illustrates the most basic version of this practice. The child draws the feeling face, writes the emotion label and strength, writes the thought in the bubble, and records the event associated with the distressing thoughts and feelings. The following transcript illustrates the process.

THERAPIST: You have really shared a very important part of yourself. Let's see if together we can catch your thoughts and feelings connected with it. How does this sound?

SHAUN: OK, I guess. If you think it will help.

THERAPIST: Let's check it out. First, write in what happened that troubled you.

SHAUN: (*Pauses and tears up.*) My dad called me a lazy loser. He said I was a disgrace to the family name.

THERAPIST: That really hurts. When he said that how did it make you feel?

SHAUN: (*Cries*). Like I'm a nothing. I'll never be anything. He hates me.

THERAPIST: Those are really painful things to be going through your mind. Let's put them in the thought bubble, OK?

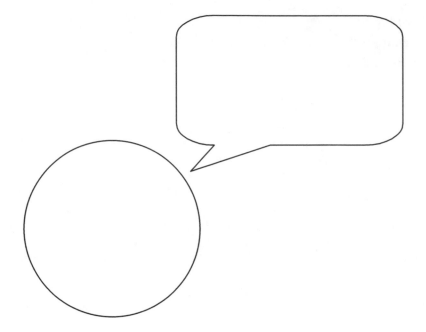

EVENT

_____

FEELING TYPE

_____

FEELING STRENGTH

_____

FIGURE 6.3. Basic Cartoon Thought Record. From Friedberg and McClure (2002). Copyright by The Guilford Press. Permission to photocopy this figure is granted to purchasers of this book for personal use only (see copyright page for details).

SHAUN: OK. (*Writes them in.*)

THERAPIST: Now, when your dad said these hurtful words to you, and "I'm a nothing. I'll never be anything and he hates me" went through your mind (*points to words in the thought bubble*), how did you feel?

SHAUN: Really shitty.

THERAPIST: Let's put that down.

SHAUN: We can?

THERAPIST: Sure.

SHAUN: (*Writes it on the thought record.*)

THERAPIST: Now what type of face did you have?

SHAUN: One like this (*draws a sad face with tears on the record*).

THERAPIST: How strong was your shitty feeling?

SHAUN: What do you mean?

THERAPIST: Remember how we did the feeling faces on a scale of 1–10?

SHAUN: Oh yeah. I felt pretty shitty. Maybe a 9.

This transcript illustrates several salient points. First, Shaun and his therapist completed the thought diary when he was distressed, thereby making the task psychologically valuable for him. Second, the therapist gently guided Shaun through the process. Third, like most children, Shaun initially confused his thoughts with his feelings; the therapist corrected Shaun without criticizing him. Finally, the therapist prompted Shaun to write down the distressing event, feeling, and thought.

Board games, as described in Chapter 9, are another viable medium for identifying thoughts and feelings. Children enjoy board games and respond well to their engaging nature. Berg (1986, 1989, 1990a, 1990b, 1990c) has created a series of cognitive-behavioral board games that we have found quite useful. Game cards reflect important areas in children's lives and are prompts to identify thoughts and feelings as well as guides for developing coping statements and problem-solving strategies. For homework assignments, children can create their own game cards.

Identifying Thoughts with Adolescents

With older children and adolescents, identifying thoughts becomes somewhat more routine. The basic task is similar to identifying thoughts with adults. The standard DTR may be applied. Although the DTR is used, we recommend completing the DTR in parts rather than as a whole. Dividing the task into parts simplifies the work and likely promotes greater compliance (J. S. Beck, 1995).

Integrating the thought record into the session content augments its application. Youngsters should readily realize why they are completing the DTR, how the DTR relates to the presenting problem, and what the outcome will be. Thought records are often done in session while youngsters are describing their distressing circumstances and the thoughts and feelings associated with them. In our clinical experience, we have found many adolescents appreciate seeing their thoughts and feelings written down in words. By writing the teenager's words down verbatim on the DTR, the therapist honors the child's expression through his/her uncensored recording.

The following transcript of a session with Ally, a 16-year-old girl, illustrates the way you might integrate a thought record into your work with adolescents.

ALLY: When my mother tells me what to do I just go wild. I'm furious. She's on me all the time.

THERAPIST: This sounds like a really important problem for you and your mom. Let's put it down in a thought record if that's OK with you?

ALLY: Whatever.

THERAPIST: I'll take that as a yes. What set off your feelings?

ALLY: My mom was yelling at me to help my sister clean her room and told me I couldn't stay out with my friends on a school night.

THERAPIST: We'll write that in the situation column (*writes*). Now, how did you feel?

ALLY: Pissed off. Furious. Really over the edge. She always does this.

THERAPIST: Those are some strong feelings. Write those down in the feeling column. We need to rate these feelings. How should we rate them?

ALLY: I don't know.

THERAPIST: We need a way to tell how strongly you feel about these emotions. Some people use a 1–10 scale, others a 1–5. Still others use a 1–100 scale. Which one do you want to use?

ALLY: 1–10, I guess.

THERAPIST: Which should be high and which one low?

ALLY: 1 is low.

THERAPIST: OK. So how furious?

ALLY: An 8, I guess.

THERAPIST: So, pretty furious? What made you an 8?

ALLY: I was seeing red. I was screaming and yelling. I was on the edge. I slammed the bedroom door.

THERAPIST: What went through your mind?

ALLY: My mother's unfair. She is such a bitch. I can't wait to move out when I'm old enough.

THERAPIST: Good. Let's write that in the thought column.

What does this dialogue illustrate? First, the therapist guided Ally through the process in a systematic manner with emotionally potent material. Second, the therapist used the teen's language in a verbatim manner while completing the thought record. Third, the therapist made sure the feeling (furious) was scaled in intensity.

Incomplete sentence fragments may also help adolescents capture their thoughts in specific situations (Friedberg et al., 1992; Padesky, 1986). Incomplete sentence fragments are a variation of the DTR that simply require the adolescent to fill in the blank. The incomplete sentences are presented as a graduated task where initially the therapist and the teenager identify the problematic situation and feeling and then the youngster supplies his/her thought. You should collaborate with the youngster on the specific stems for the events and feelings so the task becomes individualized. Some examples of incomplete sentences for a teenager who becomes angry at limit setting are the following:

"When my teacher tells me to come to class on time, I feel mad and _____ goes through my mind."
"When my parents give me a curfew, I get furious and I think _____."
When my brother goes through my stuff, I get mad and _____ pops into my head."

Incomplete sentences allow for considerable flexibility and creativity. The fragments might be constructed to tap the hot spots in adolescents' lives. As a teenager becomes more familiar with the task, the therapist can use incomplete sentences that include more blank spaces for the youth to complete. For instance, a more complex form of the incomplete sentence technique looks like this:

"When mom and dad _____ I feel _____ and _____ goes through my mind."

As you can see, this incomplete sentence fragment resembles the first three columns of the DTR. Accordingly, this incomplete sentence procedure is a graduated form of the DTR. DTRs could be assigned subsequently as a next therapeutic step.

USING THE CONTENT-SPECIFICITY HYPOTHESIS TO GUIDE IDENTIFYING THOUGHTS AND FEELINGS

We can use the content-specificity hypothesis to determine whether we have elicited the most meaningful cognition from the child. For instance, the following thought records illustrate how therapists and children may miss meaningful thoughts. In each of the examples, the reported thought is disconnected from emotional currents and reflects peripheral cognitions.

Sample Thought Record 1

Event: Mom was sick in the hospital.
Feeling: Worried (9)
Thought: I miss her.

Sample Thought Record 2

Event: Got a 79 on a math test.
Feeling: Sad (8)
Thought: I didn't do well.

Sample Thought Record 3

Event: Did not get invited to a party.
Feeling: Sad (8)
Thought: It would have been fun.

In the first thought record, the thought (I miss her) is connected to the situation but does not match the emotional intensity. We are left wondering how missing Mom is related to a high level of worry. For instance, what is the danger or threat about missing Mom? What is dangerous about Mom being in the hospital? The thought is not inaccurate or distorted. Rather, it reflects reality. Therefore, a reasonable assumption can be made that a more meaningful thought lies behind this unsettlingly realistic but probably sanitized report. Sample Thought Record 4 illustrates how the thought record might look after further processing.

Sample Thought Record 4

Event: Mom was sick in the hospital.
Feeling: Worried (9)
Thought: I won't be able to handle school on my own. Things will
    overwhelm me.

In Sample Thought Record 2, the thought "I didn't do well" is a sur-
face cognition that has more distressing thoughts concealed beneath it.
The therapist might direct his/her questioning to identify the child's possible self-critical views (e.g., "What does getting a 79 on the test and not
doing well mean about you?"), negative views about others (e.g."What
do you guess others will think of you now?"), and/or pessimistic views of
the future (e.g., "How do you expect this grade will affect you?"). Sample
Thought Record 5 shows the new thought record.

Sample Thought Record 5

Event: Getting a 79 on a test.
Feeling: Sad (8)
Thought: I'm stupid and my teacher won't like me anymore.

In Sample Thought Record 3, little insight is gained into the psychological significance regarding not being invited to the party and/or missing out on the fun. Using the content-specificity hypothesis, you might
ask questions such as the following:

"What would missing out on the fun mean to you?"
"What is it like to not be invited to a party you want to go to?"
"What does not being invited mean about you?"
"How do you expect others will see you if they knew you weren't in-
    vited?"

Following more in-depth processing, Sample Thought Record 6 illustrates
a more meaningful thought diary.

Sample Thought Record 6

Event: Did not get invited to a party.
Feeling: Sad (8)
Thought: I'm the most unpopular kid in school.

AVOIDING CONFUSION BETWEEN
THOUGHTS AND FEELINGS

We teach children and their families a crude and simplistic way to discern thoughts from feelings (Friedberg et al., 1992). First, we tell them that thoughts are the things that go through your mind and they usually take shape as sentences or phrases (e.g., "Something bad is going to happen to me.") Then we tell them that feelings are your emotions and typically can be communicated in one word (e.g., "scared"). Thoughts represent subjective judgments, evaluations, conclusions, explanations, and/or appraisals (e.g., "I'm incompetent"). Feeling sad, pissed-off, frustrated, confused, and so on are rather objective descriptions. They are simple, descriptive labels that represent the child's report of his/her feeling state. Since feelings are objective descriptions, they should not be challenged, tested, or questioned in cognitive therapy. For instance, we might respond with a statement such as "It makes perfect sense that you would feel scared if you thought something bad was going to happen to you and you won't be able to handle it. What we need to figure out is whether something bad will happen to you and you won't be able to handle it."

HELPING CHILDREN AND ADOLESCENTS
COMPLETE A DAILY THOUGHT RECORD

Children and adolescents need some direct instruction when completing a DTR. Children need to know how to fill in the event or situation. The situation is an objective description of what is happening. Events are commonly some environmental or external circumstance (e.g., I lost my keys.) Occasionally, especially in the case of anxiety, the event might be an internal stimulus (e.g., I blushed, I'm sweating). The situation is the event the child is explaining or making judgments and conclusions about. It is important that you check to make sure the situation is a relatively objective description of the distressing circumstances and does not contain hidden automatic thoughts.

Figure 6.4 shows a thought record in which the situation contains an automatic thought. The description is rather subjective and contains potentially overgeneralized labels of the teacher and the child. It is unclear what happened to shape the child's belief that the teacher dislikes him, thinks he is dumb, and is mean. Moreover, after reviewing the thought record, the therapist may conclude that the belief "He doesn't like me" may in fact be secondary to the conclusions mistakenly recorded under the situation column. You will need to devote more time

Situation	Feeling	Thought
My teacher is mean and thinks I am dumb.	Sad (8)	He does not like me.

FIGURE 6.4. Example of a thought record with embedded automatic thoughts in the situation column.

to sorting out the relevant beliefs with this child as well as helping him to clarify the situation. Figure 6.5 shows an example of a thought record where the situation is objectively identified and the automatic thought is placed in the proper column.

Completing the feeling column is also somewhat more difficult than initially meets the eye. First, children need to access their feeling vocabulary. Second, children need to rate their feelings on some scale. Rating the intensity allows you to more fully understand the nature of youngsters' emotional experiences and evaluate whether the cognition is meaningful. Moreover, the initial rating is crucial in order to determine whether any subsequent intervention is successful. For instance, the intervention should result in a lowering of the emotional intensity.

Recording thoughts and images is the third entry in the typical thought record. Youngsters need to learn to ask themselves the cardinal question "What is going through my mind?" in order to fill out this column. Further, children need to be taught the distinctions between thoughts and feelings mentioned earlier in this chapter. Finally, you need to remain mindful of the content-specificity hypothesis and evaluate whether the thought listed matches the emotional intensity reported by the child in the feeling column. In this way, you increase the likelihood you are working with the most psychologically present and pressing cognitive material.

Situation	Feeling	Thought
My teacher told me I was not paying attention in class.	Sad (8)	He doesn't like me. He was mean to tell me this. He made me feel dumb and I don't think I can do my work and he'll keep thinking I'm dumb.

FIGURE 6.5. Example of a corrected thought record.

CONCLUSION

Identifying feelings and thoughts is the cornerstone of cognitive therapy with children. As therapists, we have to teach children to attend to their emotions and inner dialogue. Therefore, we have to make the practice engaging so the youngsters will pay attention to their thoughts and feelings. In this chapter, we invited you to experiment with ways to make the self-monitoring processes come alive. Try multiple techniques and approach capturing thoughts and feelings from many angles. Put in the time and effort in this fundamental clinical task. You will be more likely to realize subsequent therapeutic dividends from your self-instructional and rational analysis interventions.

7

❖

Therapeutic Socratic Dialogues

Our therapeutic dialogues are based on the Socratic method. Three basic features characterize the Socratic method in clinical practice: systematic questioning, inductive reasoning, and constructing universal definitions (Overholser, 1994). In using systematic questioning, we recommend that you do not view all youngsters' automatic thoughts as irrational or dysfunctional (Young, Weingarten, & Beck, 2001). Rather, we encourage you to discover the database for children's beliefs and assumptions. If you adopt a gentle and curious stance, children may be less likely to see the Socratic dialogue as an inquisition. According to Overholser (1993a),

> In some ways, the process is similar to helping a child assemble a puzzle. If you hand the child a piece but the child cannot find the proper place, you do not keep handing the child the same piece. Instead, you can give the child a few other pieces. As the picture starts to develop, the child can easily place the original difficult piece. (p. 72)

There are various classes of Socratic questions (J. S. Beck, 1995; Beal, Kopec, & DiGiuseppe, 1996; Fennell, 1989). In fact, many of the techniques described in Chapters 8 through 13 can be classified into one of the following categories:

1. What's the evidence?
2. What's an alternative explanation?
3. What are the advantages and disadvantages?
4. How can I problem solve?
5. Decatastrophizing (J. S. Beck, 1995)

All these thought-testing questions invite children to evaluate their inferences, judgments, conclusions, and appraisals.

CONSIDERATIONS IN CONSTRUCTING
A THERAPEUTIC SOCRATIC DIALOGUE

A therapeutic Socratic dialogue needs to be modified based on children's responses. For example, their responses may be based on their level of distress, tolerance of ambiguity/frustration, cultural background, level of psychological maturity, or reactance to the questioning process. Unless you assess how the child is responding to the dialogue, you won't know how to modify your own responses. Figure 7.1 illustrates the pivotal issues to be considered.

This on-the-spot informal assessment can be a tricky thing. Often, we can get caught up in the questioning and neglect the level of the child's responsiveness. In these cases, we have barged ahead but not realized much success. Remaining alert to a child's overt and covert cues is essential to success. For example, 12-year-old Jonie would shift in her seat, look out the window, and respond with tangential types of responses at pivotal points in a session. By attending to her subtle cues, the therapist eventually figured out that she believed there was one correct answer to each of the questions. Instead of risking the therapist's disapproval by giving a "wrong" answer, Jonie just avoided answering all the questions!

A question we ask ourselves while initiating a therapeutic dialogue is "What is the child's level of distress?" In our experience, if the child is in acute distress, abstract dialogues peppered with multiple questions are rarely good tactics. We generally avoid questions that call for in-depth rational analysis. For example, a boy became agitated and angry in session. The therapist focused on providing support and direction (e.g., "You're at the boiling point. What has gotten you so hot? How can I help you be cooler and stay in charge?") rather than prompting extensive explanation, exploration, or discovery.

The child's ability to tolerate frustration and ambiguity is a second important issue for us. With children who do not handle ambiguity well, we begin with more concrete, simple questions (e.g., "When Jason took your hat and you made fists with your hands, what went through your mind?"). For youngsters with little tolerance for ambiguity and frustration, open-ended questions may push their limits. Therefore, we begin with more narrowly defined questions and build toward more open-ended questions. Consider April, who was furious because her mother controlled the way she dressed. After several unsuccessful passes through more abstract, open-ended questions ("What would you like to happen?"; "How would you like Mom to change?"), she profited from

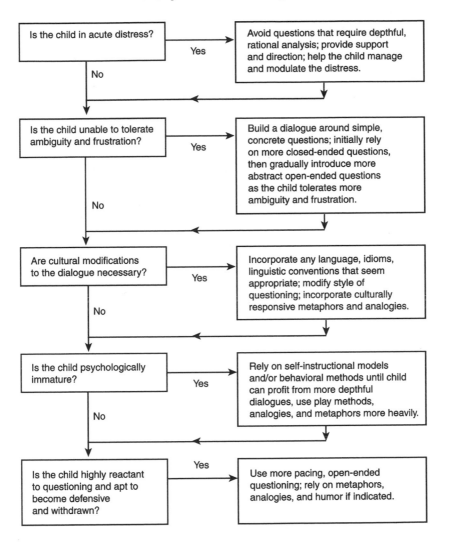

FIGURE 7.1. Flow chart for Socratic dialogues.

choices that helped her narrow her responses (e.g., "Would you like Mom to scream and yell, ground you, or talk with you like you are a young woman?").

Language is shaped by cultural background, so the same questions may be perceived differently by people from various cultures (Tharp, 1991). In these cases, you will want to check out how the child is experiencing your questions (e.g., "What is it like for you when I ask these questions?"). Additionally, you will want to make sure the metaphors and analogies you use fit the child's cultural background (Friedberg & Crosby, 2001). Finally, if appropriate, you might want to include the child's own idioms in your dialogue. The storytelling techniques described in Chapter 9 can be especially culturally responsive ways to test thoughts.

For example, the Tracks of My Fears exercise explained in Chapter 12 can be quite engaging for many children but for those who have never ridden on a train it may fall flat. For children in Chicago or New York, trains and subways make the train metaphor viable. In Dayton, Ohio, where we don't have subways, we often talk about a roller coaster at King's Island Amusement Park as a type of train. Giving children the opportunity to make the metaphors and analogies personal, familiar, and reflective of their background will increase cultural responsiveness.

Including children's idioms in your dialogue is an important but also a tricky issue. For some youngsters, their individual language forms a boundary between children's and adults' worlds. In these situations, don't trespass! There is nothing more disturbing to an adolescent than an adult therapist trying to act and talk like an adolescent!

When you make the metaphors and language in your therapeutic dialogues more culturally meaningful, don't be afraid to ask youngsters what is compelling and psychologically present about the metaphor. Your curiosity will show respect for the child's background and context. I (RDF) remember the first time I heard a youngster use the word "phat"— I thought the word was "fat." When I demonstrated my ignorance, the youngster chuckled and then generously clued me in.

You will need to adjust your Socratic dialogues to the psychological maturity level of the child. For immature youngsters, reliance on playful and metaphorical strategies is a good way to go. These youngsters may embrace puppet play, crafts, and analogies. For instance, experiential exercises such as the Thought–Feeling Watch craft activity discussed later in this chapter (see also Chapter 9) is a good device. I (RDF) was working with a 6-year-old boy who was having trouble in school because he was hitting, biting, and kicking other children. Rather than relying on purely verbal persuasion techniques, I played school with him using toy figures. In one sequence, the boy play figure kept biting the other kids and the biter became isolated and lonely. The play yielded a productive dialogue (e.g., "What happened to the boy?"; "Is this a good thing or a bad thing?") in which the child was able to see that biting resulted in negative consequences.

Finally, many children are exquisitely sensitive to questioning. Questions from adult authorities indicate that they have done something wrong. Consequently, they become defensive and withdrawn when questioned. Here you need to make sure you are scaffolding a dialogue that is well paced and does not make the child feel like he/she is facing a barrage of questions. You can vary your questioning style and ask questions with declaratives (e.g., "Tell me how you know you are a failure."; "Let's see what other reasons there might be.") rather than pester the child with question after question.

HINTS ABOUT CONSTRUCTING A SOCRATIC DIALOGUE

When developing a Socratic dialogue, avoid asking questions you are sure you know the answer to. Socratic questioning is not only an opportunity to guide the client but also a chance to demonstrate your curiosity. Crafting questions you know the answer to may not prompt genuine guided discovery. Rather, youngsters may think you are asking them a question just to hear the answer you want! Sometimes, unfortunately, we therapists act like real "know-it-alls" and use Socratic processes to show off (e.g., "I can use my questions to show how wrong you are!"). Therapeutic momentum suffers when we act so presumptuously. Thus, we encourage you to use the Socratic questioning process to genuinely promote greater understanding of the client's database for his/her beliefs. Moreover, don't presume you know the basis on which youngster's beliefs are formed (Rutter & Friedberg, 1999).

Rutter and Friedberg (1999) offer a skeletal outline of the Socratic dialogue process. The outline breaks the exchange down into its constituent parts in a five-part process: (1) elicit and identify the automatic thought, (2) tie the automatic thought to the feeling and behavior, (3) link the thought–feeling–behavior sequence together with an empathic response, (4) obtain collaboration from the client on steps 1–3 and agreement to go forward, and (5) Socratically test the belief.

Let's take an example and see if you can follow along with the five steps. Suzy, a 14-year-old, was auditioning for the choir. While she was singing, several audience members left the auditorium. Witnessing this, Suzy became dismayed and thought, "My singing is so awful I've made people leave." Read the following exchange and see if you would ask similar questions.

SUZY: I knew I shouldn't have auditioned for choir.

THERAPIST: What goes through your mind about auditioning? [Step 1: Identifying the automatic thought]

SUZY: I made a fool of myself.

THERAPIST: I see. What makes you see yourself as a fool? [Step 1 continues]

SUZY: Only an awful singer would drive away the audience.

THERAPIST: So you saw people leaving, thought it was because you were an awful singer, and that made it foolish to try out.

SUZY: Yes.

THERAPIST: How does that make you feel? [Step 2: Tying automatic thought to feeling and behavior]

SUZY: Depressed and ashamed.

THERAPIST: I think I understand now. Let me check out my understanding. It sure does make sense that you would feel ashamed and depressed if you thought your singing was so bad it chased people out of the auditorium. I guess it would make you not want to try out again. [Step 3: Connecting thoughts, feelings, and behaviors in an empathic way]

SUZY: Exactly.

THERAPIST: Does it sound like we're getting a good handle on the things that are upsetting you?

SUZY: Yes.

THERAPIST: What we need to do now is figure out whether people left because you sang so awfully and looked foolish up there. Are you willing to check this out? [Step 4: Obtaining collaboration and agreement to go forward]

SUZY: Do you think it would help?

THERAPIST: Let's give it a try. From time to time, we'll check to see if we are being successful. How does that sound?

SUZY: OK.

THERAPIST: Hmm. Let's see here. How convinced are you that people left because you were an awful singer? [Thought testing begins]

SUZY: Pretty convinced.

THERAPIST: On a scale of 1–10, with 10 being absolutely certain and 1 being totally unsure, how certain are you?

SUZY: A 9.

THERAPIST: So, pretty certain? What makes you believe that they left because of your singing?

SUZY: I don't know.

THERAPIST: That is a tough question. Have you ever left a performance?

SUZY: I guess. I've gone to the bathroom or to the snack bar.

THERAPIST: Did you leave because the show stunk?

SUZY: No, I was hungry or I had to go.

THERAPIST: That makes sense. Did you come back?

SUZY: Yes.

THERAPIST: I see. Now, let's get back to you. What time did you go on?

SUZY: Between 5:30 and 6:00 P.M.

THERAPIST: And how long had the audition been going on?

SUZY: Since 3:00.

THERAPIST: Any scheduled breaks?

SUZY: None that I know of.

THERAPIST: When is lunch?

SUZY: About noon.

THERAPIST: And dinner time is usually around?

SUZY: 5:30 or 6:00.

THERAPIST: What do you make of that?

SUZY: Maybe some people might have been hungry.

THERAPIST: That's interesting. Did you leave the audition at any time?

SUZY: Yeah, I had to go to the bathroom and I got a pop.

THERAPIST: How awful was the performer?

SUZY: Not awful. I wasn't even paying any attention to him.

THERAPIST: That's interesting. What do you make of that? Did your leaving have anything to do with him?

SUZY: No.

THERAPIST: So is it possible that other people leaving had nothing to do with you?

SUZY: I'm not sure. (*Doubt begins to appear.*)

THERAPIST: Let's continue. Was anything else happening at school that afternoon? Any basketball games or club meetings?

SUZY: I think there was a game that night.

THERAPIST: Were there any players, cheerleaders, or fans in the audience?

SUZY: Eddy plays. Julie and Erika are cheerleaders. I don't know. Maybe some of the people were basketball fans. Why?

THERAPIST: I'm just thinking about all the possibilities. What time was the game?

SUZY: 6:00, I think.

THERAPIST: So if they were going to get ready to go to the game, what time would they leave?

SUZY: About 5:30 or 5:45.

THERAPIST: That would be right about the time you went on, right?

SUZY: Yes. That's right. Huh. (*Doubt grows.*)

THERAPIST: You noticed people leaving. Did you notice if people came back?

SUZY: Let me think. I'm not sure. Yes. I am pretty sure people came back.

THERAPIST: Before you were done singing?

SUZY: (*Laughs.*) Yes.

THERAPIST: I think you know what my next question is.

SUZY: Yeah. If I was so awful, would they have come back?

THERAPIST: Now, you are chewing things over! One more question. Did everybody leave? Was there a mass exit?

Were you able to follow the questioning process? During the thought-testing phase, the therapist guided Suzy through an examination of alternative conclusions. Moreover, the therapist decreased her all-or-none thinking and catastrophizing. Through this process, Suzy learned to "chew things over."

UNIVERSAL DEFINITIONS

Children and adolescents often define themselves in very idiosyncratic ways. Overholser (1994) wrote that "universal definitions are important because language and definitions influence our perceptions, descriptions, and understanding of the world" (p. 286). For example, what therapist hasn't encountered the perfectionistic child who gets all A's in school yet becomes depressed and upset at any perceived flaw in him/herself? For this child, any mistake means he/she is incompetent or stupid. In therapy, we work to broaden these youngsters' narrow definitions.

Consider the following example. Gretchen is a 16-year-old girl who is depressed. Her history includes severe trauma marked by sexual abuse. She is highly self-critical, perfectionistic, and pessimistic. At Session 8, the therapist elicited Gretchen's belief "I am a worthless person."

THERAPIST: When I hear you say "I am a worthless person," I really understand how painful your depressed feelings are.

GRETCHEN: I really believe it. I think about it all the time.

THERAPIST: It almost defines you.

GRETCHEN: It does?

THERAPIST: How worthless do you see yourself?

GRETCHEN: Totally. I'm shit.

THERAPIST: I see. What makes you define yourself in this way?

GRETCHEN: I don't know. I just do.

THERAPIST: It is hard to come up with specifics. I know that it is painful to think about. I'm wondering if I can push you just a bit. May I?

GRETCHEN: OK.

THERAPIST: What are the things you base your definition of your worthlessness on?

GRETCHEN: I guess the fact that I'm depressed a lot.

THERAPIST: (*Writes.*) Anything else?

GRETCHEN: I don't know. I don't have tons of friends. I'm not going to win the most popular award.

THERAPIST: (*Writes.*) We've also talked a lot about how your dad abused you. How much does this enter into your definition?

GRETCHEN: Yeah, it's there.

THERAPIST: That's a difficult one (*writes.*). What other things are there?

GRETCHEN: I think I'm pretty clumsy. I also seem to drop stuff and trip and you know.

THERAPIST: I see. We'll write that down too (*writes.*). Anything else you want to add?

GRETCHEN: (*Looks at list.*) No.

THERAPIST: OK. Let's see. Which of these things do you think in your own mind most defines your worthlessness.

GRETCHEN: My sexual abuse.

THERAPIST: This is the part that most contributes to your self-definition. Let me ask you kind of a different question to give us some more angles on your definition. Who do you know who is completely worthy?

GRETCHEN: My best friend, Emily.

THERAPIST: What makes her worthy?

GRETCHEN: I guess she just is.

THERAPIST: I know it's hard to think of the special things that make Emily seem so worthy to you. But I was wondering if you would be willing to do that.

GRETCHEN: Well, she is a really good student. She gets mainly A's and B's. She has a lot of friends. People trust her and tell her things. She's a good friend.

THERAPIST: (*Writes.*) What else?

GRETCHEN: She works after school in her family's store. She tried out for gymnastics but didn't make it. And that didn't seem to bug her. That really impressed me.

THERAPIST: (*Writes.*) I've been writing these things down on paper [see Figure 7.2]. Now I want to ask you some things when we view this and rate how much of the things you see in Emily you have. How about rating them on a 1–5 scale? 1 could be not having any of the characteristics and 5 could be having a lot of each one. Are you willing to do this?

GRETCHEN: I guess so.

THERAPIST: OK. Let's start at the top. Remind me what type of student are you?

GRETCHEN: (*Smiles.*) Straight A's mostly. I got one B last year.

THERAPIST: So how much of a good student are you?

GRETCHEN: A 5.

THERAPIST: (*Writes.*) Where would you rate yourself on having lots of friends?

GRETCHEN: Maybe a 2.

THERAPIST: (*Writes.*) When you think of the friends you are close to, how good a friend would you rate yourself to be?

GRETCHEN: I think I'm a pretty good friend. Maybe a 4.

Good student gets A's and B's	5
Lots of friends	2
Is a good friend—people trust her	4
Works after school	4
Handles negative things well	3

FIGURE 7.2. Gretchen's definitional criteria.

THERAPIST: (*Writes.*) Do you have a job after school?

GRETCHEN: I don't get paid. I volunteer at the hospital.

THERAPIST: Is that still work?

GRETCHEN: (*Laughs.*) Yes.

THERAPIST: So where would you put yourself on this one?

GRETCHEN: 4, I guess.

THERAPIST: (*Writes.*) How about handling negative things?

GRETCHEN: I'm not good at that. Maybe a 1.

THERAPIST: Can I ask more about that? Have you had a lot of negative stuff happen to you?

GRETCHEN: Too much, I think.

THERAPIST: I would agree.

GRETCHEN: I have to deal with my depression, my parents breakup, and my dad's abusing me.

THERAPIST: Those are some big issues for a 16-year-old girl to deal with. Have you kept up with your schoolwork and volunteering even though you were abused and felt depressed?

GRETCHEN: Yes.

THERAPIST: Even though you were struggling with these strong feelings and painful stressors, were you an OK daughter, sister, and friend?

GRETCHEN: I think so.

THERAPIST: So what does that mean about your ability to handle negative things?

GRETCHEN: Well, it's not a 1 . . . but it's not a 5 either. Maybe a 3.

THERAPIST: OK. (*Writes.*) Let's take a look at what we have. On this side, we have all the characteristics that you say make Emily worthy. On this side, we have how you rate yourself on these same characteristics. What do you make of this?

GRETCHEN: I'm not sure.

THERAPIST: Let me ask you this. Would a totally worthless person have any of these characteristics?

GRETCHEN: No.

THERAPIST: So they would all be 1's.

GRETCHEN: Yes.

THERAPIST: How many 1's do you have?

GRETCHEN: (*Laughs.*) None.

THERAPIST: So what does that mean about your worthlessness?

GRETCHEN: Maybe I'm not as worthless as I thought.

THERAPIST: You still are unconvinced, aren't you?

GRETCHEN: I know this in my mind but I feel worthless in my heart.

THERAPIST: That tells us something. We're missing an important part that goes into your self-definition. Do you have an idea about what it is?

GRETCHEN: The abuse?

THERAPIST: Let's deal with that one. Remember you said the most powerful part of the definition was that you were sexually abused by your father?

GRETCHEN: I know it is.

THERAPIST: Let's take a look at this list of characteristics you used to define Emily's worthiness. What do you notice?

GRETCHEN: I'm not sure.

THERAPIST: Where on the list is not being sexually abused?

GRETCHEN: It's not there.

THERAPIST: What do you make of that?

GRETCHEN: (*Pause.*) I don't know.

THERAPIST: If being sexually abused absolutely determines worthiness, would it be left off the list?

GRETCHEN: (*Pause.*) Maybe I just forgot it.

THERAPIST: That's possible. Would you like to add it on now?

GRETCHEN: OK. Let's put it on.

THERAPIST: (*Adds to the list.*) What do you notice now?

GRETCHEN: I'm not sure.

THERAPIST: How many items are on your list?

GRETCHEN: Six.

THERAPIST: How many of them have to do with being sexually abused?

GRETCHEN: One. Maybe being sexually abused doesn't totally mean I'm worthless. It's one of six other things. So there are other things that make up my worthiness too.

We will go through the pivotal points in this example transcript systematically. First, the dialogue is well paced. The therapist did not pepper Gretchen with questions in an interrogative style. Second, the therapist asked how worthless Gretchen saw herself to be. The therapist then built the Socratic questioning around this all-or-none self-definition. Third, the therapist focused on the evidence for Gretchen's painful self-description ("What are the things you base your definition on?"). Fourth, based on past sessions, the therapist guessed that Gretchen's sexual abuse contributed to her harsh self-definition ("How much does this enter in your definition?"). The choice to ask this type of question is based on several considerations. Most importantly, you want to help the child feel comfortable disclosing that this is part of her definition. Further, by asking a "how much" rather than a "does" question, you are implicitly communicating that it would be rather common for the sexual abuse to be part of her definition. Finally, the dimensional "how much" question begins to counter her categorical all-or-none thinking process. It lays the foundation for subsequent thought testing.

The next step in the process is a particularly key one. Asking which of the characteristics most powerfully shapes the definition yields an important clinical edge. When you know the foundation of the belief, you can design the dialogue to explicitly test that foundation.

In the next phase, Gretchen was asked to consider a broader perspective ("Who do you know that is completely worthy?") After identifying her friend Emily, Gretchen was asked to specify what made her girlfriend worthy. The Socratic dialogue then switched from this objective third-party perspective back to her own subjective self-appraisal. Here, Gretchen rated herself on the same characteristics she used to determine Emily's worthiness. This is another critical point in the exchange. By electing to have Gretchen rate herself on the same characteristics as Emily rather than checking whether or not she had similar traits, you are addressing her all-or-none thinking. You are prompting dimensional rather than categorical thinking. Second, by doing so, you are further laying the groundwork for thought testing. Remember that earlier in the dialogue Gretchen shared that she saw herself as totally worthless. Therefore, if she rates herself as having any one of these characteristics to any extent, you have helped her cast doubt on her conclusion (i.e., How can someone be *totally* worthless if he/she shares any characteristic to any degree with a worthwhile person?)

You would expect a client to have difficulty rating herself on these dimensions. As the Socratic dialogue illustrates, you may have to help her with some of her judgments. Not surprisingly, Gretchen needed guidance in assessing her academic status, work, and coping.

In the next crucial phase of the dialogue, the therapist asked Gretchen to draw conclusions based on the data they had collected. The first pass through the questioning yielded few results ("What do you make of this?"). This question was too abstract and required a tremendous amount of synthesis from Gretchen. Consequently, the therapist narrowed the questions ("Would a totally worthless person have any of these characteristics?"; "How many 1's do you have?"; "So what does this mean about your worthlessness?"). While more successful than the abstract questioning, this line of inquiry still hit a psychological wall.

The therapist knew the crucial piece of evidence was still not addressed (i.e., sexual abuse). The therapist began with a specific question ("Where on the list is not being sexually abused?") The therapist then followed up with a summary or synthesizing question ("If being sexually abused absolutely determines worthiness, would it be left off the list?"). As this point, Gretchen paused and claimed she just forgot to put it on the list. The therapist alertly accepted this response and simply placed it on the list. It is important to note that the therapist did not argue with Gretchen or now come to believe therapy was stuck. Rather, the therapist hoped that the previous work promoting dimensional thinking was about to pay off.

After the therapist included the sexual abuse item on the list, Gretchen was asked another synthesizing question ("What do you notice now?"). Unfortunately, this abstract question came too early and was unproductive. The therapist stepped back and proceeded more systematically ("How many items are on your list?"; "How many of them have to do with being sexually abused?"). After reviewing this information, a seed of doubt crept into Gretchen's consciousness. At this point, Gretchen was able to assume a broader perspective and consider that her worth was not totally determined by her abuse history. In fact, other characteristics more powerfully shaped her self-definition.

This dialogue shows that even though the therapist made several missteps during the questioning, the process was successful. You do not have to construct a perfect Socratic dialogue! Second, the effectiveness of the Socratic dialogue was propelled by a sound case conceptualization and grasp of the technique. Third, Gretchen was not peppered with questions. Overall, the dialogue was nicely paced. Fourth, the focus was on casting doubt rather than on achieving absolute refutation and disputation. This emphasis was best illustrated by not discounting Gretchen's confusion or dismissing her omissions (e.g., "Maybe I just forgot it."). Although the therapist clearly was promoting depthful cognitive processing, Gretchen seemed to feel heard throughout the dialogue.

METAPHORICAL AND HUMOROUS QUESTIONS

Metaphorical, analogical, and humorous questions come in very handy with children and adolescents. Most of the techniques presented in the creative applications (Chapter 9), depression (Chapter 11), anxiety

(Chapter 12), and disruptive behavior (Chapter 13) chapters make liberal use of metaphors and humor. The key to success with metaphors is to use ones that are part of the child's world (Beal et al., 1996). In humorous disputes, the butt of the joke *should never be the child*. Rather, the target of humor should always be the belief. In this section, we will describe some metaphorical, fun, and humorous ways to test children's thoughts.

Beal et al. (1996) suggested a cute *Three Little Pigs Question* to decrease a child's demand that people change to suit him/her. They asked the question, "If the three little pigs had demanded that the wolf act differently, where would that belief have gotten them?" (p. 222). You could use this question with a youngster who demands that his younger brother leave him alone and not butt in when he is with his friends.

Not surprisingly, logical disputes challenge children's (illogical) beliefs and causal reasoning. *Empirical disputes* ask the client to use data and information to develop new beliefs (e.g., "What is the evidence?"). *Functional disputes* emphasize the costs and benefits of thoughts, feelings, and behaviors (e.g., "What are the advantages of thinking you are a dork?"). In Beal et al.'s paradigm, rational alternative beliefs are coping statements that counter inaccurate or maladaptive thoughts (e.g., "Even though some kids don't like me, I still have many friends. I don't need everyone to like me to be popular.").

Styles denote how the questions are delivered (Beal et al., 1996). A *didactic style* is characterized by direct teaching. The *Socratic style* is marked by questions that guide children's discovery. The *metaphorical style* involves broadening the child's perspective through the use of metaphors and analogies. Finally, the *humorous style* encourages the child to laugh at the inaccuracy of his/her thoughts.

In our practice, we tend to rely on logical, empirical, and functional disputes that are delivered in Socratic, metaphorical, and humorous ways. With adolescents, we generally emphasize the Socratic method. Younger children have greater difficulty with the Socratic method (Overholser, 1993a). If you combine a metaphorical and/or humorous approach with logical, empirical, and functional questions, it may be more appealing to younger children.

Overholser (1993b) discussed five types of analogies for clinical use. Analogies could be based on medical, mechanical, strategical, relational, and natural concepts. The *Tracks of My Fears* exercise described in Chapter 12 is an example of a mechanical analogy (e.g., "Anxiety is like a train that passes through various stations such as thinking, emotion, and interpersonal relationships."). When working with disruptive youth, we often use sports analogies that contain strategies to help them stop, relax, and think (e.g., "A teacher is like a referee in a basketball game. He can blow his whistle and call a foul."). Like Kendall et al. (1992), we make ample use of relational analogies with children—for example, we say things such as therapists are like coaches, the child is the captain of the treatment team, and youngsters are like detectives sorting through clues and evidence.

My Butterfly Thoughts is an exercise that makes use of a natural analogy. My Butterfly Thoughts uses the butterfly analogy to illustrate the concept of change. Children readily learn that caterpillars transform into butterflies. The analogy is a way to plant the seed that personal metamorphosis can occur. The butterfly analogy and related worksheet make self-instructional work fun. By using the butterfly analogy, you can avoid more direct questioning. For instance, instead of saying "What other way can you work at this?" or "What else can you say to yourself?," you can ask youngsters this question: "How can you change your caterpillar thought to a butterfly thought?"

Therapists begin by introducing the butterfly concept. The following example shows how you might introduce My Butterfly Thoughts:

> "Do you know what a butterfly is? You see, a butterfly starts out as a caterpillar. Then it *changes* into a butterfly. Isn't that cool? A caterpillar turns into a butterfly. It is really important to know that the way you explain what happens to you can change. The things that you say to yourself when you are feeling badly like 'I'm no good.' 'No one likes me,' or 'I will make a fool of myself' are your caterpillar thoughts. They haven't yet changed into butterfly thoughts. I want you to try to turn these caterpillar thoughts into butterfly thoughts."

Certainly, you can augment the explanation with pictures, cartoons, and drawings of caterpillars and butterflies.

The Butterfly Thoughts Worksheet is presented in Figures 7.3 and 7.4. In the first two columns, the child records an event and its accompanying feeling. The third column, labeled "Caterpillar Thoughts," provides a place for writing down the inaccurate or dysfunctional thoughts. The fourth column, labeled "Butterfly Thoughts," offers children the opportunity to come up with coping counterthoughts.

Ms. Stakes Sweeps is a humorous way to teach youngsters that mistakes are simply a part of life rather than a catastrophe. The central cartoon character in the Ms. Stakes Sweeps exercise is a kind, bespectacled female figure. In her dialogue with the children she shares her view that mistakes are part of being human (even her name is backward). The Ms. Stakes Sweeps exercise is presented in Figure 7.5.

Ms. Stakes Sweeps begins with an introductory text followed by several questions presented in a stepwise fashion. The questions are posed

Event	Feeling	Caterpillar Thought 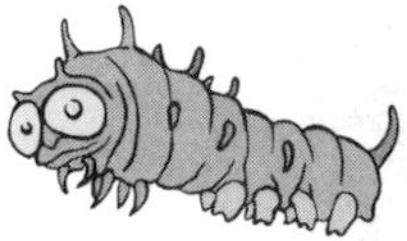	Can This Caterpillar Thought Change into a Butterfly Thought?	Butterfly Thought 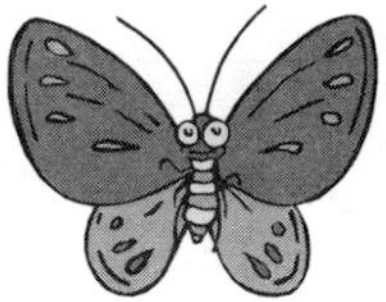

FIGURE 7.3. Butterfly Thoughts Worksheet. From Friedberg and McClure (2002). Copyright by The Guilford Press. Permission to photocopy this figure is granted to purchasers of this book for personal use only (see copyright page for details).

119

Event	Feeling	Caterpillar Thought	Can This Caterpillar Thought Change into a Butterfly Thought?	Butterfly Thought
I forgot to do my chores and Mom and Dad got mad at me.	Sad	They hate me because they think I'm lazy and spoiled.	Yes!!	I did forget to do the chores. I need to do better at reminding myself. They are disappointed in me but they still love me.

FIGURE 7.4. Sample Butterfly Thoughts Worksheet.

simply and include sentence stems for children to complete, forced-choice questions for children to circle, and open-ended questions.

The *Thought Digger* exercise (Friedberg et al., 2001) is a good example of a fun way to do thought testing and Socratic questioning. In Thought Digger, children are encouraged to become archeologists who dig for clues. We urge the youngsters to act out a digging motion when they ask themselves questions. Further, we use the term "thought digger" as a kind of therapeutic shorthand to cue youngsters (e.g., "Are you being a thought digger?"). Finally, the Thought Digger diary makes the Socratic questioning process easier for children because common questions to test inaccurate thoughts are provided on the worksheet. The youngster simply has to circle the one that best fits the situation and the inaccurate thought.

The *Thought–Feeling Watch* is a craft-like activity described in Chapter 9 around which therapists could build a Socratic dialogue. After the child enjoys the craft activity and completes his/her watch, you could initiate a therapeutic Socratic dialogue. Look over the dialogue below to see how you might engage in a playful and therapeutic Socratic dialogue.

THERAPIST: That's a really cool-looking watch. Let me ask you a question. What happens to the hands on a watch?

KIRA: They move around.

THERAPIST: Exactly. They move all over the place. Do the hands ever stop?

KIRA: Sometimes. If the watch is broken or the batteries run out.

Hello, I'm Ms. Stakes Sweeps. My job is to help you learn that mistakes are not horrible. You know, mistakes are part of life. In fact, they are even part of my name!! If you worry too much about making a mistake, it can stop you from trying new things or even keeping on doing the things you need or want to do.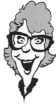

Many times children punish themselves too much for their mistakes. They may fear what parents, friends, and teachers say about mistakes. Do you ever punish yourself for your mistakes? Circle one.

YES   NO

Write down the way you punish yourself for your mistakes.

The way I punish myself for my mistakes is _____

_____

_____.

Do you ever worry what others think about your mistakes? Circle one.

YES   NO

When I make a mistake, I worry my parents will think _____

_____

_____.

When I make a mistake, I worry my teachers will think _____

_____

_____.

When I make a mistake, I worry my friends will think _____

_____

_____.

Now, do you know what a contest is? Have you ever been in a contest? Another name for a contest is called a sweepstakes. That kind of sounds like my name, doesn't it? I am going to give you some tools so you can win the Ms. Stakes Sweeps.

The tools I am going to give you are questions. Here they are:

What are the good parts of making a mistake? _____

_____

(continued)

FIGURE 7.5. Ms. Stakes Sweeps Worksheet. From Friedberg and McClure (2002). Copyright by The Guilford Press. Permission to photocopy this figure is granted to purchasers of this book for personal use only (see copyright page for details).

FIGURE 7.5. Ms. Stakes Sweeps Worksheet *(continued)*.

If there are any good parts of making mistakes, how terrible could making a mistake be? Circle one.

Not terrible   Kind of terrible   Totally terrible

Can you learn anything from making a mistake? Circle one.

YES   NO

If you can learn something from making a mistake, how terrible could making a mistake be? Circle one.

Not terrible   Kind of terrible   Totally terrible

Can you be really good at something and still make a mistake? Circle one.

YES   NO

If you can be really good at something and still make a mistake, how terrible is making a mistake? Circle one.

Not terrible   Kind of terrible   Totally terrible

Name someone you really admire and like who has made a mistake.

_____

If someone you admire and like makes mistakes, how terrible is making a mistake? Circle one.

Not terrible   Kind of terrible   Totally terrible

Do most boys and girls in your class use their erasers? Circle one.

YES   NO

If most boys and girls use their erasers, how terrible is making a mistake? Circle one.

Not terrible   Kind of terrible   Totally terrible

THERAPIST: So it is kind of unusual for the hands on the watch to stop moving?

KIRA: Yes.

THERAPIST: Do the hands on your Thought–Feeling Watch move?

KIRA: Yes, they do. See? (*Shows watch.*)

THERAPIST: I can see that they do. Look at them move. What do you suppose it means that hands on your watch move from feeling to feeling?

KIRA: I dunno. I made it the right way?

THERAPIST: Yes, you did make it the right way. But I have another question. Do the clock hands stay on one feeling?

KIRA: No. You could move them around.

THERAPIST: So if the watch is working correctly, the hands move from feeling to feeling?

KIRA: Yes.

THERAPIST: So does that mean that feelings are kind of changeable or kind of unchangeable.

KIRA: Changeable, I guess.

THERAPIST: When you are feeling really sad, do you ever think it is changeable?

KIRA: No, not really.

THERAPIST: So when you are feeling really sad, it's almost like your watch is stuck on one hour.

KIRA: Yeah.

THERAPIST: So, do you guess that it's the feeling that *really* won't change or more the way you are thinking about things that are happening to you so it makes it seem that the feelings won't change? It kind of makes it seem like your watch is stuck on one feeling.

What does this example teach us? First, the watch is a mechanical analogy that helps illustrate changeability. Second, the analogy is made concrete by the craft activity. Third, due to the analogy and the craft activity, the dialogue aimed at thought testing did not seem like an interrogation.

The use of *toy telephones* can also propel a Socratic dialogue (Deblinger, 1997). Introducing the telephones into therapy may provide you with the necessary distance from the child to carry out a Socratic dialogue. A child who may feel pressured and peppered by a traditional Socratic dialogue may readily engage in one over the "phone." We recall a youngster who was not very invested in therapeutic dialogues and would reluctantly respond with "I don't know" answers in session. When the telephone play was introduced, he almost forgot he was in therapy and responded more freely. The telephone may have diminished his sense of being interrogated. Additionally, a child can "hang up" on the therapist with impunity during telephone play.

CONCLUSION

Constructing a Socratic dialogue is more than playing "Twenty Questions" or trying to get the child to think what you think. Humor, metaphor, and playfulness are the cinder blocks you use to build Socratic dialogues with children and adolescents. The questions help you guide youngsters' discovery of heretofore hidden "truths." As you now progress through this book toward techniques and specific applications to particular disorders, we encourage you to develop creative and dynamic Socratic dialogues.

8

❖

Commonly Used Cognitive
and Behavioral Techniques

This chapter introduces you to the common cognitive and behavioral techniques we use with children and adolescents. The tools vary in complexity and in the level of rational analysis required from the youngster. We begin with our conceptualization of basic cognitive-behavioral tools and then discuss skill acquisition and application. Explanations of relatively straightforward behavioral tasks and basic cognitive self-instructional tasks follow. The chapter concludes with more complex cognitive and behavioral interventions.

DIMENSIONS OF COGNITIVE-BEHAVIORAL TECHNIQUES

Ellis (1962, 1979) classified cognitive-behavioral interventions along elegant and inelegant dimensions. In making this distinction, he was addressing the depth of rational processing involved in treatment strategies. *Inelegant techniques* focus more on changing thought content through self-instructional interventions. *Elegant techniques* tap more sophisticated reasoning processes to change thought content, process, and structure through more in-depth rational analysis. We do not see elegant techniques as superior to inelegant ones. Rather, we view each type of strategy as useful in particular situations. Elegant and inelegant techniques are both functional interventions!

There is a time and a place in the therapy process for *both* elegant and inelegant strategies. Inelegant strategies generally are preferable early in the treatment process. Inelegant strategies are often functional with highly distressed individuals and individuals who are in immediate crisis. We rely on more inelegant approaches with younger children, children who are less verbal, and children who are less cognitively sophisticated. Conversely, elegant strategies are typically employed later in treatment subsequent to the success of inelegant strategies. Older children who are more verbal and able to acquire and apply more abstract skills profit from more elegant strategies. Since elegant strategies require more effortful cognitive-emotional processing, they should not be counted on at times of crisis or during intense emotional distress. However, elegant procedures likely serve the generalization process since they focus more on changing the thought process as well as the thought content.

SKILL ACQUISITION (PSYCHOEDUCATION) VERSUS SKILL APPLICATION (PSYCHOTHERAPY)

Proficient cognitive therapy requires us to help our clients apply their acquired skills in the context of negative affective arousal (Robins & Hayes, 1993). We find that when many youngsters become upset they forget to apply their skills. Many times they will say something like "I was too worried and nervous to do the thought diary." The perfect time to do cognitive techniques is when the child is nervous.

In our minds, psychoeducation is marked by *skill acquisition* while psychotherapy is marked by *skill application*. In psychoeducation, youngsters are taught psychologically related concepts and information (e.g., models of anger, ways to manage anger such as relaxation, reattribution). In psychotherapy, clients are encouraged to call on these skills when they are emotionally distressed. All the techniques described in this chapter need to be *both* acquired and applied.

Skill acquisition is generally uncomplicated. The skill is taught in a graduated, clear manner to youngsters and their families. Most clients readily acquire specific skills. However, skill application is tougher to achieve. When supervising therapists, I (RDF) have found that they often back away from applying a cognitive-behavioral intervention when the youngster is emotionally aroused. Yet when a child practices coping skills in an emotionally charged situation, he/she will feel a genuine sense of mastery. For instance, a tearful young girl disclosed how sad she felt because she thought her father did not love her as much as his new stepdaughter. The therapist talked the girl through the distress but failed to use a thought diary or to otherwise record the new thoughts the child used to cope with the situation. While this experience was momentarily helpful, the therapist lost the opportunity to reinforce the application of acquired skills and facilitate greater generalization. Children need *in vivo* opportunities to practice their acquired skills.

BASIC BEHAVIORAL TOOLS

Relaxation Training

Relaxation training is a behavioral technique that can be applied to a variety of problems such as anxiety and anger management. Progressive muscle relaxation (Jacobson, 1938) involves alternatingly tensing and relaxing specific muscle groups. Readers are encouraged to read texts on relaxation training for in-depth coverage (Goldfried & Davison, 1976; Masters, Burish, Hollon, & Rimm, 1987), as well as to read specific resources for relaxation training for children and adolescents (Koeppen, 1974; Ollendick & Cerny, 1981). This section will briefly highlight some pivotal issues in relaxation training.

Goldfried and Davison (1976) suggest that during the muscle tension phase, muscles should be tensed three-quarters of the way rather than fully strained. Beidel and Turner (1998) recommend that relaxation sessions with children should be brief and include only a few muscle groups. Goldfried and Davison (1976) also propose that the therapist's speech patterns be soft, melodic, warm, and paced slower than conventional speech patterns. A monotonous and somewhat boring tone can facilitate the child's relaxation. Goldfried and Davison (1976) advise that 20 seconds of muscle relaxation should follow 5–10 seconds of muscle tension. Wording in relaxation scripts should match youngster's developmental level. Koeppen (1974) and Ollendick and Cerny (1981) have crafted very inventive, developmentally sensitive relaxation scripts for youngsters that include robust metaphors and analogies (e.g., bite down on a jaw-breaker).

Making relaxation more engaging is a major consideration for us. Wexler (1991) offers several inventive forms of relaxation practice. *Ten Candles* is a personal favorite. In this relaxation exercise, Wexler invites the client to imagine 10 lit candles in a row. The youngster is instructed to blow out each candle one at a time with his/her exhales. This technique is a good one because the way you blow out candles matches the way you inhale and exhale during relaxation. Additionally, visualizing blowing out a candle prompts youngsters to more effortfully exhale. Finally, the visualization keeps youngsters cognitively "busy" and engaged. If they are working on visualizing the candles, they have less mental space to ruminate.

Anxious youngsters may squirm and fidget. If the muscle relaxation does not quiet down the restlessness and fidgety behavior, you could try using each instance of fidgety behavior as a cue for deeper relaxation (e.g., "As you notice your foot tapping, you get more and more relaxed. As you shift your position in the chair, it is a signal to relax even more."). Shortening the relaxation sessions will also help. Finally, employing a sports metaphor may be helpful (Sommers-Flannagan & Sommers-Flannagan, 1995). For instance, watching a basketball player calm him/herself before taking a foul shot, or a tennis player ready him/herself for a crucial point may teach youngsters how to focus their relaxation efforts. You can bring in videotape vignettes of these sports moments and view them with your younger clients.

Systematic Desensitization

Systematic desensitization (SD) is a counterconditioning procedure used to decrease fears and anxiety. As originally designed by Wolpe (1958), SD involves pairing anxiety-producing stimuli with a counterconditioning agent (typically, relaxation). The temporally contiguous presentation causes the anxiety to be inhibited by its opposite or reciprocal (relaxation). Hence, the term *reciprocal inhibition* is typically used. Several components are included in the SD procedure. In order to conduct a systematic desensitization, anxiety hierarchies must be developed and training in a counterconditioning agent must be accomplished.

The first step in SD is breaking the fear down into constituent pieces. Each component of the fear is then ranked. As Goldstein (1973) noted, "Using the information gathered from the patient, clusters of anxiety-producing stimuli are isolated and arranged in hierarchical order" (p. 227). Anxiety hierarchies are constructed by establishing Subjective Units of Distress (SUDS) (Masters et al., 1987). SUDS reflect different levels of fear intensity associated with each fear. Common hierarchies are ranked from 1–100 in severity and intensity. Children may profit from rating scales with less variability; rating scales from 1–10 may be preferable.

In order to fully understand the nature of individual children's fears and subsequently implement an effective SD, you need to fully recognize all the aspects of children's fears. Accordingly, you need to elicit the interpersonal, cognitive, emotional, physiological, and behavioral components embedded in the fear. You should ask questions such as, "What makes _____ a 3?"; "What goes through your mind?"; "Who was there?"; "What do you do at a 3?"; and "How does your body feel at a 3?" Each scene can be written on an index card. Young children may enjoy drawing the scenes. After the scenes are detailed, they are hierarchically arranged.

After the fear is compartmentalized and hierarchically arranged, the procedure begins with the lowest item on the hierarchy. The child is instructed to relax and invited to imagine a pleasant scene. When the child is relaxed, the first item is presented. If the child experiences anxiety, he/she is instructed to gently lift one finger. When anxiety is reported, the child is told to stop imagining the scene and return to the previous pleasant scene. As children gain mastery over the scene, they move up the hierarchy until the highest level of fear is attenuated.

Morris and Kratochwill (1998) offer useful guidelines for systematic desensitization. First, they recommend that each anxiety-producing scene should be presented three or four times. Initial presentations represent practice trials. Morris and Kratochwill (1998) suggested that the anxiety-producing scene be initially presented for at least 5–10 seconds. The duration should be extended in subsequent presentations (e.g., to 10–15 seconds). Finally, Morris and Kratochwill proposed that the child experience a relaxation period lasting approximately 15–20 seconds between each presentation.

SOCIAL SKILLS TRAINING

Teaching social skills follows a characteristic cognitive-behavioral process (Beidel & Turner, 1998; Kazdin, 1994). First, the child is taught the skill through direct instruction. Often, psychoeducational material is presented to the youngster along with modeling of the particular skill (e.g., empathy). Graduated practice follows skill acquisition, for rehearsal facilitates application. Frequently, graduated practice or rehearsal involves role playing. Feedback is given to the youngster so he/she can maintain proper skill development and correct faulty skills. Finally, the child experiments with his/her skills in real-world contexts and then receives positive reinforcement for his/her efforts.

Multiple content areas may be covered under the social skills training umbrella. For instance, youngsters can learn new ways to make friends, manage their aggression, handle teasing, give and receive compliments, and make requests for help. We commonly teach children empathy skills in which youngsters try to become better at perspective taking. Through therapy, children also may acquire problem-solving skills for interpersonal situations and learn to develop a medley of alternative ways for thinking, feeling, and acting.

Empathy training and *teaching perspective taking* are components in many social skills packages. Generally, *empathy training* involves listening for feelings, identifying and labeling feelings, accepting feelings, and communicating the acceptance of feelings (LeCroy, 1994; Wexler, 1991).

Group work is especially useful for empathy and perspective training. The group allows for *in vivo* practice of empathic and perspective-taking skills. For instance, when an insensitive or offensive remark is made, a teaching moment is realized. Consider the following dialogue with an aggressive teen.

ANGELA: I'm tired of hearing Cassie's shit. She thinks she has to deal with more than anyone else. I've got a lot of crap coming down on me too.

THERAPIST: I can see you're frustrated, Angela. But I'm also wondering how do you think Cassie feels after sharing her story about the violence in her home and neighborhood and then hearing what you have to say.

ANGELA: I don't care how she feels.

THERAPIST: Well, that's an excellent example of what we need to do in group.

CASSIE: That's right. She needs to watch her mouth.

ANGELA: I don't need to watch anything.

THERAPIST: OK, both of you need to stop for a minute. Now, Angela, take a breath and ask yourself what problems are bringing you to therapy.

ANGELA: I get into fights at school and home.

THERAPIST: Good. Anybody in the group know what's going on here?

JENAE: She's getting into a fight right now.

THERAPIST: Thanks, Jenae. So Angela, I know you are good at getting *into* fights. How good do you want to be at getting *out* of them?

ANGELA: I'm not afraid of her.

CASSIE: You ought to be.

THERAPIST: Hold on girls. Time-out. Do you see how easy it is to just do what you are used to doing? Angela, I want you to try something. You're smart. I want to see if you can tell me how Cassie feels when you say you're tired of hearing about her troubles.

ANGELA: Pissed off. She's probably ready to go off on me. But she better stay level.

CASSIE: I'm not afraid of you.

THERAPIST: Cassie, what was it like to hear Angela say you were pissed off?

CASSIE: I don't care.

THERAPIST: Was it better or worse than when she said she was tired of hearing about your family troubles?

CASSIE: Better, I guess.

THERAPIST: Angela, can you try one more thing?

ANGELA: What?

THERAPIST: Can you just say how you think Cassie is feeling and drop the warning about staying level?

ANGELA: She's pissed off because she thinks I don't respect her.

THERAPIST: Cassie, is that right?

CASSIE: She's right.

THERAPIST: What's it like to hear Angela say that?

CASSIE: I like it. It felt pretty good.

THERAPIST: What has this done to your anger, Cassie?

CASSIE: It's less.

THERAPIST: How about you, Angela?

ANGELA: Less, I guess.

THERAPIST: For the rest of you in the group, what did Angela and Cassie do to avoid a fight?

What is the value of this exchange? First, the therapist used the conflict as a teaching moment in which he walked the girls through empathy training. Second, both Cassie and Angela practiced their acquired skills with each other. Third, the therapist used short, clear instructions to illustrate pivotal points.

Assertiveness training is a major component of social skill building. Children are taught various techniques such as broken record, fogging, and empathic assertion (Feindler & Guttman, 1994). These skills enable youngsters to make and respond to requests, defuse volatile situations, and manage conflict with peers, siblings, parents, and authority figures. Moreover, assertiveness training teaches youngsters how to make and respond to invitations, greet others, give and receive compliments, and ask for help. The ingredients of the social skills training help inhibited children engage in social interactions and prompt greater social facilitation. The particular skills for disinhibited or explosive aggressive children emphasize negotiating conflict in a more self-controlled, peaceful manner.

Role Playing

Role playing is a technique that facilitates social skill training and elicits important thoughts and feelings. You want the role plays to be as realistic as possible. In order to get good background information on the character they are role playing, you need to ask children specific questions. If you are role playing a friend, parent, or teacher, you need to know things about the character you are playing. Ask the child for examples of things these people might say, ways they react, mannerisms they use, things they enjoy or do not enjoy to give you insight into your character. Further, most likely, if a problem calls for a role-playing intervention, the circumstances are distressing for the child. Thus, you need to address these distressing elements in your simulated role play.

Contingency Management

Contingencies represent the relationship between behaviors and consequences. Contingency management specifies the type of rewards that depend on the specific occurrences of particular behavioral responses. New, more adaptive behaviors are promoted by the delivery of rewards for their emergence, while problematic behaviors are diminished by the removal of or nonoccurrence of these reinforcers.

Contingency management begins with identifying what behaviors you want to see more often and what behaviors you want to see less often. Thus, the nature of expected behavior, its frequency, and its duration need to be clearly expressed (e.g., "Johnny will study in a quiet room for 20 minutes at a time, 3 days per week."). Once the target behavior is identified, contingencies are established by specifying if–then type arrangements. For example, if Johnny studies in a quiet room for 20 minutes at a time, something good will follow (e.g., the family goes to a movie that Johnny chooses).

Shaping behavior also involves rewarding initial small steps toward a goal to establish behavioral momentum. For example, maintaining eye contact with an adult while receiving a command or directive may be an initial goal for a noncompliant, inattentive child. Once the child maintains eye contact, other behaviors are identified and rewarded (e.g., acknowledgment of the directive, movement toward compliance). Developing accomplishable graduated tasks is a crucial ingredient in shaping behavior.

Youngsters lose confidence in those individuals who make but break contingencies. Further, they are left with a sense of helplessness associated with continued noncontingency.

Pleasant Event Scheduling/Activity Scheduling

Pleasant event scheduling is used to increase the level of positive reinforcement in a child's daily routine as well as to activate an inactive child
(A. T. Beck et al., 1979; Greenberger & Padesky, 1995). Pleasant event
scheduling makes use of a schedule that resembles a daily planner. Generally, days of the week are listed across the page and times of day are
listed down the left-hand side of the page. This type of grid yields blank
spaces that correspond to specific times of day and days of the week.

Therapist and child collaboratively schedule several pleasant activities during the week. The idea is to increase the level of reinforcement in
the youngster's life. Moreover, when the child realizes some pleasant
activity during the week, his/her depression may lift. It is important to assign these activities and obtain the child's and family's commitment to follow through with them over the week. Depressed youngsters will lack
motivation to engage in pleasant activities. Thus, considerable effort will
be necessary to help the youngster complete the task.

With older children and adolescents, the youngster is simply invited
to record his/her pleasant activities in the spaces that correspond to the
time of day he/she did the activity. You also may request the child to rate
his/her mood prior to and after the activity.

Pleasure Prediction/Anxiety Prediction

Pleasure-prediction and anxiety-prediction techniques follow naturally
from the activity-scheduling process (J. S. Beck, 1995; Persons, 1989). In
pleasure predicting, a child plans an activity and then predicts how much
enjoyment he/she will derive from it. Following the activity, the child then
rates how much actual fun he/she actually experienced. You can work
with the youngster to compare his/her actual level of enjoyment to his/her
expected level of pleasure. Since depressed youngsters will characteristically underestimate how much fun they will have, comparing better than
expected pleasure levels tests their pessimistic predictions. In instances
where pessimistic predictions are accurate, therapeutic advantage may
still be realized. For instance, if a depressed adolescent predicted a low
level of enjoyment and then realized a similar level of low pleasure, you
could test the assumption that prediction of fun determines action (e.g.,
"Do you have to want to do something in order to actually do it?").
Moreover, the mere fact that a depressed adolescent follows through despite predicted anhedonia and actual dissatisfaction represents an important message about the youngster's self-efficacy perceptions. The following dialogue shows how to process these issues with a depressed teenager.

JEREMY: See, I told you going to the game with my friends would be a 3.

THERAPIST: So you went to the game and it was kind of in the middle, just like you predicted.

JEREMY: Yep.

THERAPIST: What made it a 3?

JEREMY: It was just kind of blah.

THERAPIST: Blah?

JEREMY: You know I looked at some of the other guys with their girl-friends and cheerleaders. I don't have that. It reminded me of what I don't have, how much of an outcast I am.

THERAPIST: I see. So those were the negative things that went into the 3. What were the fun things?

JEREMY: Well, my friends and I kind of joked around.

THERAPIST: How would you have felt if you stayed at home alone?

JEREMY: I don't know.

THERAPIST: Do you think you would have joked around with your friends?

JEREMY: Obviously not.

THERAPIST: Then you wouldn't have had that fun. How much would you have thought you were an outcast if you were sitting alone in your room?

JEREMY: Pretty much I guess.

What does this dialogue teach us? First, the therapist went right after Jeremy's belief that motivation must precede action. Second, the therapist helped Jeremy attend to the positive aspects of his actions ("How would you have felt if you stayed at home alone?" "How much would you have thought you were an outcast if you were sitting alone in your room?").

Anxiety prediction is quite similar to pleasure prediction. While depressed youngsters typically underestimate pleasure, anxious children typically overestimate their level of distress. They expect circumstances to be more stressful than they actually are. Thus, we invite youngsters to predict their anticipated level of anxiety, perform the task, and then rate their actual anxiety. This simple yet effective technique prompts youngsters to see that their predictions often inflate a situation's stressfulness. In instances where the predicted rating is lower than the actual rating, children learn they can approach the task even though they anticipate and experience anxious feelings.

Basic Problem-Solving Interventions

Problem solving consists of five basic steps (Barkley et al., 1999; D'Zurilla, 1986). Step 1 involves identifying the problem in specific and concrete terms (e.g., "My sister keeps taking my things even though I tell her not to."). In Step 2, the child is taught to generate alternative solutions. You must be careful not to preempt the brainstorming phase. Step 3 is an evaluation of options. In this step, therapists and children carefully evaluate the short-term and long-term consequences of each option. Children should write down the long-term and short-term consequences of each option. Problem solving can be somewhat of an abstract task, so recording the process on paper concretizes the procedure. In Step 4, after deliberate consideration of each solution, you and the child plan to implement the best solution. Finally, rewarding successful experimentation with alternative solutions characterizes Step 5. If the child tries out a new solution, he/she is instructed to reward him/herself. The reward could be a covert self-reward (e.g., "Congratulations, I tried something new.") or a tangible reward (e.g., some small prize or token).

In *Switching Channels* (Friedberg et al., 1992), problem solving is introduced by a game in which youngsters are given $100 in play money. They must choose music CDs from various categories in order to exhaust exactly $100. The exercise is designed to promote children's flexibility, stimulate problem solving, broaden understanding of multiple solutions, and cast doubt on the common adolescent belief that "I can only choose among desirable alternatives." The music selected for the exercise was purposely chosen to reflect unattractive options for the youngsters. Thus, by completing the exercise, youngsters gain practice in choosing among undesirable alternatives.

Castro-Blanco (1999) suggested another priming alternative for problem solving. He recommended telling jokes or sharing stories with children that contain a problem-solving situation. Certainly, most jokes or stories contain a dilemma that needs to be resolved. The joke or story serves as a template against which the youngster matches/compares his/her problem-solving strategy. The joke serves as a stimulus for discussion and generating alternative problem-solving strategies.

Time Projection

Time projection (Lazarus, 1984) is a problem-solving-like intervention designed to put space between a distressing emotion and the subsequent response. Accordingly, time projection works to decrease impulsive behavior and rash emotional decision making/responding. In general, time projection invites youngsters to consider how they would feel about the same situation at various points ranging from the immediate to the long-range future. For instance, you might ask "How will you feel about this in 6 hours? What would you do differently? How will you feel in 1 day? In 1 week? In 1 month?" You can progress all the way up to 1 year or possibly 5 years. At each time interval, you should be sure to ask what the child would do differently. As a keen reader, you realize it is highly unlikely that children will feel identically today to the way they will feel in 5 years about the same situation. Thus, if their feeling is at all changeable, rash decisions based on impulsive emotional responding (e.g., suicide, violence, running away from home) are clearly unproductive.

Evaluating Advantages and Disadvantages

Evaluating the advantages and disadvantages of certain choices, behaviors, and decisions is a straightforward problem-solving intervention that may help youngsters obtain a broader perspective. In general, advantages/disadvantages prompts youngsters to examine both sides of an issue and act in a way that serves their best interests.

Four basic steps are involved in listing the advantages and disadvantages. In Step 1, the issue about which the youngster wants to get greater perspective is defined (e.g., doing homework in front of the TV). In Step 2, the child lists as many advantages and disadvantages that he/she can think of. You may need to prompt or coach the youth through this process so he/she fully considers each side of the issue. Figure 8.1 shows a sample listing of the advantages and disadvantages youngsters might develop for doing homework in front of the television.

In Step 3, you and the child review the advantages and disadvantages. You might ask questions such as "What makes this an advan-

Doing my homework in front of the television

ADVANTAGES	DISADVANTAGES
It makes it more fun.	It is harder to concentrate.
I get to watch more TV.	It takes me longer because I take more breaks.
I don't get as bored.	I don't have a good place to write or put my books/papers.

FIGURE 8.1. Example of advantages/disadvantages.

tage?"; "What makes this a disadvantage?"; "How long does this advantage/disadvantage last?"; "How valuable/important is this advantage/disadvantage?" We recommend you review each advantage and disadvantage in depth before proceeding to Step 4.

In Step 4, the youngster arrives at a conclusion after considering all the advantages and disadvantages. We recommend helping the youngster account for *both* the advantages and the disadvantages in his/her conclusions. It is important to remember that the goal is for youngsters to mindfully contemplate both sides of an issue.

BASIC SELF-INSTRUCTIONAL TECHNIQUES: CHANGING THOUGHT CONTENT

In general, self-instructional/self-control interventions emphasize changing internal dialogue without in-depth rational analysis. The focus is on replacing maladaptive thoughts with more adaptive, productive thoughts (Meichenbaum, 1985). We consider self-instructional techniques to be inelegant tools that are nonetheless useful in various circumstances.

Generally, self-instructional interventions include preparation, encounter, and self-reward phases (Meichenbaum, 1985). In each stage, youngsters are coached to develop new guides or rules for their own behavior that will help them navigate their way through distressing situations. The goal is for them to construct new covert speech patterns that prompt more adaptive behaviors.

In the preparation stage, you encourage the youngster to ready him/herself for the distressing situation. Optimally, the self-instruction involves a calming yet strategic statement (e.g., "I know this will be hard but I have practiced walking away from a fight. Just remember to stay in control."). Self-instruction accentuates a task focus. The child is taught to attend to important tasks necessary for negotiating his/her way through stressors.

In the encounter stage, the child is schooled in developing self-monologues that decrease his/her stress while he/she is experiencing the uncomfortable circumstances (e.g., "This is just what I guessed would happen. I'm getting jumpy and angry. I have a plan. Now I need to use it. I'm going to keep my hands folded in back of me."). After the child applies the coping strategy, he/she enters the self-reward phase. The child is taught to deliver covert kudos to him/herself for following proper self-instruction (e.g., "I worked hard to stay in control. I'll pump myself up for being in control.").

BASIC RATIONAL ANALYSIS TECHNIQUES: CHANGING THOUGHT CONTENT AND PROCESS

Decatastrophizing

Decatastrophizing is useful for modulating children's dreadful predictions (J. S. Beck, 1953; Kendall et al., 1992; Seligman et al., 1995) by working to decrease children's tendency to overestimate the magnitude and probability of perceived dangers. It is typically implemented through a series of sequential questions including "What's the worst that could happen?"; "What's the best that could happen?"; and "What's the most likely thing that could happen?" (J. S. Beck, 1995). Many cognitive therapists add a problem-solving component to these questions (e.g., "If the worst thing that could happen is highly probable, how would you cope with it?").

In our clinical experience, adding a problem-solving component augments the decatastrophizing procedure. When the child expects the worst and confidently believes it is highly probable, helping the child craft a problem-solving strategy may be a complementary intervention. For example, if a child believes the most probable event is catastrophic but is able to build a reasonable problem-solving strategy, a further window for Socratic questioning is opened. Accordingly, the question "How catastrophic can this be if you can develop a problem-solving strategy?" may follow.

Test of Evidence

A test of evidence (TOE) is a common procedure that requires in-depth rational processing. A TOE prompts children to evaluate the facts supporting their beliefs and the facts disconfirming their beliefs. The TOE is a useful strategy to test overgeneralizations, faulty conclusions, and ill-founded inferences. However, for the TOE to work, the child must possess several skills.

The TOE requires youngsters to access the facts that support their belief. Helping children access the reasons for their conclusions is a first task for you in conducting a TOE. Questions such as "What convinces you 100% that your thought is true?"; "What convinces you beyond a shadow of a doubt?"; "What facts absolutely support your conclusion?"; and "What makes you absolutely certain?" will facilitate this process.

Second, therapists and youngsters must search for contrary evidence. In this phase, you assist youngsters as they try to consider facts that cast doubt on their conclusions. Youngsters may need a significant amount of help constructing disconfirming evidence, especially if they are depressed.

Questions such as "What makes you doubt your conclusion?"; "What facts make you less certain about your conclusion?"; and "What things shake your belief?" are useful.

Third, you urge the child to chew over alternative explanations of the facts used to absolutely support his/her conclusions. As you readily recognize, any alternative explanation of the facts that initially absolutely supported the conclusion casts doubt upon the thought's accuracy. Beneficial questions here might include "What is another way of looking at _____ other than your conclusion?"; "What's another way of explaining _____ in addition to your conclusion?"; or "What else could this mean in addition to your conclusion?"

In the final phase of the TOE, you encourage youngsters to derive a conclusion based on the facts supporting their thought, the facts disconfirming their thought, and the plausible alternative explanations for confirming facts. Optimally, children's new conclusions account for both the confirming and the disconfirming evidence. Moreover, these new interpretations also include a problem-solving component. After forming this new conclusion, you school children to rerate their feelings so they can judge the impact of the new interpretation.

Padesky (1988) suggested several guidelines in fashioning a TOE. First, columns should be labeled clearly as "Facts that completely support my thought" and "Facts that do not completely support my thought." Second, when youngsters begin to generate a list of evidence, you should be careful not to preempt their confirming evidence. Frequently, TOEs fall flat because of unexpressed reasons that buttress children's conclusions. Third, you need to check the evidence for feelings and thoughts that are disguised as facts (e.g., "I'm an idiot."). If there are feelings and thoughts embedded in the Facts columns, you should extract them, discuss them with the youngster, and then decide whether the thought mistakenly considered as a fact is a more primary automatic thought than one being listed.

Reattribution

Reattribution promotes youngsters' appreciation of alternate explanations. Reattribution prompts children to ask themselves "What's another way of looking at this?" Reattribution is useful when children gravitate toward assuming too much responsibility for events beyond their control, applying global labels, and making inaccurate generalizations about dissimilar situations.

Completing a *Responsibility Pie* is a common reattribution technique used successfully with adults (Greenberger & Padesky, 1995) and adolescents (Friedberg et al., 1992). A Responsibility Pie is based on the notion that there can only be 100% of anything. Each event is explained by a number of factors that uniquely contribute some amount to the whole. The task for the therapist and the youngster is to slice the pie into pieces that correspond to the degree that each explanation causes the event to occur. The youngster's reasoning task is to determine how much each factor accounts for his/her conclusion.

The process begins with the youngster listing the possible reasons for a distressing event. The child should be allowed to include his/her overly personalized explanation in the list, but this factor should be recorded last. This process honors the child's explanation by incorporating it in the list, but fosters mindful deliberation by including it later in the process. After the child has listed possible explanations, the therapist and the youngster allocate a piece of the pie to each cause. Each slice accounts for a certain percentage. The child carves him/herself a portion after all the other causes have been accounted for.

The following example illustrates how a Responsibility Pie may be used with a teenager suffering from excessive guilt.

THERAPIST: Portia, we seem to have captured the belief "It's all your fault that your father drinks." Are you willing to check out whether this belief is accurate?

PORTIA: I think so.

THERAPIST: OK. We're going to do a Responsibility Pie.

PORTIA: A what?

THERAPIST: A Responsibility Pie. We have to figure out how much of a piece of responsibility you have. The way we start is to list all the things that may have contributed to your father's alcoholism in addition to your being a bad daughter. What else might cause your dad to drink?

PORTIA: His job is hard.

THERAPIST: OK. What else?

PORTIA: His father and mother were alcoholics.

THERAPIST: You have two. What else?

PORTIA: He gets really depressed sometimes.

THERAPIST: Can you think of anything else?

PORTIA: He goes out with his drinking buddies a lot.

THERAPIST: Anything else?

PORTIA: No, that's all I can think of.

THERAPIST: Let's slice the pie. (*Draws the pie* [see Figure 8.2].) Have you ever cut up and divided a pie or cake?

PORTIA: Sure, I do that a lot.

THERAPIST: So you know you can only have 100% of anything. So we have to divide the pie into pieces. How much do you want to give to your dad's job?

PORTIA: Umm, 20%.

THERAPIST: All right, I'll write that down. How much do you give to the fact that his mom and dad were alcoholics?

PORTIA: I think that may be a big reason. Maybe 30%.

THERAPIST: How about his depression?

PORTIA: Umm, 10%.

THERAPIST: OK. I'll put that down. How about his drinking buddies?

PORTIA: That's a big one too. Maybe 30%.

THERAPIST: OK then. Now we have to include you. How much do you have?

PORTIA: I guess 10%.

THERAPIST: OK. I'll put that down. Now take a long look at this pie. What slices would you want to change?

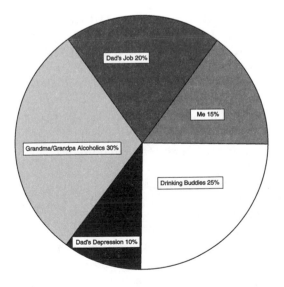

FIGURE 8.2. Portia's Responsibility Pie.

PORTIA: I think I'll give myself a little more. Maybe I'm 15% and his drinking buddies may be 25%.

THERAPIST: We'll change that one. Now as you look at this pie that you divided, what does this mean about your responsibility?

PORTIA: Well, it's not as much as I first thought. There are a lot of other things going on.

THERAPIST: Let's write that down. As you read your conclusion, what does it do to your sense of guilt?

PORTIA: It makes it less.

THERAPIST: Do you think if we talked about the 15% of responsibility you see yourself having that it might decrease too?

PORTIA: Maybe.

THERAPIST: Are you willing to try it and see what happens?

Several important elements of reattribution are illustrated in this dialogue. First, Portia allocated percentages to each cause. Second, Portia's responsibility was included but her contribution was considered last. Further, before reaching a conclusion, Portia was given the opportunity to modify her calculations. Finally, Portia's self-allotment of responsibility was not tested until after the pie was completed.

BASIC EXPOSURE THERAPY: DEVELOPING SELF-CONFIDENCE THROUGH PERFORMANCE ATTAINMENT

In exposure, the child encounters the aversive stimuli, endures the affective arousal, rehearses various coping skills, and earns genuine self-confidence. Exposure techniques are most often associated with treatment of the anxiety disorders and anger management. However, principles of exposure can be used in any therapeutic circumstance where you want the child to practice skills in the context of negative affective arousal. Indeed, Silverman and Kurtines (1997) suggest that exposure may be considered a common factor in many successful psychotherapies.

Confidence gained through authentic performance attainments is sturdy and enduring (Bandura, 1977). If a client doesn't have the chance to demonstrate the application of skills in situations where strong emotions run high, his/her therapy runs the risk of being merely an intellectual exercise and an isolated experience.

Fewer than expected behavior therapists use exposure in their clinical practice (Barlow, 1994). How can this be? We believe several factors may contribute to this finding. First, some therapists have not received supervision or training in this approach, and therefore feel unprepared to do exposure. Additionally, therapists may hold several inaccurate beliefs about exposure therapy that limit their clinical practice.

Therapists may believe that "my role as a therapist is to help the child feel better, not worse, in therapy." These therapists see exposure as being unnecessarily upsetting for the child. Indeed, some therapists may see the intervention as cruel. In fact, after hearing about an exposure trial, one therapist asked, "How could you do that to this child?" These therapists are overlooking the fact that exposure, while uncomfortable in the short term, offers long-term benefits.

Virtually all therapists want therapy to be a "safe place." Ironically, this principle sometimes limits therapists' use of exposure because they see it as dangerous. This idea could not be more off-target. If a therapist wants to promote affective expression in a structured, truly supportive environment, exposure, or performance-based treatment, fits the bill. There is no greater opportunity to express your feelings than when you are facing your fears. Thus, rather than making therapy an unsafe place, exposure helps make therapy a safe place by facilitating a client's emotional expression and subsequent coping with distress.

Another belief that may prohibit exposure practice is that it will damage the therapeutic relationship. Many of our supervisees mistakenly think that if the child becomes anxious, he/she won't trust or like the therapist anymore. However, this belief is founded on the philosophy that productive therapy relationships only allow for positive feelings in therapy or toward the therapy. In short, the conviction is that therapy must always be comfortable. However, most forms of psychotherapy do not adhere to this principle. If therapy is totally comfortable, positive change is less likely to occur. Thus, young clients must be free to experience both negative and positive emotions in therapy.

Exposure actively promotes experiencing negative feelings. In doing so, it minimizes and demystifies them. When you encourage youngsters to experience these negative feelings and coach youngsters through them, you promote genuine trust between therapist and child. Rather than damaging the therapy relationship, exposure can build stronger relationships. For example, we worked with a young boy who was the object of his peers' teasing. The client dreaded school and was hypervigilant during the school day as he looked for bullies. After we taught the youngster some self-control skills, we began graduated exposure involving puppets who were teased. As the therapist role-played the teaser delivering hurtful taunts, the youngster gained practice in coping with the teasing. The therapeutic relationship became stronger through the puppet role playing. By accurately enacting the scenario, the therapist demonstrated that he really understood what was going on in the boy's life and how hard it was for him to manage these stressors.

Therapists also shy away from exposure due to their sense of their own self-efficacy and tolerance for negative affect. I (RDF) often tell my students and supervisees that performance-based treatment is the most experiential form of treatment. If you want to deal with a client's raw feelings, exposure is for you! Many therapists will fear they will not be able to manage the level of a youngsters' distress. Sometimes this fear is reality-based. If you don't have skills to design and implement an exposure trial, it makes sense not to do one until you have read enough and have been supervised sufficiently to carry out the treatment.

Some therapists do have the skills and experience to implement the exposure, yet avoid exposure due to their intolerance of client's affect. We too find it hard to see a youngster in distress. Commonly, our hearts are torn when we see a child tremble and tear up at having to say hello to a new friend. Nonetheless, overcoming these reactions and maintaining a therapeutic focus is crucial in exposure training. If as therapists we are so intolerant of a child's anxiety that we help him/her avoid it by never allowing him/her to feel truly anxious, how can we expect him/her to accept his/her own anxiety?

Exposure is relatively technically complex but nonetheless commonsensical. A parent whose child tumbles off a jungle gym and then subsequently fears the monkey bars knowingly encourages the child to try the playground equipment again in a firm but gentle manner. Exposure is based on the same principle. If children face the fear they have come to dread, the fearsome qualities of the circumstance become attenuated and their behavioral flexibility is increased.

There are several guidelines for the effective use of exposure (Craske & Barlow, 2001; Persons, 1989). First, you must remember not to terminate the exposure session until the child's anxiety decreases. A 50% decline in children's anxiety is suggested as a crude rule of thumb (Beidel & Turner, 1998). Removing the child from the exposure session prior to his/her realizing a decline in responsiveness may counterproductively sensitize the child to the anxiety. Moreover, it further reinforces the child's avoidance and escape behavior. Finally, premature removal will run the risk of reinforcing the child's beliefs that it is necessary to avoid anxiety and that he/she is incapable of managing distress.

Second, effective exposure is comprehensive (Persons, 1989). Exposure treatment should address all the elements embedded in a child's fear. The exposure should be multimodal and incorporate physiological, cognitive, emotional, behavioral, and interpersonal components. Thus, you need to fully assess these components prior to implementing an exposure and subsequently address them in the treatment package.

Finally, repeated exposure is indicated (Persons, 1989; Craske & Barlow, 2001). A one-shot exposure treatment session is not likely to produce enduring change. Thus, repeated practice in exposure is necessary. Children need to do exposure between sessions as well. Parents, teachers, and/or other caregivers need to be educated about the nature of exposure and trained in contingency-management procedures so that they may reinforce the child's efforts.

CONCLUSION

Even before you read this book, you were probably impressed with the wide variety of cognitive-behavioral techniques and methods. We encourage you to mindfully select the techniques based upon the principles of case conceptualization (Chapter 2). Implement each technique with an appropriate level of collaborative empiricism (Chapter 3). Feel free to inventively modify the techniques, as will be suggested in the next chapter. Further, augment the technique with homework assignments (Chapter 10). Finally, titrate each intervention to suit the client's presentation (Chapters 11, 12, 13) and embed them within a family context (Chapter 14).

9

❖

Creative Applications
of Cognitive-Behavioral Therapy

In this chapter we present several creative applications of cognitive therapy. The chapter begins with storytelling and follows with descriptions of various play therapy applications. We also explore the use of cognitive-behaviorally based games, storybooks, and workbooks. Further, a variation of problem solving involving mask making is presented, and interventions based on doing crafts are suggested. The chapter concludes with a cognitive-behavioral exercise designed to eliminate excessive self-blame.

STORYTELLING

Storytelling with children is a therapeutic modality that is positively regarded by clinicians from the psychodynamic (Brandell, 1986; Gardner, 1970, 1971, 1975; Trad & Raine, 1995), Adlerian (Kottman & Stiles, 1990), and strategic–Ericksonian (Godin & Oughourlian, 1994; Greenberg, 1993; Kershaw, 1994) traditions. Until recently, cognitive therapy has ignored the potential usefulness of storytelling with children (Costantino, Malgady,& Rogler, 1994; Friedberg, 1994). Storytelling can be a very effective form of covert modeling. Lazarus (1984) remarked that storytelling "instills basic psychological realities" (p. 104).

Stories are clearly the "stuff" of childhood. Children's play has a natural narrative theme. Tea parties, wars, domestic struggles in dollhouses, and heroic ninth-inning home runs witnessed by imaginary roaring crowds are ministories with plots, characters, and dialogue. Young chil-

146

dren's natural interest in pretense, imagination, and pretend play make storytelling especially natural for them (Trad & Raine, 1995).

In contrast to a psychodynamic approach to storytelling, which focuses on symbolic meaning and interpreting intrapsychic conflict, the main emphasis in the cognitive-behavioral approach is placed on children's problem solving, perceptions of relationships, views of the environment, and self-statements. Examining a child's invented characters' thought patterns, problem solving, and emotional reactions can be very productive (Stirtzinger, 1983; Trad & Raine, 1995). Focusing on the internal states of characters, such as their wishes, fears, and motivations, uncovers children's inner worlds (Kershaw, 1994; Trad & Raine, 1995). Discerning the skills that the character must build to solve the problem or conflict in the story can direct clinicians' subsequent therapeutic efforts (Kershaw, 1994). Moreover, investigating the elements that block productive solutions is a clinical priority (Gardner, 1986; Kershaw, 1994). The story information may reflect children's perceptions of internal and external constraints on their problem solving. Kershaw (1994) noted that when solutions are included in children's stories, therapists are well advised to examine whether or not the solution is effective, adequate, and appropriate. Finally, the ease and effectiveness of conflict resolution within the story may reflect children's perceived sense of competence or control (Bellak, 1993; Rotter, 1982).

We follow Gardner's (1970, 1971, 1972, 1975, 1986) basic procedures for therapeutic storytelling. The child is encouraged to tell a story that he/she has never heard before into a tape recorder. Children are told that the story should have a beginning, middle, and end, and a lesson or moral. The lesson typically directs the clinician's attention to the most psychologically present theme (Brandell, 1986). The therapist then follows the child's story with one of his/her own that offers a more adaptive coping response or a more productive resolution.

Gardner (1972) offered some suggestions for children who have difficulty constructing a story or maintaining its flow. He recommended "graduated storytelling" in which the therapist starts the story, pauses, and then prompts the child to continue it; when the child falters, the therapist can pick up the story thread, pause, prompt again, and so on. Lawson (1987) also lists several ideas for therapists to consider that may invite children into the therapeutic process to make storytelling a more welcomed technique. Lawson (1987) advises therapists to speak slower than normal and in a lower tone to more fully engage children. Additionally, Lawson suggests including "kinesthetic and auditory predicates" in the introductions to stories. For example, incorporating various sensory modalities for children (e.g., "The wind blew and whistled through the woods . . . ") may engage children.

Attending to the way significant others are represented and described in the story may be quite therapeutically effective. Several authors (Bellak, 1993; Kershaw, 1994; Trad & Raine, 1995) suggest questions to consider when you are exploring children's stories, such as the way parental and peer figures are described. Are parental figures nurturant, competent, available, rejecting, loving, or menacing? Are peers described as friendly, hostile, competitive, or competent? Further, do these separate characters reflect the child's competing motivations?

The general emotional climate of the story may also be quite revealing. For example, does it have a hostile tone? The atmosphere of the story is important and may reflect a child's conception of the world (Bellak, 1993; Gardner, 1986; Stirtzinger, 1983). Where does the story take place? Action that takes place in a wasteland or a dark rain forest is much different than action that takes place in a crowded city or a warm woods (Bellak, 1993).

We have several tips for constructing a therapeutic alternative story. Generally, effective stories fill gaps in children's temporal ordering, prompt reattribution, and correct inaccuracies in children's understanding of causal antecedents (Russell, Van den Brock, Adams, Rosenberger, & Essig, 1993). Children must be able to identify with the behaviors, cognitions, feelings, and motivations represented in the therapist's story. Further, children should see the characters' abilities as similar or potentially similar to their own capacities, skills, and options.

The child's identification with story characters can be enhanced in several ways. In the therapist's stories, we recommend creating a conflict that parallels that of the child's story, but where characters are successful in overcoming or meeting their challenges (Gardner, 1986; Mills, Crowley, & Ryan, 1986). When children recognize that the problem in your story corresponds to their own dilemma, the story's impact is enhanced (Mills et al., 1986). The central character in your story represents a metaphor or covert model for the child (Callow & Benson, 1990). Thus you choice of characters will depend on the individual child, the problem, and the surrounding circumstances or context.

For instance, Davis (1989) found that abused children typically share stories about animals such as bunnies that have few inherent defenses. In these cases, therapeutic stories should offer a competing but parallel figure who has some natural defense. For example, a turtle is a good character because it has a protective shell. Turtles are particularly valuable story figures because they make choices about retreating into their shell or revealing themselves. Moreover, they allow for flexible reasoning since they rarely totally abandon their shells (i.e., completely remain within their protective cover).

Frogs and mice are personal favorites. Frogs may typically be seen as inert types who rarely venture beyond their own lily pad. Thus, they are natural metaphors for inhibited and fearful children. Moreover, their "hidden" capacity to spring from lily pad to lily pad can communicate ways in which their latent resources can be assessed. Mice, on the other hand, offer other opportunities for therapeutic storytellers. Children seem to readily identify with mice, perhaps because they are so small and ostensibly helpless. Accordingly, they must negotiate life's tricky impasses by using their wits. Mice characters are covert "models" who can teach children that successful resolution of conflicts does not depend on size and strength.

Animals or characters that can transform themselves can offer hope, illustrate change, and decrease rigid thinking. For instance, story characters who change from one state to another, such as caterpillars, swans, and/or dalmatians, can be quite useful. Themes involving emotional growth and skill acquisition can be gracefully woven around narratives that detail the metamorphoses of these characters from a negative circumstance to a more sanguine situation. For example, therapeutic stories about a dalmatian who is teased about being ordinary yet eventually gains his spots may communicate a variety of therapeutic messages.

The following is a sample story that offers a more adaptive resolution to a young child's fear of independence.

> Once upon a time, a long, long time ago in a place far, far away, there lived a little seal. This seal's name was Hickory. Hickory was afraid that if he did things for himself his mom and dad would stop caring for him. He thought the more he did for himself the more things would be expected of him.
>
> Many times Hickory would ask his dad to get him some fish even though he could get them himself. If Hickory forgot something at school, his mom always agreed to get it for him. Sometimes Hickory would ask his mom and dad to carry him to the next rock rather than swim himself. His mom and dad got very frustrated and did not know what to do.
>
> Hickory was afraid. He thought growing up was dangerous. He knew what it was like to be a little seal but he did not know what it would be like to be a bigger seal. One day at seal school, he met a sea lion. The sea lion, named Regis, saw that Hickory was scared about doing things for himself. Regis and Hickory became friends.
>
> On a sunny afternoon, Regis asked Hickory why he asked others to do things for him that he could do on his own. Hickory said he was scared to. Regis suggested he try it and see what happens. So there was a big iceberg out on the ocean. Regis said, "Do you think you can swim to that all by yourself?" "I'm afraid to," said Hickory. "What are you

afraid of?," asked Regis. Hickory replied, "Will you take care of me if I make it?" "Sure," Regis smiled.

So Hickory went out to the edge of the water and dove in. While he was swimming out to the iceberg, he worried: "What if I make it and he asks me to do more?"; "I really like being taken care of."; "If I don't do this, I am sure Regis won't make me do this again." As these thoughts raced through his mind, Hickory swam slower and slower.

He heard Regis shouting from the shore. "You can do it, Hickory. I will be right here on the shore when you come back." This helped Hickory. He swam a little more. More voices from the shore shouted. It was his mom and dad. They were cheering for him. "Swim, Hickory, swim. Every time you look back we'll be here. No matter how far or fast you swim, we'll always be right here waiting for you." This made Hickory feel warm and strong. He easily reached the iceberg and even sat there in the sun having a nice fish snack and looking back at the shore where Regis and his mom and dad were waiting. He stayed on the iceberg for a little while enjoying his snack and the view.

What are the helpful elements in this story? First, the story pinpoints Hickory's beliefs about independence (e.g., If I do things for myself, my mom and dad won't care for me. The more I do for myself the more will be expected of me.). Second, Hickory is a coping model. He did not easily accomplish his goals; he had to struggle to make things work out for himself. Third, the story yields simple lessons or counterimages (e.g., People will love you if you can do things for yourself. Growing up is not dangerous and has its own rewards.).

Creating a storybook to accompany the storytelling technique is also productive (Kestenbaum, 1985). Kestenbaum suggested using a loose-leaf notebook or three-ring binder when building a volume of stories. Children may add new stories each week. Reviewing these stories will give them a tangible form of progress. Additionally, a section could be added where the therapist and child note what has been learned from each story. In fact, Goncalves (1994) suggested that homework assignments based on stories potentiate their impact. We invite children to experiment with strategies embedded in the story. Youngsters might then record their experiments in the binder alongside the appropriate story.

PLAY THERAPY APPLICATIONS

In cognitive-behavioral play therapy, therapists are active, goal directed, and use the play to modify problematic thought, feeling, and behavior patterns (Knell, 1993). Play is the medium by which inaccurate internal dialogues are elicited and more adaptive coping methods are taught.

You can use play to help teach a difficult skill, such as dividing the Responsibility Pie (discussed in Chapter 8), by using clay to explain the process. For example, a chunk of clay can be divided into separate pieces, each of which represents a perceived portion of responsibility. Children are then able to see a concrete, visual depiction of the responsibility allocation process. The following dialogue personifies the process.

THERAPIST: We've listed all the things you think caused Pearl to ignore you. Now what we need to do is figure out which of these things are the biggest reasons. Let's play with some clay to figure it out. How does that sound?

LEAH: Can I use the clay?

THERAPIST: Sure.

LEAH: This is sticky.

THERAPIST: What we need to decide is how much of this blob of clay we should give to each reason you come up with for why Pearl ignored you.

LEAH: (*Rolling the clay into a large ball.*) OK.

THERAPIST: Let's use this plastic knife to cut off the pieces. How much should we give to Pearl being tired?

LEAH: This much. (*Cuts off about 20%.*)

THERAPIST: How much should we give to Pearl and Susan talking together and not hearing you?

LEAH: That's big. (*Slices off about 40%.*)

THERAPIST: Let's see. What was our next one?

LEAH: She was in a hurry to get to her seat before the teacher came in.

THERAPIST: That's right. Slice off how much for that one?

LEAH: (*Slices off about 30%.*)

THERAPIST: What's this little slice left?

LEAH: How much she doesn't like me?

For therapists who do not like clay (it can be messy!), a similar procedure can be done with a cardboard circle and a pair of scissors. The child generates a list of explanations and then cuts from the circle the piece that corresponds to the amount allocated by the child. The reason is written on each piece of the pie. Thus, the child owns a tangible way to track the reattribution process.

Puppet play lends itself nicely to cognitive therapy applications, promoting Socratic dialogues and self-instructional procedures. Puppets can be purchased or made in session. In our work with youngsters in the Preventing Anxiety and Depression in Youth program, we made liberal use of sandwich bag puppets (Friedberg et al., 2001). Sandwich bag puppets are simple to make: the child draws a character or pastes one made from colored paper on the bottom of a brown sandwich bag. The following transcript shows how therapists can use puppets in self-instructional training.

THERAPIST: Which puppet would you like to play, Estella?

ESTELLA: I'll pick the wolf.

THERAPIST: Let's see—I'll pick the lamb.

ESTELLA: He's cute. I have one like that at home.

THERAPIST: Let's put on a puppet show. What should it be about?

ESTELLA: I don't know. I just want to play.

THERAPIST: How about we do a puppet show about being angry?

ESTELLA: OK. What will we do?

THERAPIST: What could the wolf and the lamb argue about?

ESTELLA: Maybe the wolf is mad because the lamb acts like she is better than her.

THERAPIST: OK. Let's start.

ESTELLA: Grr, I'm going to eat you up and bite you because you think you are so special. I hate you. You stupid lamb.

THERAPIST: You are scary. I am going to run away.

ESTELLA: I'll catch up with you because I am strong and fast.

THERAPIST: What makes you so mad at me?

ESTELLA: I don't know. Grr. (*Tries to bite the lamb.*)

THERAPIST: I am so scared and confused.

ESTELLA: Good!

THERAPIST: Estella, this is a good place to see if we can teach the wolf some of the tools we have been learning. Pick a puppet that can be the teacher.

ESTELLA: This looks like a teacher. (*Picks a bear.*)

THERAPIST: Do you want to be the bear and teach the wolf to work with her mad feelings and make friends?

ESTELLA: No, you do it. I'll just be the wolf.

THERAPIST: How about we both do it?

ESTELLA: OK.

THERAPIST: (*Putting on the bear puppet.*)

ESTELLA: Grr. I don't like you, you stupid lamb.

THERAPIST: Oh no, here we go again.

ESTELLA: I'm going to chase you.

THERAPIST: (*as the bear now*) Now, wait a minute, Wolf. How are you feeling?

ESTELLA: Mad. I'm going to get that lamb.

THERAPIST: Wolf, what do you want to show the lamb?

ESTELLA: That I'm in charge. She's no better than me. If she doesn't want to be my friend then I will bite her.

THERAPIST: I see, Wolf. You want to make friends with her but guess that she thinks she is better.

ESTELLA: Yes. I will get her.

THERAPIST: How do you guess Lamb feels?

ESTELLA: Scared, grr. (*Laughs.*)

THERAPIST: She sure does. Look at her tremble. How much does she look like she wants to be friends?

ESTELLA: Not that much.

THERAPIST: Estella, what can Wolf say to herself to cool off her angry feelings.

ESTELLA: I forget.

THERAPIST: Well, what have we learned that we could teach the wolf?

ESTELLA: The things I say to myself.

THERAPIST: Give it a try.

ESTELLA: Now, Wolf, don't let the anger boil. Turn down the heat on your angry stove.

THERAPIST: Great. How does it work for the wolf?

ESTELLA: No good. He's still angry. Grr. I'm going to get that lamb.

THERAPIST: Here, you be the bear and use more self-talk to calm down the wolf.

ESTELLA: Don't boil over. Put out the fire in you.

In this example, Estella and her therapist took the opportunity to replace maladaptive statements with the coping statements learned earlier in therapy. The puppet play also promoted acquisition of additional coping statements (e.g., "Don't boil over. Put out the fire in you.").

Popular children's games also lend themselves nicely to cognitive-behavioral play therapy. Simon, Jenga, Connect Four, and Life are just a few games that can be serviceable tools. Childhood games are good tools because they usually involve a problem-solving component and, since they usually involve some performance pressures, they are emotionally arousing. Cognitive therapists use such games as a stimulus to identify thoughts and feelings, correct maladaptive thinking patterns, and improve social skills.

Often, therapists wonder whether they should "let" a child win games. Letting a child win or not depends on what you are trying to teach the child. If the youngster has low frustration tolerance and is a poor loser, the child needs practice in tolerating defeat. For instance, Sunny would kick the table and pout when she lost at checkers. Letting her win wouldn't teach her anything, whereas her defeats were learning opportunities where she could apply her coping skills. If the child is timorous and lacks self-efficacy, discrete "tanking" by the therapist may be in order. For example, Benny thought he was no good at playing Nerf basketball and would not permit himself to take a shot. The therapist deliberately missed several shots, which enabled Benny to find his courage to take a long shot. However, letting the child win must not be transparent. Therefore, balance is often indicated. Game play should reflect life's contingencies: sometimes you win and sometimes you lose.

Cheating during a game is another dilemma that concerns therapists. We do not allow cheating during the game play. Allowing cheating sends the wrong message to the child. Moreover, the child's cheating behavior is also frequently embedded in his/her presenting problems. Allowing the child to cheat means you are colluding with the child's dishonest behavior. Thus, we recommend you elicit and modify the maladaptive beliefs associated with the cheating. The following dialogue exemplifies the process.

THERAPIST: Dennis, you moved my piece back two spaces and you moved your game piece ahead a place. Is that what the game card said?

DENNIS: I don't remember.

THERAPIST: I see. Do you think it is fair?

DENNIS: I don't know. (*Puts head on table.*)

THERAPIST: Does this happen sometimes when you play with your friends?

DENNIS: Sometimes.

THERAPIST: What popped into your head when you moved my piece?

DENNIS: I don't know.

THERAPIST: What was it like seeing me move ahead of you?

DENNIS: Bad.

THERAPIST: When you felt bad, what went through your mind?

DENNIS: I hate to lose.

THERAPIST: What would it mean to lose?

DENNIS: You're better than me.

THERAPIST: So you feel bad when you think you might lose and the thought "I'm better than you" went through your head. So you moved your piece ahead of mine?

DENNIS: (*Tears up, nods.*)

THERAPIST: How did it work out for you?

DENNIS: Not good.

THERAPIST: Can we make a plan together so first you learn that losing a game is not so horrible and there are ways to help yourself feel better when you lose so you don't feel forced to cheat?

This dialogue contains several helpful hints. First, the therapist limited the cheating. Second, the therapist did not punish or ridicule Dennis but rather helped him identify the thoughts and feelings that mediated the cheating. Third, the therapist linked cheating in the therapy session with Dennis's social skills problems. Finally, the therapist initiated a problem-solving process.

GAMES, STORYBOOKS, WORKBOOKS, AND MAKING MASKS

Games

Berg (1986, 1989, 1990a, 1990b, 1990c) has developed a series of attractively designed and packaged games that focus on a variety of childhood problems. Each game includes a set of cards specifically targeted to the psychologically salient issues embedded in each problem area. A manual that guides the novice through the game is included, along with tokens, spinners, game pieces, dice, and a game board. More recently, several storybooks and videos have been developed to augment these games.

Storybooks

There are several cognitive-behaviorally oriented storybooks that can be helpful for a variety of children. For example, Waters's (1980) *Rational Stories for Children* contains six stories for children and accompanying guidelines for parents. The stories include themes such as accepting oneself, building frustration tolerance, coping with fearfulness, managing anger, problem solving, and cognitive restructuring. Each children's story includes illustrations; the parent guide includes handy psychoeducational material. Waters (1979) also wrote *Color Us Rational*, a collection of stories in coloring-book form. The 12 stories in the book reflect Ellis's (1962) 12 basic irrational beliefs (e.g., It is easier to avoid problems than confront them, I must be approved by everyone, etc.). Children can color the accompanying pictures while the therapist and/or parent reads each story to them. *Homer the Homely Hound Dog* (Garcia & Pellegrini, 1974) tells the story of a self-critical dog who learns to be more self-forgiving. Catalogues from the Institute for Rational-Emotive Therapy, *Childs work/Childs play* and Western Psychological Services are some resources that offer additional storybook materials.

Workbooks

There are several cognitive-behaviorally based workbooks for children and adolescents. Vernon (1989a, 1989b, 1998) offers a series of exercises that are developmentally sensitive and separated by age/grade level. These exercises offer a wide range of activities, including crafts, stories, and experiments. Each exercise and activity includes a series of questions to guide therapists through the process. Moreover, Vernon includes discussion and processing questions. Each exercise also informs the therapist about the materials needed to complete the exercises.

Kendall's (1990) *Coping Cat Workbook* is a clever collection of techniques and exercises for treating anxious children. The *Coping Cat Workbook* is engaging and includes delightful cartoons and exercises. The *Coping Cat* series is widely applied and has enjoyed considerable empirical success (Kendall & Treadwell, 1996; Kendall et al., 1997). The *Coping Cat* is suitable for children from about age 7 to about age 13, depending on their psychological maturity.

Therapeutic Exercises for Children (Friedberg et al., 2001) is a set of cognitive-behavioral techniques, exercises, and activities for children ages 8 to 11 who are primarily experiencing anxiety and depression. The workbook contains guidelines for therapists and helps scaffold forms of Socratic dialogue with children. *Therapeutic Exercises for Children* includes illustrations and text that is engaging for youngsters.

Kendall's (1988) *Stop and Think Workbook* is an inventive way to work with impulsive children. The workbook includes numerous exercises that promote children's sequencing, planning, and problem-solving skills. Similarly to the *Coping Cat Workbook*, Kendall includes Show That I Can (STIC) assignments. Role-playing exercises and illustrations enliven the material.

Fed up and frustrated with limited progress with their young clients, therapists understandably may overrely on workbooks for answers. In our experience, this strategy rarely works. It is usually best when the workbook exercise emerges naturally from the session content and is presented in an engaging manner. The following exchange illustrates the way a workbook exercise is integrated into session content.

JUSTIN: Things are always my fault. I'm always to blame for everything.

THERAPIST: How do you feel when you think everything is your fault?

JUSTIN: Really bad.

THERAPIST: Mad, scared, sad, or worried?

JUSTIN: More sad, I guess.

THERAPIST: That makes a lot of sense. If you believe everything is your fault, you'd feel really sad. What we need to figure out now is how much you are to blame for everything. Are you willing to do that?

JUSTIN: I guess so.

THERAPIST: Well, I have this exercise that might help. Are you willing to check it out?

In this example, the therapist elicited Justin's automatic thoughts and feelings. After identifying these problematic thoughts and feelings, the therapist introduced a workbook exercise. The exercise gracefully flowed from the session content and was directly connected to Justin's presenting problems.

Making Masks

Making masks is a fun way to teach problem solving. Creating a personalized mask is an activity that can augment the traditional problem solving procedure explained in Chapter 8. Mask making combines covert modeling and problem solving into a craft-oriented exercise. Moreover, mask making is also similar to the superhero modeling used by Kendall and his colleagues (1992).

The child is asked to choose a hero or model (e.g., a sports figure,

story character, TV star, family member, teacher). Next, the child is told
to find a picture of his/her hero, to cut it out, and to paste it on a face-
shaped piece of cardboard. If the hero's picture is unavailable, the child is
invited to draw his/her own rendition of the hero on the cardboard or
simply to write the hero's name on the mask. The child should cut out eye
and mouth spaces on the mask. Finally, the child glues the completed
mask to a paint stirrer, popsicle stick, or tongue depressor, which serves
as a handle.

Then you ask the child to go through the problem-solving process as
if he/she were his/her own superhero. The child has to pretend that the
hero is doing the problem solving. The following transcript illustrates
how you might use mask making.

THERAPIST: So you've pasted Harry Potter's face on your mask.

KYLE: Yes, I love those books.

THERAPIST: OK. Now we're going to do the problem solving in a different
way with this mask. I want you to pretend you are Harry Potter and
see how many strategies you can come up with to solve the problem.

KYLE: What will the problem be?

THERAPIST: Let's pick a problem you have been struggling with.

KYLE: Umm . . . picking a partner in school for a project.

THERAPIST: OK. Put the mask up to your face and imagine you are Harry
Potter. What would you do, Harry, to pick a partner for your social
studies project?

This example illustrates several pivotal points. First, Kyle picked a
favorite character to identify with. Second, Kyle selected an important
problem to focus on. Third, rather than putting Kyle on the spot to generate alternative solutions, the mask making gave Kyle the opportunity to
play Harry Potter and discover what Harry might do in the situation.

THOUGHT–FEELING HOOPS

Thought–Feeling Hoops is a play activity that involves pairing identifying
thoughts and feelings with shooting a basketball. The activity provides an
experiential and fun way for children to learn basic self-monitoring skills.
Thought–Feeling Hoops is an ideal accompaniment to the thought records described in Chapter 6.

In order to do this exercise, you need a basketball hoop and a ball,
although even a crumpled-up ball of paper and an empty wastepaper bas-

ket will do. When playing Thought–Feeling Hoops, the child is instructed to share his/her thoughts and feelings before and after he/she takes his/her "shots." This practice enables the children and you to connect situations, thoughts, and feelings. Moreover, therapists are also able to use this exercise to illustrate the inaccuracy of children's predictions. Thought–Feeling Hoops provides an opportunity to explore fears of negative evaluation and performance pressures associated with generalized anxiety and social anxiety. Children's fears of risk taking may also be treated through this activity. Finally, Thought–Feeling Hoops may address children's tolerance for negative emotions such as frustration and disappointment.

Using Thought–Feeling Hoops to connect situations, feelings, and thoughts is a relatively straightforward task. As the child prepares to shoot, ask him/her to define the event or situation (e.g., "What's happening?"). The child responds by saying, "I'm going to shoot the ball." Next, ask the youngster how he/she is feeling (e.g., "anxious") and what is going through his/her mind (e.g., "I'll miss and you'll think I can't play."). After the child shoots the ball, ask him/her to record his/her situations, thoughts, and feelings in one of the various thought diaries discussed in Chapter 6. In sum, the child tells the therapist the situation, feeling, and thought, shoots the ball, and then records these elements in a thought record.

Thought–Feeling Hoops can also be used to test children's inaccurate predictions. Prior to shooting, the child predicts that he/she will make or miss the basket. By shooting, the child is actually testing out his/her prediction. If the child predicts that he/she will miss and he/she subsequently makes the basket, you can process this experience using questions such as:

"What was it like to see your prediction not come true?"
"Do you make other guesses about how well you do?"
"How often do these come true?"
"How often are your predictions inaccurate?"
"Do you think your estimates may be off about other things also?"

If a child predicts he/she will miss the shot and in fact does, you have yet another opportunity to intervene. In this instance, the child can be helped to see that while he/she missed one shot, he/she also has a chance to shoot again. Further, you can help the child explore whether the consequences of his/her missed shot occurred (i.e., Were they laughed at or criticized for missing the shot?).

Thought–Feeling Hoops can tap children's fear of negative evaluation and performance worries. Shooting baskets is just the type of activity socially anxious children dread. Therefore, the exercise can be used as a graduated exposure trial. Some children may fear the task's "public" nature. Other youngsters may become anxious about missing shots or looking foolish. You can elicit the children's negative predictions and use the activity as a behavioral test of accuracy. The following transcript illustrates the way therapists may process this activity.

THERAPIST: Jimmy, you look nervous about shooting.

JIMMY: No, I'm not.

THERAPIST: What's going through your mind right now?

JIMMY: I dunno. Maybe the ball will not make it to the backboard or it will bounce out of the hoop.

THERAPIST: How do you feel about that?

JIMMY: Nervous.

THERAPIST: So when you think the ball will bounce funny and you feel nervous, what do you expect to happen?

JIMMY: Maybe you'll laugh and think I'm no good at basketball.

THERAPIST: If I laugh and think you are no good at basketball, what will happen?

JIMMY: I'll feel embarrassed.

THERAPIST: What do you expect I will think?

JIMMY: That I'm a doofus and I don't know how to play. That I look funny when I shoot.

THERAPIST: That's pretty scary. Would you be willing to shoot some baskets with me and see if we could put these thoughts to rest?

JIMMY: OK. (*He shoots and the ball goes in.*) Yeah, two points!

THERAPIST: Try another shot.

JIMMY: (*Shoots and misses.*)

THERAPIST: Tough luck. Now hold on a second. What did you guess I would think?

JIMMY: That I'm a doofus and I look funny when I shoot.

THERAPIST: Do you want to check this out and ask me?

JIMMY: Well, what did you think?

What is important about this dialogue? First, the therapist used the game to help identify Jimmy's thoughts and feelings. Jimmy felt comfortable disclosing his negative predictions and the feelings associated with them. Second, the game provided a nonthreatening opportunity to test out the predictions. Jimmy was able to check out his predictions in a here-and-now context.

What other therapeutic possibilities present themselves in this exercise? The therapist might elect to provide Jimmy with feedback disconfirming his negative expectations (e.g., "No, I did not think you are a doofus."). Another strategy would be to help Jimmy prepare for the possibility of negative feedback (e.g., "Suppose I did think you were a doofus. What would that mean? How would you know if I was right? How does my opinion define who you are?"). In this way, you could help Jimmy develop ways to cope with teasing if other children mocked him.

PRIMING EXERCISES

Thought–Feeling Bookmark

The Thought–Feeling Bookmark and the Thought–Feeling Watch are craft-oriented activities designed to increase children's perceptions of changeability. The Thought–Feeling Bookmark is a priming technique that also includes a self-instructional component. The bookmark metaphor contributes to the priming function. The essential point is to help children realize that where they place a bookmark in a book changes over time and with activity. Similarly, thoughts and feelings change with time and activity. The bookmark metaphor is presented to children in a manner similar to the example presented below.

> "Do you like to read? I like books too. How do you keep your place in a book? I use a bookmark. You know, there is something special about bookmarks. When you read a book, you are turning pages. You are moving from the old page to a new page. The bookmark also changes as you read. It moves from one part of the book to another part. How is this like your thoughts and feelings? That's right, your thoughts and feelings change too."

Decorating the bookmark with a coping statement serves the self-instructional function. Creating the Thought–Feeling Bookmark is simple and fun. The material needed to make the bookmark includes colored cardboard/construction paper, pens, markers, crayons, ribbons, glitter, glue, confetti, and a hole punch. Encourage children to decorate their bookmark any way they wish. You can then instruct them to write down a simple coping thought on the bookmark such as "Things change," "I can handle challenges," or "Feelings change."

Thought–Feeling Watch

The Thought–Feeling Watch is a craft activity that serves as a self-monitoring device as well as a priming intervention. The Thought–Feeling Watch helps children realize that feelings change and acts as a prompt for identifying maladaptive thoughts. The wristwatch metaphor is central to this exercise. Feelings are equated with hands on a wristwatch. Accordingly, the watch metaphor cogently communicates that like time, feelings always change. The hands on the wristwatch symbolize the "clock time," while the hands on the Thought–Feeling Watch signify the "emotional time."

You might present the Thought–Feeling Watch in a manner similar to the one presented below.

> "I really like watches. Do you? The thing that I like about watches is the way they move. The hands never stay still. Have you ever noticed that? Take a look at a watch or clock. The only time the hands do not move is when the watch is broken. The hands on a working clock move even during a long day. Together we are going to make a Thought–Feeling Watch to remind us that thoughts and feelings change. Instead of numbers on the watch, we'll draw feeling faces on it."

The Thought–Feeling Watch can help youngsters capture the thoughts and images that shape their feelings. For instance, the child could be asked to write down his/her thoughts when the hands on the watch point to different feelings. Additionally, the therapist and the child could play a game in which the child moves the hands of the watch to different feelings and then role-plays a situation in which these feelings arise. Finally, the child could learn to turn the hands of the clock to different feeling faces and practice developing coping thoughts when these feelings occur.

Making the Thought–Feeling Watch is easy. You and the child will need colored paper, pens or markers, brass grommet clasps, Velcro dots, and a glue stick. You can precut the colored paper into a medium-sized circle for the watch face, a pointer shape for a watch hand, and a long narrow rectangle measured to the size of the child's wrist for the watchband. The child draws mad, sad, scared, and happy faces on the medium-sized circle at 12:00, 3:00, 6:00, and 9:00 o'clock. The watch hand, watch face, and watchband are attached by the metal grommets. Finally, the Velcro dots are glued to the ends of the wrist strips. Figure 9.1 shows the materials and a completed Thought–Feeling Watch.

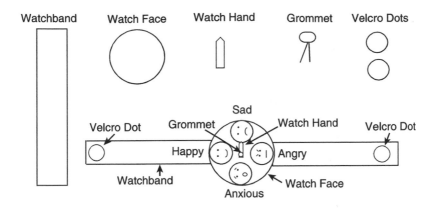

FIGURE 9.1. Thought–Feeling Watch diagram.

Since the Thought–Feeling Watch is a nonverbal craft, it may be especially useful with children who are initially hesitant to express their feelings. For instance, after completing the watch, the child could point to the feeling on his/her watch instead of having to say it aloud. Additionally, since the child draws his/her own feelings on the watch, he/she is more likely to identify with his/her own drawings than with preprinted feeling faces. Thus, the Thought–Feeling Watch may click with relatively unexpressive children.

Taking Command or Blaming Yourself Worksheet

The Taking Command or Blaming Yourself Worksheet is a priming exercise designed to help children decrease excessively punitive attributions. The goal of the exercise is for children to learn to take control or command of their feelings without either self-blaming or avoiding personal responsibility. The worksheet has six self-statements enclosed in a thought bubble (see Figure 9.2). Underneath each thought bubble are the options "Take Command" and "Blame Self." The child is then asked to draw a line from the thought to either option, showing whether the thought is a way to take command or to blame him/herself.

You should set up the exercise with a brief discussion about the difference between taking command and self-blame. You can ask the child if he/she blames him/herself for the bad things that happen to him/her. The child can then be asked for examples of the way he/she blames him/herself. After these instances of self-blame are elicited, you can process these

Draw a line to show if the thought is a way to TAKE COMMAND or a way to BLAME YOURSELF.

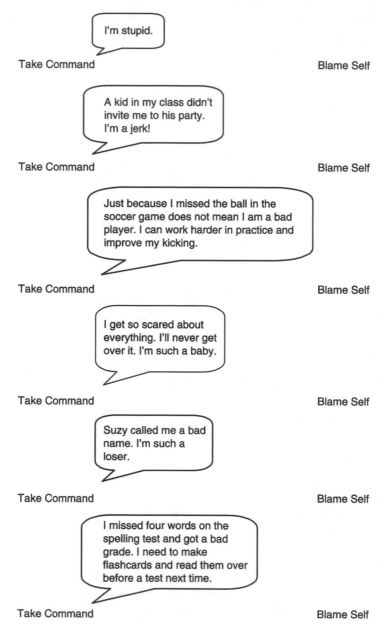

FIGURE 9.2. Taking Command or Blaming Yourself Worksheet. From Friedberg and McClure (2002). Copyright by The Guilford Press. Permission to photocopy this figure is granted to purchasers of this book for personal use only (see copyright page for details).

self-blaming statements with the child. For instance, you might ask the following key processing questions:

"How does blaming yourself help you?"
"In what ways does blaming yourself help you?"
"How does blaming yourself hurt you?"
"What do you gain by blaming yourself?"
"What do you lose by blaming yourself?"
"What else could you do if you didn't blame yourself?"
"What could you do instead of blaming yourself?"

Making the distinction between not blaming themselves and avoiding responsibility is the next step in the process. Then, you can explore the notion of taking command or responsibility. Having the child define taking command is a useful strategy. You might ask the child the following questions:

"What does 'taking command' mean?"
"What does 'taking charge of yourself' mean?"
"When do you take charge?"
"When do you take command?"
"What things do you take command over?"
"How do you feel when you take charge or take command?"
"What is the difference between taking command and blaming yourself?"

After you and the child have fully processed the terms, you can collaboratively introduce the task. For instance, you may say:

"This worksheet can help you find the difference between blaming yourself and taking command. Here's how to do this worksheet. Do you see the thought bubble with the thought in it? Underneath each thought bubble are choices titled 'Take Command' or 'Blame Self.' You need to decide whether the thought in the bubble is either a way to take command or blame yourself. After you choose, draw a line from your choice to the thought bubble. Do you understand what to do?"

The therapist and child should discuss the item so the child has an opportunity to explain each response and the therapist has an opportunity to clarify any confusion. Further, after the task is completed, the child and the therapist should each summarize the task to add closure. You might ask the following questions to facilitate closure:

"What was it like to do this worksheet?"

"What did you like about this worksheet?"

"What didn't you like about this worksheet? What did you learn from this worksheet?"

From the Taking Command or Blaming Yourself Worksheet, the child will begin to determine what events are in and what events are not in his/her control. The Taking Command or Blaming Yourself Worksheet enables youngsters to discern the difference between destructive self-blaming and adopting corrective feedback leading to productive change.

CONCLUSION

Children and adolescents may not immediately engage with traditional techniques. In this chapter, we presented various ways we have modified some traditional cognitive approaches. We encourage you to try out our ideas and make them your own through your adaptations. Storytelling, play therapy, craft activities, puppet play, and board games are just some ways you can enliven therapy. The key part is making the therapy fun. While you may work with children who have distressing and difficult emotions, the therapy does not necessarily have to be morose and humorless. In fact, in our experience, we find that if children and adolescents see the sessions as too clinical, the session becomes less therapeutic. We encourage you to use the skills presented in the chapters on case conceptualization and the session structure to formulate and focus a creative intervention strategy. Enjoy experimenting with the techniques. The adventuresome spirit is contagious and children will catch onto the coping skills approach.

10

❖

Homework

Homework promotes skill acquisition and application in real-world contexts (Spiegler & Guevrememont, 1998). Children need to rehearse their new skills outside therapy. Moreover, homework is both a practice and a process. Care needs to be directed both at *what* tasks are assigned and *how* these tasks are prescribed. As mentioned in Chapter 4, children can react strongly and negatively to words like "homework"—more than likely some children will bristle at the mere mention of the "H" word. To combat this problem, homework assignments should be cleverly designed to engage kids. Consequently, this chapter will offer ways to develop effective homework assignments.

Assigning homework may seem straightforward, but it is a demanding task for most therapists. When you assign homework, you have to plan ahead rather than react and respond. However, unexpected things happen within session and therapy may not go in the direction you plan. For instance, we were working with an anxious young girl and planning for her to identify her thoughts surrounding some test anxiety and fears of disapproval. As the session progressed, a more central issue involving anger toward her sister popped up. We needed to hastily but deliberately develop a new homework assignment to address the emergent issue. A good homework assignment advances therapy's momentum and builds on what has happened in a session.

GENERAL CONSIDERATIONS IN ASSIGNING HOMEWORK

There are several issues to consider when assigning homework (J. S. Beck, 1995). First, children may not respond to the term "homework." Kendall

et al. (1992) used the inventive term "Show That I Can" assignment
(shortened to the acronym "STIC" assignments). In the Prevention Anxiety and Depression in Youth program, which features a mouse mascot
named "Pandy," we refer to homework as mousework. Additionally, we
have also referred to homework as "building your tool kit." Burns (1989)
recommends calling homework "self-help assignments." In any event,
you should pick a word or phrase for homework that will motivate children.

   Homework should be assigned and developed collaboratively. The
homework tasks become the child's own, thereby increasing the child's
level of responsibility and the possibility of compliance. The following exchange illustrates a collaborative approach to homework assignments.

DESMOND: I can't make myself stop and think things over.

THERAPIST: You just react and your feelings take charge of you?

DESMOND: That's right. My feelings cast a spell on me.

THERAPIST: Would you like to learn to become more powerful than your
   feelings?

DESMOND: Sure. How?

THERAPIST: Let's see if together we can form a plan. What if I taught you
   how to write down your thoughts and feelings when you are upset
   and you practiced these skills over the week?

DESMOND: How would that help?

THERAPIST: We'd have to keep track of how these things worked, but for
   many youngsters writing down their thoughts and feelings allows
   them time to pause and think things out.

DESMOND: How much do I need to write?

THERAPIST: That's kind of up to us and the plan we form.

DESMOND: How many times a week will I have to do this?

THERAPIST: Let's decide that together after I show you your thought diary.

   In this exchange, Desmond and his therapist worked together on the
homework assignment. The therapist introduced the idea of homework
after Desmond identified a troubling issue. The therapist worked diligently to include Desmond in the task assignment (e.g., How much
should he write? How many times should he do it?). Finally, the therapist
used the term "practice" rather than "homework" to engage the youngster.

   A second major consideration is connecting homework assignments to the child's presenting complaints. The closer the connection between the homework assignment and the presenting complaint, the more meaningful the assignment will be to the youngster. Explaining the connection between the homework and the child's problems so that he/she clearly understands the association is a key therapeutic task. Tying the homework to the presenting problem also keeps you "honest." If you remain mindful about linking assignments and problems, you are less apt to apply homework in a cookbook or rote manner.

Compliance requires knowing what is expected. For youngsters to complete a homework assignment, they must be able to understand it. Misunderstanding the task is a major reason for noncompliance. Therefore, specificity is important in assigning homework. Many times homework is assigned in a vague and cryptic manner (e.g., "Let's keep track of your thoughts."). Children may not know what this task entails and may have numerous unanswered questions. How do I keep track of my thoughts? What thoughts should I keep track of? When should I keep track of my thoughts? How often? Why should I do this in the first place? If children are unsure about a task, they may be less willing to do it. Thus, delineating the details involved in homework tasks is important.

The following transcript shows how homework may be specified with a youngster.

THERAPIST: We captured your thought that "I need to be liked by everybody or else I'm worthless." What do we need to do next?

MAE: Make everybody like me? (*Laughs.*) No. I don't know.

THERAPIST: It makes sense that if you believed your worth depends on whether everyone liked you, you would feel tons of pressure.

MAE: I do, it's awful.

THERAPIST: So do you think it would be a good idea to see if your worth totally depends on everybody liking you? Together let's see if we can create a way to test this thought. What we have to do is define your worth. OK. When you're in school and you need to define something, what do you do?

MAE: Look it up in a book or something.

THERAPIST: That's right, ask the experts. Who are the experts about your self-worth?

MAE: Me, I guess.

THERAPIST: Anybody else?

MAE: My friends, my parents. I don't want to ask them if they think I'm worthy. That's lame.

THERAPIST: How about asking them a question like "What makes a person worthy?"

MAE: OK.

THERAPIST: Who will you ask?

MAE: Mom, Dad, my aunt, my friends Tessa, Mary, Brian, and Kyle.

THERAPIST: Writing things down will really help. So after you talk with your family and friends, write down what they say. It may help you keep track and remember the definitions. . . . Then I want you to write down your own list. You define "worthiness" for yourself. Write down all the things that define worthiness. Let's start one now. What is it that makes a worthy person?

MAE: If they are kind.

THERAPIST: Write that down.

MAE: (*Writes.*) Then what will we do next week with this stuff?

THERAPIST: We'll compare all the definitions, see how much of each characteristic you have, and then try to make a conclusion about whether everybody liking you absolutely determines your worthiness.

This exchange embodies several pivotal points. First, homework was not merely prescribed, it was agreed upon! Second, the tasks involved in the behavioral experiment were explicitly delineated (e.g., "Who are the experts about your self-worth?"; "Writing things down will really help."). Finally, the specific task was directly linked to Mae's distressing belief (e.g., "I need to be liked by everybody or else I'm worthless.")

Homework tasks need to be broken down into discrete, graduated steps that lead to a goal that can be realistically accomplished (J. S. Beck, 1995; Spiegler & Guevremont, 1998). Even small tasks can initially appear overwhelming to young children. Following this strategy for homework assignments will help them feel that the task is manageable. Simple assignments are obviously to be preferred over complex ones. Beginning the homework assignment in session supplies a graduated approach to the task. First, you explain and demonstrate the assignment. The child is provided with a model and relieved of the burden of trying to figure it out for him/herself. Second, by beginning the task in session you jump-start the homework process. The child can see what it takes to do the homework and gets a headstart toward completion. After all, completing an already begun assignment is much easier than starting a fresh task all by yourself. Devoting session time to homework assignments and collaborating on the first steps of the assignment explicitly communicates the significance of homework to the child. Finally, by beginning the assignment in session, you gain a glimpse into the difficulties the child may experience in successfully completing the task.

The following transcript shows a way to work with an adolescent as he begins homework in session.

THERAPIST: Let's see if we can start you off listing questions that help you test the upsetting thoughts that cross your mind. You already have written some thoughts in your thought diary. Which one is listed first?

ANDRE: "Whatever I do is never enough so I might as well do nothing."

THERAPIST: What question can you ask yourself to test that belief?

ANDRE: I can't think of any.

THERAPIST: I bet that is what happens when you are at home or school over the week. The thought just jumps into your mind and you don't have any questions ready to cast doubt on it. That's what this experiment is all about: coming up with questions to show yourself you can question your automatic thoughts. Let's think about our work together and begin to write down some questions that have been helpful in the past. Then we'll put them in your therapy notebook. What questions did we come up with today that seemed helpful?

ANDRE: I liked the question "What's another way of looking at things?"

THERAPIST: OK, that's a start. Let's write that one down. How about another one?

ANDRE: Umm. What's the evidence?

THERAPIST: You've got two now. How many do you guess you can write for next week?

ANDRE: Probably three more.

The dialogue emphasizes several therapeutic strategies. First, the therapist teaches Andre the skills necessary to do the homework task in session. Second, Andre's initial difficulty is normalized rather than criticized (e.g., "I bet that is what happens when you are at home or school over the week."). Third, by completing two questions in session, Andre is now faced with a simplified, graduated task.

During the homework assignment in session, the therapist should fully and effortfully process the task with the youngster. Potential obstacles to completing the task should be addressed (e.g., "What might get in the way of you doing this task?"; "How might you avoid this assignment?"). Additionally, the child's expectations regarding the task's helpfulness can be explored (e.g., "How do you suppose this will be helpful?"). Finally, you may want to seize the opportunity to check on the child's perceived ability to do the homework (e.g., "What seems hard about this?"; "How much of this can you do?").

Due to the necessity of beginning the task in session, you should not leave the assignment to the last few minutes of a session. You should allocate enough session time to begin the task as well as to process it with the child. Rushing to assign homework during the last moments of a session creates time pressures that will squeeze out the possibility for effective therapeutic processing.

Allowing enough time for the assignment and processing of homework creates greater likelihood of homework compliance. When you assign homework, try not to hurriedly give the youngster the task as you are closing down the session (e.g., "By the way, do three thought records before we meet next Thursday."). Throwing in the homework in this way gives children the message that the assignment is an add-on rather than a central therapeutic piece. Additionally, the thrown-in assignment is likely to be disconnected from the youngster's pressing issues. Finally, collaboration is compromised when homework is hastily assigned at the close of a session.

Following up on homework assignments in the subsequent session is a must! When therapists forget to check in regarding the homework they assign, children learn that homework is not important. They think, "If my therapist doesn't think enough of this assignment to see what happened, then why should I do it?" Second, homework review emphasizes out-of-session work as pivotal to the process. Third, by checking homework, the therapist can discover the thoughts and feelings accompanying compliance and noncompliance. Frequently, these samples of behavior reflect children's presenting problems. For instance, a child's failure to complete a homework task may be shaped by perfectionistic beliefs (e.g., "Unless I can do it perfectly, I won't even try."). These beliefs likely pervade other areas of functioning and accordingly may become grist for the therapeutic mill.

HOMEWORK NONCOMPLIANCE

Noncompliance offers an opportunity for discovering the motivations and reasons that underlie the child's behavior. We try to find out what got in the way of completing a task. Many times, we simply ask the child: "What's up with you not doing your therapy homework?" Often, when I (RDF) teach supervisees to process noncompliance, they are reluctant to approach the task. When I ask them what their objection is, they indicate they worry that the child will feel criticized or put down. This belief seems founded on the idea that if you process homework with a young client, you naturally have to act like a punitive schoolteacher. The point in working through noncompliance is not to punish the child or to belittle him/her. Rather, processing noncompliance provides another therapeutic avenue for problem solving, thought testing, and behavioral intervention.

Children's noncompliance may be due to several factors. Difficulties with the task, poor assignment by the therapist, and/or psychological difficulties on the part of children and their families (J. S. Beck, 1995; Burns, 1989) are common culprits. Regardless of the source of the noncompliance, it should be a central focus in therapy. Figure 10.1 helps you figure out the basis for the noncompliance. Noncompliance can be decreased through active steps.

By assigning graduated tasks and beginning the work in session, therapists gain a sense regarding whether the child understands the task. Most simply, does the child have a clue about what the assignment is? Does the child know what he/she is supposed to do? What are the therapist's expectations? The task may be too complex or too abstract for the younger child. Moreover, the task may exceed the child's skill levels in various areas. If the task demands writing or reading, the youngster's noncompliance may reflect skill deficits, as well as avoidance of potential embarrassment or shame about his/her low skill level. Further, a homework assignment requiring alternative coping responses to distressing thoughts is premature for a youngster who has yet to learn to identify feelings and thoughts. Thus, the child is ill equipped to complete the task. In these circumstances, we suggest simplifying the initial task, teaching skills necessary to complete the undertaking, or redesigning the assignment to match the child's capacities.

A third issue in understanding noncompliance is determining whether the homework assignment is psychologically meaningful, relevant, and appropriate. Multicultural considerations may come into play here. For example, does the language used in the homework assignment present a cultural barrier for the child? Does the behavioral task violate any of his/her cultural norms? For instance, is the therapy moving toward achieving greater autonomy while less autonomy is valued within the youngster's culture?

Remaining mindful about whether the child's environmental context supports homework is important. In the simplest sense, do parents/caregivers encourage the youngster to complete his/her homework? Some parents will actively encourage and reinforce therapeutic homework while others will be less involved. Teaching parents to reinforce and praise their children for working on therapeutic tasks is a first step. For

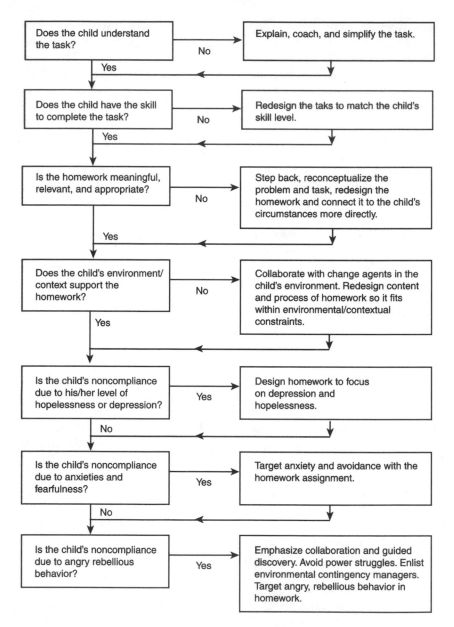

FIGURE 10.1. Decision tree for processing homework noncompliance.

instance, developing a contingency plan with parents can facilitate homework compliance (e.g., "If Kyle does three thought diaries when he feels guilty, what can you do for him in return?"). In this way, therapy homework becomes part of the family routine.

However, there may be instances when parents/caregivers do not support the child's therapeutic homework. In these instances, we recommend that you consider several questions. What prevents the family from supporting the homework? Are there cultural prescriptions? Do family members gain from the child's distress? Are the parents/caregivers attentive to the child's efforts?

Consider the following example. After three sessions, Mandy, an 11-year-old girl, was progressing well in therapy. She was learning to separate herself from her parent's marital conflicts and to contain her sense of responsibility to emotionally support her father. She attended sessions regularly and was compliant with homework. However, her therapy took an unexpected and sudden turn for the worse. She became more agitated and noncompliant with therapy tasks. Contingency plans with the parents failed. As we worked through the issue, it became clear that Mandy's distress served a vital function for her parents. Dad wanted Mandy to take care of him. As long as Mandy was in turmoil, Dad and Mom's marital relationship difficulties could be avoided.

Another example is also illustrative. Micah was a highly anxious child who feared losing control of his emotions. He worried that he might have a "panic" attack on a school bus trip or in an airplane. Treatment initially provided good and rapid results. Micah quickly invested in self-monitoring and self-instructional tasks. However, like therapy with Mandy, therapy with Micah abruptly stalled and homework compliance lessened. It seemed that Micah's father also had a rather severe anxiety disorder and he took solace from the fact that he and Micah shared the same vulnerabilities. As therapy progressed, Micah's father unwittingly discouraged his progress. We addressed this issue with the family. Then the father confessed, "I was starting to feel really alone in my own anxiety. As Micah started to conquer his fears, I felt worse about myself. I focused on myself and thought I'll never get over my own fear."

Effective homework assignments are emotionally meaningful. When children and their families perceive tasks as banal and unrelated to their circumstances, noncompliance becomes more likely. As previously mentioned, linking the assignment to the presenting problems is a potent way to make homework more emotionally relevant. For example, if a rebellious and noncompliant youngster wants his mother to stop nagging him, homework assignments should be developed that meet this goal. If the youngster recognizes how better problem solving gives him more freedom, he will be more likely to become invested in the task. If the homework assignments have little apparent connection to the problems discussed in therapy, youngsters understandably will "blow off" the assignments.

Homework assignments that are custom-made to fit the individual child's needs are more compelling than generic tasks. For instance, thought diaries can be tailored to the individual child. We recommend assigning thought diaries by saying "Each time you feel sad, complete one of these diaries or each time you get in an argument at school, fill out a thought diary." We find these instructions direct children's attention to their individual difficulties and subsequently increase the assignment's relevance.

Noncompliance may also be a function of children's level of hopelessness and depression. Failure to comply with homework is relatively common in very depressed and hopeless children. Their level of distress contributes to their belief that nothing will help. Moreover, youngsters' pessimism, passivity, and low self-efficacy makes every coping effort arduous. The noncompliance due to their depression is really their pessimism, lethargy, and perceived helplessness talking. In these instances, homework assignments that are graduated and that emphasize increased self-efficacy are good strategies. For example, simplifying pleasant event scheduling by having children place stickers on the chart instead of writing on it makes the task easier for depressed youngsters.

Avoidance is a hallmark feature of anxious youngsters. Like depressed youngsters, the severity of their distress will shape anxious children's compliance. If the task assigned elicits a significant amount of anxiety, children may avoid the task simply because they feel anxious. As is often the case with depressed children, the noncompliance is a function of the child's presenting problem. Accordingly, helping the child identify and modify the thoughts and feelings surrounding the task becomes a central therapeutic issue. For example, an anxious child refused to share her feelings with her parents due to her fears of negative evaluation. Coping with these fears subsequently formed the basis of the homework assignment.

Determining whether the child's noncompliance is a function of rebelliousness and psychological reactance is another consideration. Psychological *reactance* is a construct used to explain people's tendency to try to restore their freedom when they think they are being controlled (Brehm, 1966). Accordingly, it may be useful to ascertain whether the child sees the task as controlling. If the youngster is exquisitely sensitive to perceived control, collaboration on homework becomes even more pivotal. The following transcript illustrates processing homework with a noncompliant teenager who seems reactant to perceived control.

THERAPIST: How would it be for you to capture what goes through your mind when you are angry?

STACY: I already know why I get angry.

THERAPIST: You really don't see how this can help?

STACY: It won't. It's stupid. Why should I do your worksheet?

THERAPIST: I think you enjoy shooting these ideas down

STACY: (*Shrugs.*)

THERAPIST: What's fun about that?

STACY: Seeing you get frustrated. Then I'm in charge.

THERAPIST: So what happens when you are not in charge?

STACY: You're smart, you figure it out.

THERAPIST: OK. I think you may shoot down ideas and get pissed off to take charge when things don't go your way. How does that sound?

STACY: So?

THERAPIST: How does it work out for you?

STACY: Pretty good. I'm not doing your assignment.

THERAPIST: That's true. But wouldn't you rather be doing something else than talking to me?

STACY: Almost anything else.

THERAPIST: So if we figured out a way for you to have to come to the clinic less and for you to be in charge of your thoughts and feelings more, would that be helpful?

STACY: I guess.

THERAPIST: I agree. What about if you took charge of how you captured the things that cross your mind? It seems that young people who take charge in that way seem to progress through therapy. I'm not sure that it will work for you, but I'm convinced it's worth a try.

First, note how in this dialogue the therapist asked direct, specific questions. Second, the therapist conceptualized perceived control as a central issue and worked earnestly to avoid appearing controlling. Finally, the therapist introduced the assignment as a way for Stacy to maintain control.

Collaborative problem solving can maximize homework compliance. You and the child may be able to brainstorm ways to improve homework compliance. Keeping a notebook with assignments in it, setting aside a particular time of day for therapeutic tasks, or writing a reminder note in a visible place may facilitate children's greater compliance. The following dialogue shows the collaborative problem-solving process between the therapist and child.

THERAPIST: What blocked you from doing your thought diary this week?

ISABEL: I got really busy and forgot to do it.

THERAPIST: What school homework did you have this week?

ISABEL: I had a big spelling test.

THERAPIST: Did you do the spelling homework?

ISABEL: Yes.

THERAPIST: What helped you remember to get your spelling homework done?

ISABEL: I always do my homework before dinner so I can watch TV after dinner.

THERAPIST: What a good idea—you set aside a time to do your spelling.

ISABEL: Thanks. It helps.

THERAPIST: Can you think of anything that might help you remember to do your thought diary like the way you remember to do your spelling?

ISABEL: Maybe I can do it after I do my spelling and science homework.

THERAPIST: What might help you remember to do it when you are doing your science and spelling homework?

ISABEL: Maybe when I get home from your office I could put my diary on my desk next to my school supplies.

THERAPIST: That sounds like another good idea. You could keep all your worksheets together so you can do them at the same time. I wonder how you might make sure that you bring your diary here for our next meeting?

ISABEL: I'll just remember.

THERAPIST: That's a good goal. How can we help you remember?

ISABEL: I could write a note to myself and put it on our refrigerator.

THERAPIST: What might the note say?

ISABEL: Bring diary for time with Dr. Jessica.

The exchange shows important processes and practices. First, the therapist used Isabel's success with spelling homework as a basis for success with therapy homework. Second, Isabel developed a plan for compliance rather than mere reliance on words. Finally, the therapist mindfully avoided belittling Isabel for her lack of noncompliance.

CONCLUSION

Homework shows children that they can apply their coping skills. Consistent follow-through on specific, relevant homework tasks facilitates skill application. Noncompliance is decreased by assigning psychologically meaningful tools that are connected to the child's presenting problems. Finally, the successful use of homework requires maintaining a clear therapeutic focus. If you are unclear about an assignment, expect the child to be confused. If you see homework as a peripheral, tedious task, he/she will see it that way too. So, as therapists, use this chapter to do your homework on homework!

11

❖

Working with Depressed
Children and Adolescents

Childhood depression has been a neglected area of research that has gone largely unrecognized and untreated until recently (Beardslee et al., 1993). Recognizing the signs and symptoms of depression in children and adolescents is essential in developing an effective treatment regimen. However, since depression can take many forms, it is a challenge to recognize them. This chapter will focus on unipolar depression, including the diagnostic categories of major depressive disorder, dysthymia, and adjustment disorder with depressed mood.

Cognitive therapy has shown promise in treating depressed children and adolescents (Gillham et al., 1995; Kaslow & Thompson, 1998; Ollendick & King, 1998; Reinecke, Ryan, & DuBois, 1998). By applying empirically supported cognitive techniques in developmentally appropriate ways, we have helped children and adolescents to address their depressive symptoms. By challenging depressed children and adolescents' negative views of themselves, others, the environment, and the future, cognitive therapy promotes a more accurate and balanced outlook.

SYMPTOMS OF DEPRESSION

Symptoms in Children

Children experiencing depression can exhibit symptoms in all four domains of the cognitive model, as well as in their interpersonal relationships. Affective symptoms often include a depressed or sad mood. However, some depressed children experience irritability rather than a sad or depressed mood, thus making identification of their depression more challenging. They may be described by parents and teachers as angry, irritable, easily annoyed, and "moody." Further, depressed youth frequently feel hopeless and believe that they will never feel better or their lives will never improve. Feeling hopeless is often related to suicidal thoughts or wishes to die.

Negative cognitive styles and negative attributions are also common in depressed youth (Kendall & MacDonald, 1993). For instance, 10-year-old Christy played on a soccer team. When her soccer team lost a game, Christy attributed the defeat to her own behaviors, such as missing a goal or kicking the ball out of bounds. However, when the team won a game, she still maintained a negative cognitive set (e.g., "We only won because Megan got the ball back when I messed up and kicked it to the other team."). Such cognitive styles include internal, stable, and global attributions for failures, and external, unstable, specific attributions for successes (Abramson, Seligman, & Teasdale, 1978). These children have a generally pessimistic outlook, believing that "anything that can go wrong will go wrong." Like Oscar the Grouch on *Sesame Street*, they always expect the worst.

Consistent with this negative cognitive style, depressed children frequently generalize negative events and make predictions of negative outcomes regardless of contrasting evidence. In addition, their negative interpretations of others' behaviors, the environment, or their own experiences serve to reinforce their existing beliefs regarding low self-worth. Positive events are quickly discounted or forgotten, while negative experiences are long remembered as evidence of their own inadequacies. Mary, a depressed 11-year-old girl who believed that "no one likes me," might think to herself, "Sarah did not say 'Good morning.' She hates me just like everyone else," while ignoring the fact that Jeremy and Elizabeth both greeted her when she walked into class. Relatedly, low self-esteem often accompanies depression. Thoughts related to an inability to fit in or beliefs about inadequacy are frequently present. Depressed children often find it nearly impossible to name anything positive about themselves. For instance, 12-year-old Edna could not name a single reason why a classmate would want to be her friend. Another depressed youngster, Herb, easily named several things he would like to change about himself, but could not identify anything he liked about himself.

Some depressed children seem lost in space, distracted by their own internal dialogues. Attention and concentration are additional cognitive areas that may be impacted by depression in youth. In therapy for example, depressed children often have trouble focusing on session content or completing therapy assignments. Further, seemingly simple decision making is very difficult for many children with depression. Observing the child completing self-report questionnaires sometimes reveals difficulties with decision making. For instance, 11-year-old Sabrina spent excessive time deliberating over the proper responses. We often allow children to choose a small prize at the end of sessions. When choosing, depressed children may debate the merits of particular toy choices for an extended period of time. They appear compelled to make just the right choice.

Depressed youth also experience *anhedonia*, a decreased interest or pleasure in activities. This symptom shows itself behaviorally and affectively. Games, television shows, and hobbies the child used to enjoy no longer appeal to them. The youngster reports being bored all the time or confesses that "nothing is fun anymore." Apathy, disinterest in spending time with peers, and withdrawal from others are also common with anhedonia. Invitations to visit with friends are often declined. Further, depressed youth often do not receive such invitations due to their socially withdrawn behaviors. Thus, the child's social contact is significantly decreased, leading to increased feelings of loneliness. When asked about his interests or hobbies, 12-year-old Eric commented, "I used to like miniature golfing, but now I just don't feel like going." Similarly, such children demonstrate a "lack of mirth" response (Stark, 1990). Thus, the depressed child may not respond to activities, TV shows, or humorous stories with the expected enthusiasm of a typical child.

Children referred to treatment for behavior problems, such as arguing, fighting with siblings, or talking back to adults, are often experiencing a mood disturbance. Additionally, social withdrawal is another behavioral sign of depression. Identifying the frequency of social interactions will be more meaningful than tallying the number of friends reported by the child or his/her parents. This point is illustrated in the case of Brea, an 11-year-old child brought to therapy by her mother due to recent irritability, fatigue, crying, and a drop in grades. Her mother described her as a social child with many friends. However, when asked how often she had seen her friends in the past 2 weeks, Brea revealed many fewer social interactions, thereby demonstrating a change from her previous level of functioning. Declining invitations or opportunities to spend time with peers are signs of social withdrawal. In situations with peers, such as recess or social gatherings, depressed children may not interact with the other children, but instead watch them from afar. This symptom is illustrated in 9-year-old Nicole who walked the outer fence of the playground by herself while watching her peers play ball. Predictions that an activity will be boring are also common among depressed children; such predictions thus appear linked to withdrawal. At the same time, the child's decreased involvement in pleasurable activities can serve to perpetuate feelings of isolation and depression.

Younger children may not know how to put words to what they are feeling, or may be uncomfortable doing so. Consequently, it is not uncommon for a depressed youngster under the age of 9 years to express distress through behavioral problems and acting out (Schwartz, Gladstone, & Kaslow, 1998). Such youngsters have difficulty getting along with others, including peers and siblings. Disruptive and aggressive behavior was the focus of a referral for depressed, 7-year-old Ron, who was talking back and fighting at school. Older children may be more able to identify their distressing feelings and beliefs, and thus may exhibit more typical depressive symptoms, including sad moods and self-critical cognitions (Schwartz et al., 1998). Some depressed youngsters exhibit psychomotor agitation or restlessness. These children have difficulty sitting still and are fidgety. The opposite can also occur. These youngsters do not move as much as or run around like most children. Rather, they appear tired and engage in fewer and slower movements.

The more subtle signs of depression are often hard to detect. These are frequently physical in nature. Children who are unable or unwilling to verbalize their emotional states frequently communicate their distress through recurrent somatic complaints. Younger children may lack the ability to verbalize distress and therefore make more somatic complaints than adolescents (Birmaher et al., 1996). They report frequent and unfounded headaches, stomachaches, or other physical complaints (Stark, Rouse, & Livingston, 1991). Many of these children repeatedly visit the school nurse and miss school due to physical complaints.

Problems with eating or sleeping also occur with depressed children. These children may have a diminished appetite, may gain or lose weight, or fail to gain weight at the expected rate. Youngsters suffering from depression may also have difficulty falling asleep and may wake up in the middle of the night or early in the morning and be unable to fall back to sleep. In contrast, other depressed youth sleep excessively. Edward, a 9-year-old fourth grader, frequently fell asleep in class and complained of constant fatigue, stating he did not "feel like" doing anything.

Peer problems and peer rejection comprise frequent interpersonal stressors among depressed children. Social difficulties may be the result of several factors (Kovacs & Goldston, 1991). Depressed children are often more socially withdrawn, and may appear shy. Consequently, they do not initiate or take part in many social interactions, resulting in fewer peer relationships. Some depressed youngsters lack social skills or opportunities for social interactions. They often feel more isolated, thus leading to deeper depressive feelings. Particularly for older children, if the youngster is experiencing tearfulness and crying, he/she may be teased and further isolated from peers. An irritable mood can impact peer relationships: other children may become annoyed with and avoid the irritable or pessimistic child (Kovacs & Goldston, 1991). The irritable older depressed child often has interactions with peers that involve more aggression and negativity than displayed by younger children (Speier, Sherak, Hirsch, & Cantwell, 1995).

Schoolage children suffering from depression often develop academically related symptoms, including a decrease in performance, low motivation, fear of failure, and acting-out behaviors in the classroom (Speier et al., 1995). These children are often self-critical, experience feelings of guilt, and may demonstrate delayed language development. Depressed children may present in your office with many different complaints.

Symptoms in Adolescents

Many similar symptoms also characterize depression in adolescents. Somatic complaints, social withdrawal, hopelessness, and irritability occur in depressed adolescents as well as in depressed children (Schwartz et al., 1998). However, some differences in symptom presentation have been noted. Adolescents are more able to verbalize their symptoms than young children, which helps clinicians to more readily identify the former's symptoms. Other differences in symptom presentation include adolescents' increased risk for suicide attempts, substance use, and school dropout compared to children.

Depressed adolescents tend to have comorbid psychopathology, including anxiety disorders and substance abuse (Gotlib & Hammen, 1992; Goodyer, Herbert, Secher, & Pearson, 1997; Kovacs, Feinberg, Crouse-Novak, Paulauskas, & Finkelstein, 1984; Kovacs, Gatsonis, Paulauskas, & Richards, 1989). Low self-esteem, poor body image, high self-consciousness, and inadequate coping are common in depressed adolescents. Further, these teens report inadequate social support and increased conflict with parents (Lewinsohn, Clarke, Rohde, Hops, & Seeley, 1996). Adolescents often struggle with issues of autonomy as well. Consequently, they may be less likely to seek help from parents when feeling depressed, thus leading to further isolation.

Like younger children, depressed adolescents demonstrate academic difficulties. However, those difficulties may become more severe, including truancy or dropping out (Speier et al., 1995). Depressed adolescents are increasingly argumentative, may have a delayed onset of puberty, slowed onset of abstract thinking, and mood swings. Risk taking and antisocial behavior may increase, including substance use, vandalism, unsafe sexual activity, and accidents or traffic violations. These adolescents demonstrate low self-esteem, experience weight fluctuations, and may develop eating disorders (Speier et al., 1995).

CULTURAL AND GENDER CONSIDERATIONS

With any client, assessing the individual within a cultural context is critical and likely requires consultation or additional clinical interviews with family members. A brief description of the limited research on cultural issues with depressed African American, Native American, Asian American, Hispanic American, and female clients follows.

Some community-based studies point to different symptom presentation with African American versus Caucasian youth. Specifically, a study of children ages 9–13 years suggests a more maladaptive attributional style in Caucasian children compared to African American children (Thompson, Kaslow, Weiss, & Nolen-Hoeksema, 1998). Compared to the African American youth, the Caucasian youth blamed themselves more for negative outcomes and saw events in a more pessimistic light, as unchangeable, and as causing painful effects throughout their lives.

A study by DeRoos and Allen-Measures (1998) suggested that depressed African American youth tend to experience low self-worth and isolation, whereas Caucasian children who are depressed are more likely to exhibit negative mood states and guilt. Another recent study found higher scores on self-reported measures of depression and anxiety, and higher teacher ratings of depression, in African American compared to Caucasian fifth graders (Cole, Martin, Peeke, Henderson, & Harwell, 1998). Results of this study are indicative of a relationship between age and the presence of ethnic differences, given that similar significant differences were not found in older children. Regarding clinically referred youth, most studies do not reveal significant differences between Caucasian and African American youth (Nettles & Pleck, 1994).

Gibbs (1998) noted an alarming increase in the rate of suicide in African American youngsters. Citing 1996 statistics from the U.S. Department of Health and Human Services, Gibbs noted that the suicide rate for African American male youngsters quadrupled between 1980 and 1992; the rate for African American females doubled during the same time period. Importantly, Gibbs mentioned that identification of suicidal tendencies in African American youth is more difficult because they may express suicidality differently than their Caucasian counterparts. Suicidality in African Americans seems marked by high levels of anger, acting out, and engaging in high-risk behaviors.

Although current research is insufficient and nonconclusive, high rates of suicide in Native American teenagers and drug and alcohol abuse (Ho, 1992; LaFramboise & Low, 1998) seem to support affective disturbance in these youth. Indeed, the U.S. Surgeon General (1999) indicates that between 1979 and 1992, the suicide rate among Native American adolescent males was the highest in the nation. Allen (1998) suggests that the limited literature devoted to depression in Native American youth may be a result of the nonapplicability of Western culture's diagnostic classifications to Native American children.

Ho (1992) argues that children of Asian immigrants demonstrate a high number of somatic complaints due to their internalization of psychological distress. Somatic complaints may represent a more acceptable expression of internal distress within Asian culture (Ho, 1992). Nagata (1998) noted that the sparcity of literature on depression in Asian American youth should not be seen as a sign of the absence of psychological distress among this group, but instead probably reflects a cultural hesitancy to seek mental health services within this population.

In a recent review, Roberts (2000) concluded that Mexican American youth seem to be at risk for depression. Additionally, citing statistics from the Center for Disease Control, the U. S. Surgeon General (1999) reports that there is a high risk for suicide in Hispanic youth. Further, Roberts (1992) examined the manifestations of depressive symptoms in diverse cultural groups using adolescents' responses to items on the Center for Epidemiologic Studies Depression Scale. The study examined white non-Hispanics, African Americans, persons of Mexican origin, and other Hispanics. Roberts's results indicated greater similarities than differences in the responses of these groups of adolescents. However, some differences in patterns of item endorsement reveal that the two Hispanic groups had a tendency for somatic and negative mood symptoms to cluster together. However, Roberts warned against interpreting these findings as evidence that Hispanic Americans express distress through somatic complaints or that they do not differentiate between physical and psychological distress. We urge caution in interpreting this line of research. We agree with Roberts (2000) who wrote, "It is difficult to draw any firm conclusions concerning ethnic status and risks of depression from these studies because they employ different measures of depression and they also focus on different ethnic minority clients" (p. 362).

Gender differences in depression vary depending on age, development, and cultural differences and expectations. Nolen-Hoeksema and Girgus (1995) report similar prevalence rates for depression in prepubertal boys and girls. However, girls demonstrate higher rates of depression than boys between the ages of 12 and 15 years, with these differences continuing into adulthood. Differences in cognitive styles may also exist between genders at different age levels (Nolen-Hoeksema & Girgus, 1995). Prepubescent girls demonstrate more optimistic explanatory styles than boys. In early adolescence, youngsters in general become more pessimistic. However, by late adolescence boys demonstrate more optimistic thinking than girls. Thus, girls have a tendency to become more depressed and pessimistic over time compared to boys. Several factors have been discussed in the literature as contributing to these differences (Nolen-Hoeksema & Girgus, 1995). Cultural expectations, social norms, and gender biases may all contribute to these differences. Hormonal changes, physical development, and body dissatisfaction also may be related to differences in rates of depression between boys and girls.

ASSESSMENT OF DEPRESSION

A comprehensive assessment of youngsters should gather information from multiple sources. Input from the child, parents, teachers, and other caregivers should be collected and considered. Numerous assessment instruments and structured interviews can be used. In addition, we recommend consultation with physicians to rule out physical causes for symptoms or to provide medical treatment and medication if necessary.

A variety of assessment instruments including self-report measures, interviews, observer ratings, peer nominations, and projective techniques have been used to assess the presence and severity of depression (Kaslow & Racusin, 1990). Specifically, the Children's Depression Inventory (CDI) is a popular tool, and includes both a long and a short version. In fact, the CDI is the most frequently used self-report depression inventory used with children (Fristad, Emery, & Beck, 1997). The CDI can be completed by children or adolescents prior to sessions and may be used periodically over the course of treatment to monitor changes in reported symptoms.

The Revised Children's Depression Rating Scale (CDRS-R) is another self-report rating measure that assesses depressive symptoms and global depression (Poznanski et al., 1984). The CDRS-R includes parent, teacher, and sibling forms, thus allowing the examiner to incorporate the observations of others into the assessment process. The CDRS-R has been normed on samples 9 to 16 years old, and therefore is useful with both child and adolescent populations.

Other self-report measures include the Depression Self-Rating Scale (DSRS; Birleson, 1981), the Depression Adjective Checklist (C-DACL; Sokoloff & Lubin, 1983), and the Children's Depression Scale Revised (CDS-R; Reynolds, Anderson, & Bartell, 1985). Numerous structured interviews have also been developed and used to assess depression in children. A thorough clinical interview provides important data on symptoms, as well as their frequency, intensity, duration, antecedents, and context.

We use self-report inventories and interviews to tap depressive symptoms. Some youth find it easier to communicate their level of distress through a written measure. We have found that many children who are unable to verbalize their affective distress to parents or therapists may request that the parent see their CDI. For example, Taylor is a 10-year-old boy who believed his mother "did not have any time for him." After completing the CDI and endorsing a clinically significant level of symptoms, Taylor requested us to show the inventory to his mother. Taylor was unable to verbalize his affective distress to his mother, but hoped that showing her his responses would communicate his distress.

Seamless Integration of Assessment and Therapy

We try to seamlessly combine assessment and treatment. Unfortunately, it is easy to slip into a mechanical style in which one simply administers the measures and neglects to refer back to them. However, when you discuss the process of completing self-report inventories with youngsters, you will often find that they will reveal important beliefs about emotional expression. For example, they sometimes reveal inaccurate beliefs about expressing thoughts and feelings that may be contributing to their over- or underreporting of symptoms. Further, discrepancies between the child's verbal self-report, the parent report, and therapists' behavioral observations are more readily addressed when you incorporate the results of self-report inventories into the session.

Consider 9-year-old Amanda, who appeared to be experiencing a number of symptoms of depression and anxiety (and who was reported by her mother to be sad and withdrawn), but denied such symptoms on the CDI. When asked what it was like to complete the inventory, Amanda confessed that she was afraid she had gotten some of the answers "wrong." Not content with this level of analysis, the therapist dug deeper and discovered the thought "It is wrong to say you are sad or upset." Amanda had formed this belief based on the reactions of others when she had previously expressed negative affect and pessimistic thoughts. Her father often responded to her expressions with comments such as "Don't say that, Amanda, things aren't as bad as you think," or "Don't be sad." Thus, Amanda's father had inadvertently taught her that her feelings and thoughts were "wrong" and had thus reinforced her not expressing negative thoughts and feelings.

Examining each subscale of the self-report measures is important to help tease out the specific depressive symptoms the child is experiencing, such as somatic complaints or social withdrawal. For example, upon first glance 8-year-old Billy's CDI score did not change from intake to Session 4. However, closer inspection of the two CDIs revealed that his somatic complaints had significantly decreased since intake and that he was expressing more negative feelings. This data fit with the conceptualization that Billy was developing more adaptive ways to express negative affect. In doing so, he was now able to identify the specifics of his distress, leading to greater symptoms identification on the CDI. At the same time, he was exhibiting fewer somatic symptoms. He now had the skills to put his feelings into words, and therefore did not express his distress solely through physical complaints.

Some depressed youngsters are appropriate candidates for an evaluation for antidepressant medication. For those with severe depression, or if depressive symptoms do not show improvement with psychotherapy alone, a referral for a medication evaluation should be considered. Clinicians should refer parents to a child psychiatrist or their family doctor. Obtaining a release of information will help you and medical providers clearly communicate concerns, clinical symptoms, and treatment options to facilitate the most effective intervention plan. Talking to the family about the use of antidepressant medication prior to the referral can help decrease anxiety, combat misconceptions, and increase the likelihood of follow-through.

TREATMENT OF DEPRESSION: CHOOSING AN INTERVENTION STRATEGY

All the intervention strategies presented in this chapter are suitable for use with depressed youth. Selecting an intervention to start with is driven by factors such as the youth's age, level of cognitive development, severity of depression, and prerequisite skills. First, safety must be established by assessing and, if necessary, treating suicidality in the client. This process should include assessing his/her risk for self-harm, developing safety plans, reducing his/her hopelessness, and testing his/her inaccurate thoughts related to the suicidal ideation. Second, determine the cognitive level of the child to determine how useful cognitive interventions may be. Consider the youth's language development and cognitive maturity to determine if cognitive techniques will be profitable. Third, beginning with basic techniques is usually best, given the low motivation, activity level, problem-solving ability, and hopelessness that frequently accompanies depressive states. Behavioral activation techniques will increase social interaction and reduce withdrawal behaviors. Thus, pleasant event schedules and social skills training are good initial interventions for battling depressive symptoms. Further, by presenting early interventions in small, graduated tasks, early successes can increase self-efficacy and motivation. Figure 11.1 provides a decision tree to guide you through selecting specific intervention strategies.

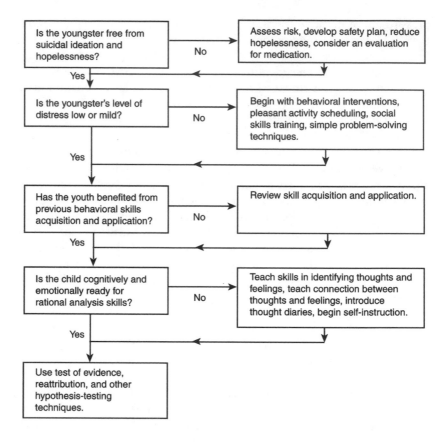

FIGURE 11.1. Choosing an intervention strategy.

SUICIDALITY WITH DEPRESSED CHILDREN
AND ADOLESCENTS

The reality that depressed children and adolescents think about and often attempt to harm themselves demands that we actively address this issue. The U.S. Surgeon General (1999) warns that suicide peaks at mid-adolescence and is the third leading cause of death for youngsters in this age group. Suicide in younger children is more rare, but its presence should be taken quite seriously. For instance, in their report of 43 cases, Kovacs, Goldston, and Gatsonis (1993) found a suicidal attempt in a child 8.3 years old. A surprisingly high number of our clients report experiencing past or present suicidal thoughts either verbally or via the CDI.

When working with depressed youth with past or present suicidal ideation, I (JMM) initially worried about "pushing them too hard" and whether they "could handle it." My tendency was to back off quickly and accept "I don't know" during Socratic questioning or less effort in homework completion. I was afraid to exacerbate their suicidal ideation. Understanding suicidal ideation as a maladaptive problem-solving strategy helped me overcome this hesitancy. Doing so made it easier for me to work with children to identify alternative strategies without fear of upsetting the child. When addressing suicidal ideation, you are essentially teaching appropriate coping skills while still empathizing with the youth's distress. By casting doubt on the use of self-harm and not shaming or arguing with the youth, you will more effectively treat suicidality. By working with youth in this way, I saw how challenging them on their beliefs actually lowered, rather than increased, the suicidality.

The U.S. Surgeon General (1999) identifies several risk factors for suicidal behavior. More specifically, for girls, the presence of depression and a history of previous suicide attempts represent risk factors. For boys, a history of previous suicide attempts, disruptive behaviors, and substance abuse are major risk factors. Additionally, Speier et al. (1995) counted hopelessness, perceived family stress, presence of firearms, poor school adjustment, peer rejection, social isolation, discovery of pregnancy, and legal problems as risk factors. Finally, citing a variety of studies, the U.S. Surgeon General (1999) warned that exposure to reports of real or fictional suicide can increase suicide risk in vulnerable young children.

Assessing Suicidality

Suicidal ideation should always be assessed at intake. You need to be comfortable about asking children about suicidal thoughts and behaviors. Your own anxiety or discomfort with the topic will be apparent to youngsters and lead to hesitancy to admit such thoughts by the youth. When assessing for suicidal ideation, we recommend directly asking youth about their thoughts and behaviors:

"When have you thought about hurting yourself?"
"When have you wished you were dead?"
"When have you intentionally cut/hit/punched/choked yourself?"

Suicidal intent is a key factor in the risk assessment. Specifically, a child who truly intends to kill him/herself is at greater risk, regardless of whether the means endorsed are truly lethal (Speier et al., 1995). For example, consider a child who consumes four or five vitamin C tablets. Although the means used by this youth is not lethal, the goal of the action

tells the true tale. If the youngster thought the vitamins would kill him/
her, then the action is much more serious than if the youngster thought
the chewable vitamins were candy. Consequently, we strongly recommend that you heavily weigh intent as a variable along with the lethality
of method, accessibility of method, and history of previous attempts.

Children express suicidality with different language and metaphors.
Thus you must assess for suicidality with those differences in mind. Some
youth will openly state "I want to die." With other children, you must inquire about possible suicidal ideation "hidden" in statements such as, "I
wish I could go to sleep and never wake up"; "I wish I was never born";
"I feel like crawling in a hole forever"; "I wish I would get hit by a car";
or "I would be better off dead." Occasionally a child may make the statement "I'm going to kill myself" as a way of expressing negative affect,
with no true intent. To assess the meaning behind any of the above statements, you must query the child, using questions such as "What do you
mean by that?"; "What would it be like if that were true?"; "How often
do you have those thoughts?"; "When have you ever done anything to try
and make those things happen?"

You will need to thoroughly assess plans for suicidal behavior and
past attempts. As with adults, a youth's history of suicidal attempts or
gestures increases the youth's risk of future suicidal behavior. Kovacs et
al. (1993) reported that more than 50% of youth who attempted suicide
once made another attempt. Further, between 16 and 30% of clinically
referred youth who thought about killing themselves actually attempted
suicide. The adolescent years have been found to be a period of particularly high risk for attempted suicide, with the risk declining after age 17
(Kovacs et al., 1993). Boys are at greater risk for suicide completion than
females (Speier et al., 1995).

Self-report inventories are often part of the initial interview with
children. They are a useful initial step in assessing suicidality. The CDI
specifically assesses for suicidal ideation on item 9. Hopelessness, which
frequently correlates with suicidal ideation, is assessed on item 2. Although scoring the entire measure prior to seeing the child is recommended, you should at least check items 2 and 9. Regardless of the child's
response on the CDI, we strongly suggest that you assess suicidal ideation
verbally. Doing so allows you to observe the child's response to such an
inquiry and may reveal a hesitancy to admit such thoughts. This is illustrated in the case of 10-year-old Daniel, who denied most symptoms, including items 2 and 9 on the CDI.

THERAPIST: Have you ever thought about hurting or killing yourself?

DANIEL: No.

THERAPIST: Have you ever wished you were dead?

DANIEL: No.

THERAPIST: If you did have some thoughts about hurting yourself, would you tell me?

DANIEL: Probably not.

THERAPIST: What would be hard about telling me?

DANIEL: Those thoughts are bad and people who do that are bad.

THERAPIST: Those thoughts are bad?

DANIEL: You should never hurt yourself on purpose.

THERAPIST: Is it possible to have those thoughts without actually hurting yourself?

DANIEL: Yeah.

THERAPIST: Actually, talking about thoughts can help kids solve problems and make them not want to hurt themselves anymore.

DANIEL: Really?

THERAPIST: You know, sometimes talking about those thoughts can be scary, but it can also help us find ways for kids to stop from hurting themselves. Have you ever had thoughts of hurting yourself?

DANIEL: Well, sometimes when I get really mad, I feel like hurting myself.

THERAPIST: Would it be OK to talk about those thoughts now?

DANIEL: I guess so.

The therapist worked with Daniel on increasing his comfort about disclosing his thoughts. In this example, we see how the therapist utilized Socratic questioning to identify Daniel's beliefs that prevented him from talking about his suicidal thoughts. The therapist then guided Daniel through a reasoning process to help him conclude that talking is helpful. Moreover, the therapist normalized Daniel's experience. The therapist should continue down this path and assess for any plan and intent (e.g., "What have you thought about doing to hurt yourself?"; "What have you done in the past to hurt yourself?"; "If you did have these thoughts, what would you try to do to hurt yourself?"; "When you have these thoughts, how likely are you to hurt yourself?").

Assessing suicidal ideation with youngsters who openly admit to suicidal thoughts can be equally challenging. Ensuring the child's safety is the primary goal. Doing so requires the involvement of parents or other caregivers. Parents should be provided with resources (e.g., crisis numbers) and armed with problem-solving strategies to help identify suicidal ideation in their children and then help their child work through these thoughts and generate alternative problem-solving solutions. The following transcript illustrates assessing for suicidal ideation in an adolescent who more openly admits to suicidal thoughts.

THERAPIST: I noticed you marked "I want to kill myself" on the questionnaire you filled out. Can you tell me more about that thought?

GINA: Sometimes when I've had a really bad day and I feel all alone, I think that no one would even miss me if I were dead.

THERAPIST: How do you feel when you have those thoughts?

GINA: Just really sad and like I want to go to sleep and never wake up.

THERAPIST: So you *feel* really sad and you *think* "No one would miss me if I were dead." What do you do when that happens?

GINA: Nothing really. Just lay on my bed and cry.

THERAPIST: What else do you do?

GINA: Well, sometimes I think about taking a bunch of my mom's sleeping pills from the medicine cabinet.

THERAPIST: Have you ever taken any pills?

GINA: No, but I think about doing it when things are going really bad.

THERAPIST: How often do you have that thought?

GINA: Well, the last time was about a week ago. I guess about once a week or so.

In this example, the therapist worked to identify the situation, as well as the thoughts, feelings, and behaviors that accompanied Gina's suicidal ideation. Through questioning, the therapist continued to identify specific suicidal plans, means, and any past attempts. The therapist will want to gain more details, such as specific antecedents to the suicidal thoughts, any history of other self-harm behaviors, and what has stopped Gina from making an attempt so far. Finally, the therapist should introduce a safety plan and discuss alternative, more adaptive problem-solving strategies with Gina.

Collaboration remains a key concept even when working with suicidal youngsters. However, since collaboration occurs on a continuum, typically much less collaboration is warranted when youngsters intend to harm themselves. At the same time, some degree of collaboration can be maintained during the problem-solving process. For example, 11-year-old Erin had been having thoughts about hurting herself. She revealed to her therapist that she had thought of choking herself on several occasions, and had attempted to do so on one occasion. Together the therapist and Erin decided that it would be a good plan to tell her mom so that together they could work to keep her safe. The therapist asked, "How should we let your mom in on what we have talked about and our plan to keep you safe?" This statement clearly indicated that the therapist intended to inform the parent, yet allowed Erin to choose how her mother was informed.

We also find checking the youngster's level of self-control to be helpful. For example, suppose 13-year-old Stan verbally reported suicidal ideation and endorsed items 2 and 9 on the CDI. You might ask Stan, "On a scale of 1 to 10, with 10 meaning you definitely will try to kill yourself and 1 being there is no chance you would try to kill yourself, where are you?" We think it is important to follow up on this answer (e.g., "What makes you a 6?"; "Do you feel safe and in control at a 6?"; "At what point would you feel not safe and out of control?"). Finally, assessing for factors that influence the scale is another good tactic (e.g., "What could happen that would make you go to a 9?"; "What would you do then?"; "What needs to happen for you to go to a 2?").

A thorough assessment of the youngster's suicidal ideation will include asking about the frequency, intensity, and duration of ideation (e.g., "How often do you think about hurting yourself?"; "How long do those thoughts last?"). All these factors should be considered in determining risk level and all will help you design interventions. Further, assessing what has stopped the child from attempting suicide in the past will help you predict future attempts. The accessibility of the method or means of suicide is also crucial. For instance, if the youth states that she has thought about taking a bottle of sleeping pills, it will be important to find out how she would get the pills (e.g., Are such pills easily available to her in her home?). Finally, frequent check-ins with depressed youth are important.

Treatment of Suicidality

Cognitive therapy treatment of suicidal youth flows from the assessment. Advising parents to remove pills, guns, knives, razors, or other potential means of self-harm from the home is often the first step. Enlisting parental involvement and cooperation is a crucial component to maintaining safety for the child. Therapists should discuss in detail with parents what will be removed and how to ensure the optimal safety level for their child. We often instruct parents to secure items in a locked box, rather than just "hiding" them, to further ensure safety. Removing both prescription and nonprescription medications from the child's access is also important, as both can be dangerous in overdose.

Developing a contract or agreement for safety with the child is a good strategy. The agreement should be specific and include alternative problem-solving strategies to increase its usefulness. Also, you must process the safety plan with the youth to ensure that the youngster is committed to keeping safe. Having the child write out the agreement can aid him/her in remembering it by making it more concrete. Further, you should supply the youth with a copy of the plan so he/she can carry it around with him/her and use it as a coping card (see Figure 11.2). Things like crisis numbers, people to talk to, and the child's reasons for not harming him/herself should be included in the plan.

The child's response to signing a contract is important. For example, 13-year-old Tony responded "What happens if I break the contract?" This response was further explored to distinguish innocent curiosity from intent to self-harm. You can ask the child questions such as "What would get in the way of you keeping the contract?" or "What might happen if you do break the contract?" Tony responded that if he broke the contract, then next time people wouldn't believe him and he might have to go to the hospital.

Because suicidality is often a maladaptive problem-solving, coping, or escape strategy, generating alternatives to self-harm is an important early intervention. You should work with the child and/or parent to develop a list of alternative problem-solving strategies. An example with 12-year-old Ryan follows.

THERAPIST: What else can you do when you feel bad and think about killing yourself besides hurting yourself?

RYAN: Tell somebody.

THERAPIST: OK. Who could you tell?

If I feel like hurting myself, I will do one or more of these:

1. Talk to my mom about my feelings.
2. Write in my feeling journal.
3. Remind myself that hurting myself is a permanent solution to a temporary problem.
4. Ask myself "What else can I try?"
5. Call the crisis hotline and talk out my feelings (555-5555).

FIGURE 11.2. Coping card.

RYAN: I don't know. I guess I could tell you.

THERAPIST: That's right. You could tell me, and I am glad you told me to-day so we can find some ways to help you stay safe. I wonder who you could tell at times when you are not with me and are thinking about hurting yourself?

RYAN: I could tell my mom. Or I could tell my teacher if I was at school.

THERAPIST: Right. So there are several people you can talk to. Also, when you think about hurting yourself, you make a guess that you can't think of any other way out. So, what have you learned in therapy that might help you with that guess?

RYAN: Well, we talked about how sometimes I make wrong guesses about what will happen in the future. So maybe I could check out what I am guessing about my problems.

THERAPIST: What tool have you learned that might help you test that guess?

RYAN: I could ask myself, "What am I guessing about how this problem will turn out?" Then I could ask myself "What is the evidence?" to see if my guess is right—like I did when we checked out my guess about making the football team.

THERAPIST: How might you remember those questions when you are feel-ing bad or thinking about hurting yourself?

RYAN: I could write them down to remember. I have been carrying around my therapy notebook, so I guess I could write them in there and then check my notebook when I think about hurting myself.

Ryan identified several people he could talk to who will be able to get him help when he feels like harming himself. Further, the therapist helped Ryan tie in previously learned skills to apply to his suicidal thoughts ("So what have you learned in therapy that might help you with that guess?"). Addressing the thoughts and distortions that contribute to the suicidality will also help in targeting and correcting inaccurate thoughts.

Time projection, described in Chapter 8, is a helpful intervention with suicidal youth. Suicidal youngsters have a narrow, foreshortened sense of time. Hopelessness blinds children to seeing the way things change over time. Time projection works to widen children's view of the future by predicting how thoughts, feelings, and events may be different in 1 day, 1 week, 1 month, 1 year, or whatever. By asking suicidal young-sters to predict how they will think or feel in the future, you are trying to help these youngsters see that suicide is a *permanent* solution to a *temporary* problem.

Suppose you are working with 14-year-old Drew who has been hospitalized after a severe suicide attempt and you want to try time projection. Drew believes that her pain surrounding her breakup with Tommy will never end so she might as well kill herself. Time projection widens her sense of time ("How will you feel in 1 week . . . 3 weeks . . . 3 months . . . 6 months . . . etc.?"). As Drew starts to see that her feelings change over time, she learns that impulsive decisions made in the heat of the moment need to be suspended or delayed (e.g., "You said your feelings about Tommy may change in 6 months, a year, or maybe 2 years. How long would you be dead? How does that work for you? It seems like you are trying to come up with a permanent solution for a problem that may be temporary.").

Persons (1989) offers a number of very handy tips for working with suicidal youngsters. For example, suppose Drew's motivation for the suicide attempt was to get Tommy back. You could use Person's elegant question, "How can killing yourself bring him back to you?" Additionally, what if Drew's motivation was vengeful and she simply wanted to make her boyfriend feel sorry and pay for the breakup. Persons astutely recommends questions along the lines of "Suppose he does feel bad, how will you be able to enjoy this if you are dead?" or "How long will he feel bad? How long will you be dead?"

Addressing the accuracy of the child's thoughts related to wanting to die is also helpful. When children are depressed they often believe things will never get better. We consider the case of Leah to illustrate this point.

THERAPIST: How often do you feel like you can't go on?

LEAH: All the time.

THERAPIST: Do you always feel like killing yourself and think that no one would miss you?

LEAH: No—only once in awhile.

THERAPIST: What is different on the days you don't feel like dying?

LEAH: Well, those days are better. No one is getting on my back, like last week when I went to the mall with Kelly, stuff like that.

THERAPIST: So every day is not 100% awful.

LEAH: No. I guess it is just once in awhile when it gets really bad I think I can't go on.

THERAPIST: What might you tell yourself on those days to help get through them?

LEAH: I could remind myself that things usually get better and I can handle whatever the problem is.

THERAPIST: That sounds like a good idea. Let's come up with a plan to help you do that.

The therapist worked with Gina to help her objectively identify the temporary versus permanent nature of her depressive feelings by challenging her distortion that she *always* feels like dying. Ideas can then be written on coping cards for the youth to carry with him/herself. Whenever Gina has thoughts of self-harm, she can take out the card and choose a coping strategy from the list.

Suicide may also reflect helplessness about dealing with angry feelings (Persons, 1989). Being angry and unskilled in coping with this feeling can really impact youngsters. Amy is a 17-year-old young woman who was hospitalized for depression. Her depressed mood improved and her suicidal ideation decreased over her period of hospitalization. Nearing her discharge, she had an angry falling out with her parents and then became suicidal again. In her case, suicidal ideation worked as a way to avoid the conflict at home. As long as she was suicidal, she could stay in the hospital and not have to manage her angry feelings toward her parents.

Trevor, a very depressed 16-year-old boy, used his suicidal ideation to express his anger. Whenever he would get mad, he would tell his parents he would kill himself. We worked with Trevor to help him develop problem-solving options ("What else could you say to your parents when you are angry?"; "How else could you let them know how much pain you are in without hurting yourself?"; "How else can you make them hear you?").

Ensuring that parents understand the seriousness of a child's suicidal thoughts is also important. Especially with younger children, parents may find it difficult to take the child's threats seriously. However, parents must attend to these threats in order to identify key warning signs of dangerous behaviors. If his/her threats are initially ignored or met with negativity, the child may simply not tell others when he/she is having such thoughts. Additionally, the child's beliefs that no one cares about him/her may be reinforced, leading to increased suicidal thoughts. Finally, if the child is trying to get help or attention, he/she may find more severe means than threats to do so (e.g., actual self-harm).

If a reasonable degree of safety for the child cannot be achieved, his/her hospitalization must be considered. If, for example, the adolescent will not contract for safety or admits intent to harm him/herself, you and his/her parents will not be able to protect the youngster.

BEHAVIORAL INTERVENTIONS FOR DEPRESSION

Pleasant Activity Scheduling

Pleasant activity scheduling is a valuable first line of defense against anhedonia, social withdrawal, and fatigue. Remember, depressed children do not find activities as much fun as they found them before they were depressed! Therefore, you will have to dig to discover pleasant activities. You may need to ask, "What did you do for fun before you were depressed?" Inquiring about what other children, siblings, or television characters might spend time doing may also spark ideas. Also, consider addressing how long the child will do the activity, how often he/she will do it, and how he/she will remember to do the assignment.

The following transcript illustrates how a therapist can work collaboratively with a depressed 8-year-old child to develop an activity schedule.

THERAPIST: Let's come up with some things that are fun to do. What kinds of things do you do for fun?

CARLA: Nothing is fun. I just sit in my room or watch TV, and that's boring.

THERAPIST: Can you think back to anything that used to be fun?

CARLA: Not really.

THERAPIST: Do you remember ever doing anything else besides sitting in your room or watching TV?

CARLA: No.

THERAPIST: Are there any kids you know who do anything else besides sit and watch TV?

CARLA: Everyone but me has stuff to do and has fun.

THERAPIST: Like who?

CARLA: My sister, the neighbors, my cousins.

THERAPIST: What kinds of things do they do besides watch TV?

CARLA: Well, my sister Josie rides her bike all the time.

THERAPIST: Have you ever gone biking with Josie?

CARLA: Yes, a long time ago.

THERAPIST: How was it to ride bikes with Josie?

CARLA: Well, it was fun then, but it would probably be boring now.

THERAPIST: What are the clues that tell you it would probably be boring?

CARLA: Everything is boring now.

THERAPIST: What are the clues that tell you there is some chance it won't be boring?

CARLA: It was fun a long time ago.

THERAPIST: So, is it possible that riding bikes might be even a little tiny bit fun?

CARLA: I guess maybe.

THERAPIST: Would you be willing to try riding bikes and see what happens?

CARLA: I guess.

As this transcript demonstrates, the therapist overcomes a common challenge of identifying activities by focusing on activities Carla engaged in prior to her depression. Naming an activity was very difficult for Carla. Indeed, it would be easy to label her as resistant or defiant. In actuality, Carla's loss of pleasure reflects her belief that "nothing is fun." Therefore generating a list of pleasant activities with her is challenging. The therapist skillfully sticks with the task without blaming Carla. Eventually, they are able to agree on an activity for her to try.

Developing a *picture schedule* to follow can be a fun approach. The therapist helps the child to create a weekly calendar. Pictures cut out from magazines or the child's own drawings of the selected activities are then placed on the appropriate days of the calendar. For example, if Carla is to ride her bike on Wednesday and Saturday, a picture of a bike can be drawn or glued to those days on the calendar. In a variation of this activity, the therapist can take photographs of the child engaging in the activity to make the pleasant events schedule a realistic model to follow. In these cases, instead of drawing or pasting pictures on the calendar, the child acts out the activity for the therapist. The therapist then takes a Polaroid photograph of the child acting out the activity. The process serves the child both as practice engaging in the activity and as a graduated step to completing the activity independently for homework. The process of acting out the activities and taking the pictures may also be fun for the depressed youngster, thus serving as behavioral activation in itself. For instance, 8-year-old Tommy was scheduled to play basketball on Saturday, so he posed with a basketball for a picture. He was scheduled to read a book with his mom on Tuesday, so he posed holding an opened book. The pictures were then taped to the pleasant activities schedule. Tommy used weather as a metaphor for his mood. A sunny day was a happy mood. The more clouds indicated sadder moods, with stormy weather being the saddest. Under the activity pictures he drew the "weather" to indicate his feelings for the day (see Figure 11.3).

Monday	Tuesday	Wednesday	Thursday	Friday	Saturday	Sunday

FIGURE 11.3. Sample pleasant activity schedule.

Ensuring that the events chosen are things children can initiate on their own helps facilitate effective completion of the activity. For some children, items that the child has control over will have a greater likelihood of being carried out and will lead to a greater sense of accomplishment. Such things may include play activities, reading a humorous story, or talking with peers. Nonetheless, it is critical to include parents in the treatment. Parents can work with the child in completing activities between sessions. If, for example, a child's pleasant activities schedule includes playing outside, parents may take the child to a park to help facilitate the activity.

Rating feelings prior to and following the scheduled activity will be particularly important for depressed children. The ratings will provide valuable information about the child's mood, most successful activities, and changes in ratings. Ratings will also provide evidence for the child that depressive feelings are temporary and changeable. Such evidence may help challenge thoughts such as "Nothing's fun anymore" or "Everything is boring" when utilizing thought testing.

Adolescents are typically more able than younger children to engage in scheduled events without the support of parents due to their increased independence. In some ways, this can increase the likelihood of success. At the same time, depressed adolescents may have isolated themselves to the point that it is difficult to generate possible "pleasant activities." These adolescents may not belong to social clubs, have few friends, and may not be involved in a sports team. Thus, you will need to be creative in identifying activities. Taking a more active role in "mandatory" activities or in family events are options. For instance, Kyle, a 15-year-old depressed boy, rarely participated in the softball or kickball games during physical education class. He usually just sat on the sidelines. For therapy homework, Kyle and his therapist decided he would become more involved in the games. First, he opted to play a position where he would have little contact with the ball, such as outfield. Successfully participating in these games and coping with the discomfort associated with participation by using his therapy skills, he gradually worked up to volunteering to play first base.

We have found that testing predictions regarding activities is helpful when adolescents do not anticipate enjoying the activity. The following transcript illustrates this process.

THERAPIST: How much fun do you think you will have playing Feeling Hoops?

BRENDA: Probably like a 3.

THERAPIST: When I asked you to play, what went through your mind?

BRENDA: I don't want to play. This is childish and stupid.

THERAPIST: What is hard about playing Feeling Hoops?

BRENDA: I stink at playing. I'm such a loser. It's never any fun.

THERAPIST: When you have those thoughts, how do you feel?

BRENDA: Really sad.

THERAPIST: OK. So you're thinking, "I'm such a loser," you feel sad, and you are guessing Feeling Hoops will only be a 3 on the fun scale?

BRENDA: Yeah, that's right.

THERAPIST: OK. How about if we try an experiment? What if you play Feeling Hoops for a few minutes and see if your guess is right?

BRENDA: I guess. (*Brenda begins playing Feeling Hoops.*)

THERAPIST: Brenda, I noticed you just smiled and laughed when the ball bounced off the rim. What was going through your mind?

BRENDA: I was just thinking, "Cool, that one was actually close to going in."

THERAPIST: So you were standing there watching the ball go through the air. It got closer and closer to the hoop and hit the rim. What is zipping through your mind?

BRENDA: I'm doing better than I thought I would.

THERAPIST: When you have that thought, how do you feel?

BRENDA: I feel kind of excited.

THERAPIST: On a scale of 1 to 10, how much fun are you having right now?

BRENDA: About a 5.

THERAPIST: Do you remember how much fun you predicted you would have?

BRENDA: A 3.

THERAPIST: So you predicted a 3, but you are having a 5 on the fun scale. What does that tell you about your prediction?

BRENDA: I was wrong—it was more fun than I thought it would be.

THERAPIST: Do you think there are other things that might be more fun than you first think they will be.

BRENDA: Yeah, maybe other things I think wouldn't be fun really would be OK.

This dialogue provides one example of how predictions can be tested with a depressed adolescent to increase success with a pleasant events schedule. Imbedded in the example is identification of thoughts and feelings before and after the activity. Next, the therapist should utilize this information to work with Brenda on identifying the link between her automatic thoughts ("I'm such a loser.") and feeling sad. The experiment also demonstrates how depressed feelings are temporary and changeable, thus combating the depressed youth's feelings of hopelessness and beliefs that things will never get better.

Social Skills Training

Making friends and initiating social interactions pose great challenges for depressed children. By teaching social skills the therapist can provide depressed children with the skills and confidence they need to initiate interactions with peers. When teaching social skills, therapists must consider the developmentally appropriate behaviors for the child. If the youngster lacks the skills to successfully interact with peers, such interactions may lead to more peer rejection and deeper depressive symptoms. This experience will reinforce beliefs about low self-worth and lead to further social withdrawal.

Essentially, the therapist teaches the youngster communication skills for initiating and responding to interactions with others. You will need to teach them to ask questions, respond to questions from others, and share interests with peers. Skills such as assertiveness, maintaining eye contact, proper facial expression, giving compliments, having a conversation, conflict resolution, and asking others to stop a bothersome behavior have all been taught in social skills building programs (Stark et al., 1991).

Skills are taught through direct instruction, modeling, and role playing, and also through stories or books. Group settings provide realistic experiences, naturally lending themselves to identifying and practicing social skills. The group can also provide modeling and feedback for the youth regarding social skills. Younger children will benefit most from concrete instruction of skills and practice. Teaching ways to approach a group of peers, join or initiate a game, and share a toy can be practiced through role plays and puppet play. Acting out positive and negative social interactions and having the child identify problem areas can also be beneficial. You can play a bully dominating and cheating at a game. The child must then identify the problem behaviors and provide alternative social behaviors.

Role playing a situation in which the depressed child must initiate an interaction with a peer is also helpful. You could play the role of a classmate, with the child assigned to initiating an interaction. Requesting to borrow some paper or a pencil, asking about an assignment, making a comment about a lesson, or complimenting the other student are all possible interactions. The following dialogue shows how to integrate social skills training in therapy.

THERAPIST: OK, Kelly, we are going to do the role play like we talked about. Remember to use the skills we talked about.

KELLY: I'll try.

THERAPIST: All right. We are sitting in homeroom and it's the first day of school. I'm a new student sitting right beside you. I'm looking through a magazine.

KELLY: Hi.

THERAPIST: (*Continues to look through the magazine as if she doesn't hear Kelly.*)

KELLY: (*Starts to squirm in her seat a little and her face begins to turn red.*) Um, Hi, my name is Kelly, what's your name?

THERAPIST: (*Looks up.*) Oh sorry, I was just reading. My name is Jessica.

KELLY: What are you reading about?

THERAPIST: It's an article about the U.S. Women's Soccer team. I'm going to try out for the school team. Do you play soccer?

KELLY: (*Appears more relaxed.*) I love soccer! Uh, um (*looks down*), do you think you would want to practice together after school sometime?

THERAPIST: Sure. OK. Kelly, how did you feel during that role play?

The role play was used to give Kelly a chance to practice initiating a conversation with a peer. The therapist made it a little challenging for Kelly by ignoring her first effort. However, the therapist balanced that difficulty by allowing Kelly to experience success. Subsequent role plays should include more challenging interactions so Kelly learns to apply her skills in a "worst case scenario." The therapist should continue to process with Kelly her thoughts and feelings before, during, and after the role play. Identifying what was easiest, hardest, and most surprising about the role play will also help in addressing maladaptive thoughts and beliefs, as well as inaccurate predictions.

Depressed adolescents will benefit from some of the same social skills training as children. Adolescents may be more aware of social skills than children but simply feel awkward or lack practice/confidence to implement them. However, adolescents will be expected to tune into more subtle social cues than young children. Thus, adolescents may need to be educated on social behaviors such as nonverbal cues in addition to more concrete skills. Reading body language, eye contact, and verbal cues are helpful skills. Further, since they are more developmentally mature, adolescents may benefit from exercises in observing and taking social cues from others. Adolescents can be instructed in ways to observe peers and imitate social behavior in situations in which they are uncomfortable or unsure of expected social norms.

A depressed adolescent may begin by noting positive social behaviors used by peers at school and how others react to them. Once the skills are identified, they can be practiced in session by role playing with the therapist. The adolescent can gradually begin testing the use of the social skills in other situations. Using popular movies or TV shows to illustrate examples of social behaviors and cues is a fun strategy. In this exercise, teens identify their favorite shows or movies and then are instructed to watch them while recording target social skills. Video clips from the shows or movies can be viewed in session to further illustrate the skill identification.

PROBLEM SOLVING

Problem solving also poses unique difficulties for depressed children. Difficulties with decision making and a sense of hopelessness may make problem solving seem like an insurmountable task for depressed youngsters. Some depressed youngsters may need to be directly taught the steps of problem solving. For other depressed youth, dysfunctional thoughts may interfere with their ability to problem solve or to carry out the identified solution. Thoughts that they are unable to solve the problem or will fail are examples of dysfunctional beliefs. Identifying the obstacles to problem solving and challenging dysfunctional beliefs will facilitate problem solving.

To aid depressed children with problem solving, we have found that distancing them from the situation is initially helpful. Having the child think of a hero or a role model, and then asking the child how that person might solve the problem is useful. Putting the child in the position of solving the problem for someone else will also generate more ideas.

THERAPIST: If your best friend, Jeff, was feeling really down because he just failed his spelling test, what could he do to help solve his problem?

MATTHEW: He could ask the teacher to give him extra practice sheets for the next test.

THERAPIST: How would that help?

MATTHEW: Well, he could practice more and maybe learn the words better next time.

THERAPIST: That sounds like a good plan. What else could he do?

MATTHEW: He could have his mom quiz him before the test.

THERAPIST: So he could practice more and have his mom quiz him. Matt, you said you were feeling down because you got a D on your math test. Can any of your ideas for Jeff help *you* solve *your* problem?

This process helps Matthew solve his problem by generalizing the solutions he came up with to help Jeff. Distancing himself from the situation helps him initially to generate steps for problem solving, and then allows him to apply those steps to his own situation. Doing so battles the obstacle that many depressed children have in seeing alternative solutions for their problems.

Identifying alternative solutions to problems forms a greater barrier for depressed youngsters. The pessimistic outlook that characterizes many depressed youth serves as an obstacle to effective problem solving and generating potential solutions. The depressed youth may only see one resolution to a problem, typically one with a negative outcome. Building skills in generating alternative solutions will significantly increase the depressed child's successful utilization of problem-solving techniques.

SELF-MONITORING

Identifying feelings and thoughts paves the way for self-instructional and rational analysis techniques. However, due to the depth of their depressive feelings, some depressed youth may have trouble capturing their thoughts and feelings. In these circumstances, you may have to become more active and directive in the self-monitoring process.

There are multiple reasons depressed children have difficulty reporting their thoughts (Fennell, 1989; Padesky, 1988). Some youngsters may be ashamed of their thoughts. Here, you should go after the beliefs that may lie beneath their nondisclosure (e.g., "What would it mean about you if you told me what was going through your mind? How do you guess I will react?"). Other youngsters may worry that their strong feelings and thoughts will overwhelm them. They predict that they will feel even more depressed and won't be able to control their feelings. In these cases, a good strategy would be to check out these beliefs (e.g., "What do you fear might happen if you told me what was going through your mind?"), and then help them gradually express small bits of their thoughts and feelings so they can gain confidence in their self-control capacities.

Further, some depressed youngsters may be too worn out by their depressed feelings. Here, the self-report measures like the CDI come in real handy! You can use the items on the CDI that the youngster endorsed as a springboard (e.g., "I see you circled that you think you are ugly. Is that a belief you would like to change?"). Finally, difficulty reporting thoughts and feelings may be due to pessimism and hopelessness. In other words, the inability to capture thoughts and feeling may be their depression talking. For these youngsters, you will need to immediately and directly target their pessimism and hopelessness (e.g., "What makes things change?"; "What causes change?"; "How does not identifying thoughts and feelings help you?").

Naming the Distortion

Naming the distortion is a simple technique that prepares the child for more advanced self-instructional and rational analysis approaches (Burns, 1980; Persons, 1989). Identifying distortions is illustrated in the example of Tracy, a perfectionistic 15-year-old who frequently uses all-or-nothing thinking and catastrophizing.

TRACY: I know I did terrible on my biology quiz. I am going to fail biology and then I will never get into a good college!

THERAPIST: Does that thought match any of the distortions we have learned?

TRACY: I don't remember them all. Can I use the list in my therapy folder?

THERAPIST: Of course. Using the list will help you remember. You should use the list often to check on yourself and see if you might be using any of the distortions.

TRACY: Oh, this is the one where I take one thing and blow it out of proportion so that everything seems bad. Catastrophizing?

THERAPIST: That's right. That is just a big word that means you are "taking one thing and blowing it out of proportion so that everything seems bad." It is kind of like telling your own fortune as being really bad, without thinking of what is more likely to happen.

TRACY: I think I do that a lot.

THERAPIST: How do you feel when you make those kinds of predictions?

TRACY: Very nervous!

THERAPIST: How do you think you were doing that with your statement "I am going to fail biology and then I will never get into a good college!"

TRACY: Well, I guess I have done well on all my homework assignments. And this was only a quiz, so it won't bring down my grade too much. Plus, I can always do extra credit.

The therapist helped emphasize how such distortions can impact Tracy's feelings (e.g., "How do you feel when you make those kinds of predictions?"). The therapist then brought the discussion back to her statement about biology ("How do you think you were doing that with your statement 'I am going to fail biology and then I will never get into a good college'!"). The skill of naming the distortion can then be added to homework assignments as part of thought records. After recording automatic thoughts, teens can identify any cognitive distortions imbedded in the thoughts.

SELF-INSTRUCTIONAL APPROACHES

Treasure Chest is an adaptation of a self-instructional task. Treasure Chest makes the analogy between forgotten/misplaced coping thoughts and buried treasure. You and the child draw or even construct a "treasure chest" in session. You and the child then develop positive coping statements that go into the treasure chest. The positive coping statements ("I'm not bad when I make a mistake, I'm just normal.") can be written down on the drawing of the treasure chest or written on cards that are placed inside the constructed chest. You then instruct the child to go to the treasure chest and pull out their positive "loot" whenever they feel low. Homework assignments for youngsters might include filling up a treasure chest by coming up with five things they like about themselves. A sample treasure chest is illustrated in Figure 11.4.

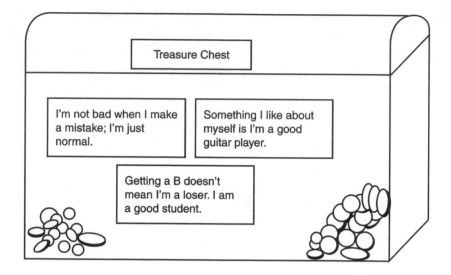

FIGURE 11.4. Sample treasure chest.

Replace Mint is another fun and creative way to teach self-instruction tools to children. Like Treasure Chest, Replace Mint makes use of analogies. In this exercise, positive coping thoughts are equated with new, shiny coins or fresh crisp dollars. Children are instructed to go to the mint and print out new emotional currencies. You could elaborate on the analogy further by encouraging the youngsters to shred their old bills (negative thoughts). For example, negative thoughts could be written down on old, worn pieces of construction paper. Then, they can be returned to the mint to be replaced. Finally, the old currency can be shredded and replaced by new currency (i.e., positive coping thoughts written on fresh crisp pieces of construction paper).

To illustrate how to use Replace Mint with children, consider the following transcript with 11-year-old Matt, who is struggling with painful self-critical thoughts. Read how the therapist describes Replace Mint and helps Matt change his currency.

THERAPIST: Do you know how money is made?

MATT: I think it comes from a big bank.

THERAPIST: Kind of. It comes from a mint.

MATT: A mint?

THERAPIST: Not the type of mint you eat. This type of mint is a place where money is printed. Have you ever seen any new, crisp dollar bills?

MATT: Yes. My uncle gave me a new dollar once. It was really clean and stiff.

THERAPIST: You know that the mint prints new dollar bills to replace the old, worn-out ones. It's like what we were talking about with your thoughts. What are some old worn-out thoughts you have about yourself?

MATT: I'm no good. Nobody likes me.

THERAPIST: Write these on the crumbled green paper. They are just like the old bills. (*Matt writes the thoughts on the construction paper.*) What do you suppose the new fresh, crisp paper is for?

MATT: Different things I can say to myself.

THERAPIST: Exactly. We're going to be a mint for new thoughts. We'll replace the tired negative thoughts with fresh new thoughts you can carry around. We'll call this game Replace Mint.

In this activity, Matt learned that worn-out thoughts could be replaced with fresh, more adaptive thoughts. Additionally, by writing the new thoughts on the construction paper, Matt has created a coping card. He can carry it with him! Finally, the experiential nature of the activity makes the abstract process more concrete. Matt can remember the task of how he took his old thoughts "out of circulation."

RATIONAL ANALYSIS TECHNIQUES

Reattribution

A *Responsibility Pie* (discussed in more detail in Chapter 8) helps the youngster view his/her responsibility in a more accurate light and prompts him/her to examine alternative explanations (Padesky, 1988; Seligman et al., 1995). The technique involves generating a list of all of the factors that may have contributed to an event. The child then assigns each factor a portion of the pie to represent the amount of responsibility that factor has for the overall outcome. Young children will not likely understand fractions or percentages but can benefit from this technique if the therapist uses a primarily visual presentation. They may color or cut out portions of the pie, using the size of the "piece" to represent the amount of responsibility.

A variation of Responsibility Pie is *Reattribution Pizza*, a game based on a popular image for many youngsters. The child uses construction paper, crayons, and scissors to make a pizza. The child then makes a menu of "toppings," which consist of the factors he/she believes are contributing to the problem or situation. The menu basically lists the factor or attribution, with the "price" being the amount of responsibility (see Figure 11.5). The child then cuts the pizza pieces in different sizes to represent the amount of responsibility he/she is attributing to each factor. "Toppings" such as mushrooms and pepperoni can be labeled with the various attributions. Figure 11.6 demonstrates how the topping labels can be placed on the pizza.

Similar to depressed children, adolescents frequently take responsibility for factors out of their control. For instance, Stephanie has finished generating a list of factors that have contributed to her parents' separation and is now assigning percentages to each factor (see Figure 11.7).

THERAPIST: So you already decided that you getting suspended from school is 20%, you not listening to your parents is 20%, and fighting with your sister is 50%. The next thing on the list is your father's drinking.

STEPHANIE: Yeah. He drank a lot and that made him really mean to us and my mom. That's probably like 40%.

THERAPIST: OK. With everything you've already listed, that makes 130%! What do you think that means?

STEPHANIE: I guess I overestimated some of the first few. I think fighting with my sister might be more like 25%, and not listening is 15%. That makes 100% now.

THERAPIST: Right, but we still have a few more things on our list. What is the next item?

PIZZA MENU

Mushrooms (My fault for fighting with her) 1/8
Pepperoni (It was raining) 1/8
Tomatoes (The other car was going too fast). 2/8

FIGURE 11.5. Pizza menu.

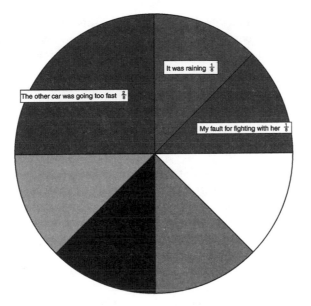

FIGURE 11.6. Reattribution pizza.

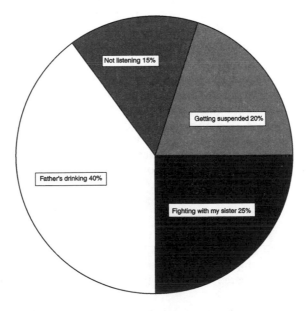

FIGURE 11.7. Responsibility pie.

The therapist and Stephanie continued this process until all items were assigned percentages. As with many depressed adolescents, Stephanie's initial tendency was to primarily blame herself for negative events. However, examining all the possible causes and evidence helped her to see more accurately what is and is not her responsibility. In doing so, she had to reassign responsibility more accurately.

Hypothesis Testing

Conducting experiments to test predictions teaches children to examine the evidence before forming conclusions. Experiments include gathering evidence for and against automatic thoughts, recording observations, and examining changes in thoughts and feelings. The results of these experiments help challenge automatic thoughts such as "Everyone at school hates me" or "I can't pass reading."

These experiments are designed to test the evidence supporting particular thoughts. In *Reporter*, you and the child work as reporters searching for a story. Cognitive distortions are "false leads" in the story, potentially leading the child astray from finding the "truth." Thus, experiments and tests of evidence are designed to find the facts without getting sidetracked by false leads.

You can teach children to work as a *Private I* or detective to check the evidence. The detective is working to uncover the truth and solve the question "Is my expectation/guess true?" The Private I technique for testing the evidence is introduced with a discussion of detectives:

> "Do you know what a detective or Private I does? A Private I looks for clues or evidence to answer questions. Private I's sometimes answer questions to figure out a mystery or to find a missing object or person. Private I's make a hunch or guess about what happened, gather the facts, put all the facts together, and them come up with an answer. In here we are going to act like Private I's to gather clues and answer the question 'Is my hypothesis/guess true?' This will help us answer questions about your problems and check the evidence and make sure it matches and fits together. So, you will be a Private I figuring out the truth about the things you say to yourself."

After introducing the Private I technique, you should illustrate it by working through an example from the child's life (see Figure 11.8). Doing so will serve as a graduated task for when the child will work more independently.

Adolescents can be taught to complete charts outlining evidence supporting and countering their hypothesis. On one side of the chart, they

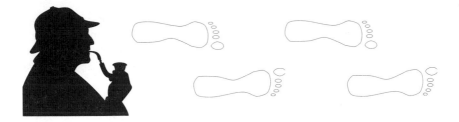

Private I's pay attention to people and things around them to get clues for their hunches. You can work as a Private I to check the clues about the things that bother you.

Write a statement about something that is bothering you to investigate. (What is your hunch?)

_____

_____

_____

What are the clues? (Remember clues can be things you do, see, hear, learn, etc.)

_____

_____

_____

Now, put the clues together. Did the clues you found show that your hunch was right or wrong? What is your conclusion?

_____

_____

_____

FIGURE 11.8. Private I Worksheet. From Friedberg and McClure (2002). Copyright by The Guilford Press. Permission to photocopy this figure is granted to purchasers of this book for personal use only (see copyright page for details).

list evidence supporting the hypothesis 100%. On the other side, they list facts not supporting the hypothesis. It is important that only facts (vs. opinions) are listed. When 15-year-old Jon identified the hypothesis "I'm stupid," he identified "I'm a failure" as evidence supporting his belief. We worked with Jon to distinguish facts from opinions. One way of doing so is to ask, "Would other people agree with that statement?" He then made a chart in which he listed the evidence for and against "I'm stupid." After completing the chart, he concluded, thanks to Socratic dialogue, "The evidence shows I'm not totally stupid, although sometimes I tell myself I am when I make a mistake."

Continuum Techniques

A continuum technique (J. S. Beck, 1995; Padesky, 1988) is a useful way to decrease children's all-or-none thinking. Depressed youngsters place themselves in either/or categories. For example, 14-year-old Jenny thought that because she received one B on her report card she was a total failure. Sixteen-year-old Albert thought that because he was not "a jock" he was completely unpopular. Finally, 12-year-old Greta believed that because the other girls made fun of her hair and clothes, she was a total loser. The continuum technique works to cast doubt on these either/or labels through rational analysis. Generally, we recommend continuum techniques with older elementary school children and adolescents.

We will begin with a general description and then suggest various adaptations. Suppose you are working with Greta. First, you draw a line with two end points (see Figure 11.9). On one end, place her label "Total Loser" and on the other end place her label "Totally Together." Then ask Greta to specifically list criteria that define each label. The next step is to

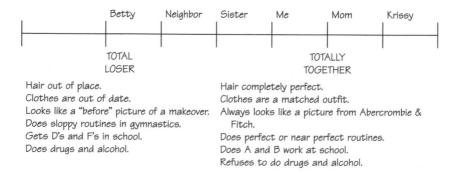

FIGURE 11.9. Greta's continuum.

place people she knows somewhere on the line. Finally, she places herself on the continuum and then makes a conclusion.

As you can see from the figure, the criteria are all or none. Very few people would likely be at the high or low end. Look at where Greta placed herself. She is about at an "above average" midpoint. The intriguing issue that arises is that she is really "behind" only her mother and the star of the gymnastic team, Krissy. With this subjective data in hand, you could ask her, "If someone was a total loser, where would she be on the line? In your mind's eye, you are a little in back of Mom and Krissy. Even if that is true, how does that make you a total loser?"

The line drawing may be too abstract for some youngsters. You could use boxes to represent each end of the continuum. For instance, you could get two shoe boxes and title the boxes "Total Loser" and "Totally Together." Then the criteria could be written on cards or pieces of paper and placed inside the box. The boxes could be positioned at separate ends of the table or floor. Names of people who fit the criteria could be placed on the table based on how close they come to meeting the criteria cards within each box. The box metaphor concretizes the concept and gives rise to meaningful metaphors/analogies. For example, you can talk to the youngster about how these categories or labels "box them in." Further, you can discuss with the youngster how this task helps them "think out of the box."

CONCLUSION

Cognitive therapy offers a range of interventions you can tailor to the client's specific symptomology and developmental level. Depressive symptoms can manifest in different ways depending on the youth's temperament, age, gender, culture, or developmental level. In this chapter we have illustrated numerous ways to creatively apply cognitive techniques to depressed children and adolescents. Remember, it is important to keep the interventions fun and engaging, especially for depressed youngsters! We encourage you to adapt the interventions provided in this chapter to meet the individual needs of your clients. Also, use your own creativity to apply cognitive techniques in new and fun ways!

12

❖

Working with Anxious Children and Adolescents

SYMPTOMS OF ANXIETY IN YOUTH

Anxiety, fears, and worries are commonplace childhood occurrences. Contemporary stressors such as academic demands, drugs, violence, and sexually transmitted diseases create pressure for children and adolescents. Mastering inevitable childhood pressures can be quite difficult.

According to the cognitive model, five spheres of functioning change when children are anxious. They will experience physiological, mood, behavioral, cognitive and interpersonal changes. Treatment naturally focuses on quieting down the distressing symptoms by providing increased coping skills.

Many anxious children experience bodily/somatic complaints. They appear uneasy, seeming at times to be uncomfortable inside their own skin. Commonly, these youngsters report profuse sweating, light-headedness, dizziness, muscle tension, stomach distress, increased heart rates, breathlessness, and bowel irregularities. Often, their physical complaints have already been assessed by a pediatrician. However, if the child has not been seen by a pediatrician and presents with some of these multiple somatic complaints, you should recommend a physical evaluation by a physician.

Worry, dread, panic, fear, and irritability are the emotional components of anxiety. Youngsters may use more colorful and poetic language to report their anxiety. They may say that they feel "fluttery" or "jittery" or "jumpy." We have heard youngsters report anxiety by saying they feel "yucky" or "weird" inside. Francis and Gragg (1995) noted that children with fears of contamination may report that they feel "germy."

Behavioral symptoms generally reflect more overt signs of anxiety. Avoidance is the hallmark of anxious symptoms. Children are usually referred because they are no longer able to avoid the circumstances they fear and/or their avoidance has come at tremendous cost (e.g., schoolwork, health problems, peer problems, family conflict). Nail biting, thumb sucking, compulsions, and hypervigilance are other common behavioral symptoms of anxiety. Children may engage in these behaviors to soothe themselves or to cope with threatening situations. Not surprisingly, anxious children are inattentive, distractable, and restless. When a child continually scans the environment, looking for and expecting danger, it is hard for him/her to concentrate and sit still. Many of these youngsters believe their very survival depends on being a moving target!

Cognitive symptoms reflect the way children package information. Anxious children's internal dialogues are punctuated by catastrophic predictions and expectations of unsuccessful coping (e.g., "Something bad will happen and I won't be able to handle it."). Their minds lock onto the potentially threatening aspects of situations (e.g., "What if _____ happens?"). They expect the worst to happen and worry about their coping capacity.

Consider this example. Jake is a highly competent but harshly perfectionistic sixth-grade student. He is plagued by awful expectations that he will misunderstand or forget to do an assignment. Consequently, he repeatedly checks his own notebook and asks his teachers for endless clarifications. He expects to be caught ill prepared and to catastrophically disappoint himself and others. In fact, Jake has rarely missed a meaningful assignment. However, this fact does little to relieve Jake's discomfort.

Kashani and Orvaschel (1990) aptly note that "anxiety exerts its most detrimental effects on the interpersonal spheres of functioning" (p. 318). Reading aloud and/or speaking in class are perceived crucibles for anxious children (Kendall et al., 1992). Additionally, being assigned to a group for a class project, being chosen for a team, unstructured social situations, and taking tests are common hot spots for anxious youngsters (Beidel & Turner, 1998). They are highly self-conscious and exquisitely sensitive to others' potential negative evaluation or scrutiny.

Casey is a 10-year-old girl who finds unstructured social situations and small group projects threatening. One day in social studies class, Casey's teacher tells the class to color each original colony a different color on a map. The teacher informs the children that they will be working with partners. At this, Casey begins to ruminate on who she will be teamed with and consequently tunes out the teacher. Her inner dialogue is filled with thoughts like "Who should I pick? Will they pick me? What if they don't want to be with me? What if I'm last? What if I'm alone?" These thoughts race through her mind, sending her into a tailspin. Before she knows it, Casey's teacher says, "OK children, pair up in work groups." Stunned, Casey now realizes that she has not paid attention to all of her teacher's instructions. This realization momentarily paralyzes her. This slight hesitation causes her to delay selecting a partner. This delay, in turn, means that everyone else pairs up, leaving her as the lone single. She now has to go to the teacher and admit that she does not have a partner and does not have a clue about the assignment. The teacher responds critically, fueling Casey's fear of negative evaluation and ridicule. She is left alone without a partner and her view of herself as an outsider is strengthened.

Parents with anxious children may be either overinvolved or underinvolved in their children's lives (Chorpita & Barlow, 1998; Kendall et al., 1991). Underinvolved parents are distant, removed, and withdrawn from their children. They may drop their child off at your office for you to "fix" and then return after your "repair" work is completed. Consequently, they may miss parental sessions and/or fail to follow through on contingency management assignments.

Overinvolved, overprotective parents want to shield their child from life's inevitable stressors. They do not trust the child's coping resources and see their child as excessively fragile. As an example of overprotectiveness, take the case of a mother whose daughter does not like the cafeteria food. She suddenly realizes that her daughter has forgotten to take her lunch to school. So she rushes with a warm sandwich in an insulated lunch bag so the child will not get upset at lunchtime.

CULTURAL AND GENDER DIFFERENCES IN SYMPTOM EXPRESSION

Silverman, LaGreca, and Wasserstein (1995) investigated worries in Caucasian, African American, and Hispanic children in grades two through six. They found that African American children worried more intensely about war, personal harm, and family. Beidel, Turner, and Trager (1994) found no ethnic differences between African American and Caucasian children on measures of test anxiety. However, a large number of African American youngsters met criteria for social anxiety. Treadwell, Flannery-Schroeder, and Kendall (1995) found that while most items on the Revised Children's Manifest Anxiety Scale (RCMAS; Reynolds & Richmond, 1985) were endorsed similarly by African American and Caucasian youth, the African American youngsters endorsed the anger items on the scale at a higher rate. Neal, Lilly, and Zakis (1993) found that most fears were similarly endorsed by African American children and Caucasian children. However, the school-fears factor was not as pivotal for the African American youngsters as for their Caucasian counterparts. Fear of getting one's hair cut was more of a concern for African American youngsters than for Caucasian youth.

Several authors (Hicks et al., 1996; Ginsburg & Silverman, 1996; Silverman et al., 1995) have found considerable similarities between anxious Caucasian and anxious Hispanic youngsters. In terms of differences, Hispanic children presented with more separation anxiety difficulties. Additionally, Hispanic children worried more about health concerns than did Caucasian children (Silverman et al., 1995). Silverman and her colleagues also found a gender difference indicating that Hispanic girls had more school worries and performance anxiety than Hispanic boys.

Our review turned up very few articles on anxiety disorders in Native American youth. Munn, Sullivan, and Romero (1999) found that Native American and Caucasian youngsters obtained similar symptom scores on the RCMAS. However, Munn et al. cautioned that these results may be limited to highly acculturated Cherokee youth.

Gender differences in anxiety disorders seem to be context-specific. Community studies reveal that anxious girls outnumber anxious boys (Beidel & Turner, 1998). However, clinic-based studies do not show significant gender differences (Treadwell et al., 1995). This is an interesting yet poorly understood finding (Castellanos & Hunter, 1999). One possible hypothesis advanced by Treadwell et al. (1995) is that once the anxious symptoms warrant clinical intervention, gender differences are less notable. A complementary hypotheses is that anxious girls outnumber anxious boys in community studies because they are socialized to be more emotionally expressive. Since (1) girls are socialized to be more emotionally expressive than boys and (2) since anxiety may be more permissible in girls, (3) there is more social tolerance for anxious symptoms in girls and (4) therefore girls must exhibit more extreme anxiety symptoms to be referred to treatment.

Due to the limited number of studies and the tendency for this line of research to confound demographic distinctions with ethnocultural variations (Beutler, Brown, Crothers, Booker, & Seabrook, 1996; Cuellar, 1998), we suggest you interpret the results cautiously. In trying to understand these findings, we have found it useful to examine the similarities and differences. For instance, what are the implications of the similarities? First, there may be common features of anxiety that cut across gender and ethnic differences. Second, the similarities may be a product of measurement techniques. Certainly, it would make sense that if measures developed on Western diagnostic/conceptual dimensions were used for all children, some similarities would emerge. Third, the ethnic children participating in the research and coming to the clinic may be more highly acculturated than children who do not participate in research or seek traditional mental health services. The differences found in symptom expression may reveal context-specific fears and anxieties (e.g., haircuts, school, neighborhood violence). Indeed, we need to address these specific contextual elements. Further, differences in anxious symptom expression (e.g., greater irritability, somatization) suggest that we should direct our attention to these treatment targets and incorporate them into our intervention plan.

ASSESSMENT OF ANXIETY

Revised Children's Manifest Anxiety Scale

The Revised Children's Manifest Anxiety Scale (RCMAS; Reynolds & Richmond, 1985) is a widely used measure of children's anxious symptomology. Thirty-seven yes/no items make up the inventory. The RCMAS produces a Total Anxiety Score; four factor scores: Physiological Symptoms, Worries, Social Evaluations, Concentration Difficulties; and a Lie Scale. Scores may be reported as raw scores, percentile ranks, and/or standard scores. The RCMAS is designed for children ages 6–19 years old.

Multidimensional Anxiety Scale for Children

The Multidimensional Anxiety Scale for Children (MASC; March, 1997) contains 39 items that factor into four subscales. The MASC is suitable for children ages 8–19 years old. The four subscales yielded by the MASC include Harm Avoidance, Physical Symptoms, Social Anxiety, and Separation/Panic. The MASC also contains a Total Anxiety Scale, an Inconsistency Index, and an Anxiety Disorder Index. A handy 10-item short form is also available.

Social Phobia and Anxiety Inventory for Children

The Social Phobia and Anxiety Inventory for Children (SPAI-C; Beidel, Turner, & Morris, 1995) specifically addresses symptoms associated with social phobia. Severity of distress is rated on a 3-point scale. There are separate parent and child versions. Beidel and Turner (1998) report solid psychometric characteristics. Beidel and Turner claim that the SPAI-C is best suited for children between the ages of 8 and 14. For children over

14, they suggest using the adult version of the scale. For younger children, they recommend relying on the parent version.

Fear Survey Schedule for Children—Revised

The Fear Survey Schedule for Children—Revised (FSSC-R; Ollendick, 1983) is an 80-item scale that taps a variety of common childhood fears. The scale possesses solid psychometric properties and is appropriate for children ages 7 through 16 (Ollendick, King, & Frary, 1989). The FSSC-R yields a Total Fear Score and five factor scores: Fear of Failure and Criticism, Fear of the Unknown, Fear of Injury and Small Animals, Fear of Danger and Death, and Medical Fears.

A WORD ON MEDICAL EVALUATIONS

Young people with anxiety disorders can present with many physical symptoms. Additionally, many medical conditions can mimic anxious complaints. Therefore, as part of the assessment process, we recommend thorough medical evaluation of the youth by a pediatrician. First, the medical evaluation can rule out any physical problem that is masquerading as an anxiety disorder. Second, the medical evaluation will reveal any coexisting physical problem that might exacerbate anxiety. Third, as therapist, you will need to know whether the client's anxiety might exacerbate a medical condition. Fourth, if the child is taking medicine for a medical condition, you will want to know what influence the medicine has on the child's anxious symptoms. Fifth, in cases of severe anxiety, medication might be indicated in order for the child to fully profit from the psychotherapy. Sixth, the data obtained from a medical evaluation will be useful in testing the child's health-related fears and anxieties. Finally, you will need medical clearance to do some forms of exposure treatment.

CHOOSING INTERVENTIONS IN ANXIETY DISORDERS

In her work with adults, Padesky (1988) suggests titrating the type of intervention to the client's level of distress. For instance, when an anxious child is in a state of low arousal, you might elect to teach the child time management techniques, or to work with the child's parents to decrease his/her caffeine intake or his/her watching of scary or violent movies. Next you might add relaxation. Finally, you might initiate problem-solving approaches.

We present techniques in this section in a graduated, sequential manner. We begin with self-monitoring techniques, then address relatively simple cognitive and behavioral interventions, and finally proceed to more complex cognitive and behavioral interventions (see Figure 12.1). It is very unlikely you will need to use every intervention we list with each child.

When you choose your intervention approach, keep in mind the stage of therapy. Early in therapy you will likely rely on self-monitoring and simple techniques. Additionally, you will want to make sure that children can identify their thoughts, feelings, and behaviors via self-monitoring before you use the other intervention tools. Finally, choice of intervention depends on what you want to accomplish. Accordingly, we designed a table that includes a menu of interventions and their rationale to guide you (see Table 12.1).

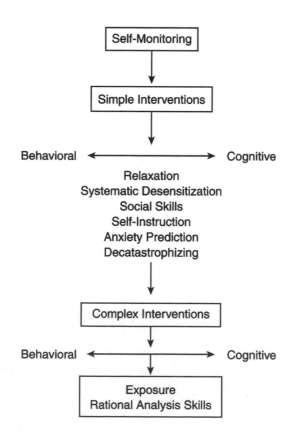

FIGURE 12.1. Recommended sequence of cognitive-behavioral strategies.

TABLE 12.1. Therapeutic Process, Tool, and Purpose

Therapeutic Process	Specific Tool	Purpose
Self-monitoring	Bubble-Up	Determines Subjective Units of Distress. Serves as a foundation for construction of anxiety/fear hierarchy.
	Tracks of My Fears	Identifies cognitive, emotional, interpersonal, physiological, and behavioral components of fear. Forms the basis for subsequent interventions.
	Fear Thermometer	Assesses "degree" of fear and anxiety. Serves as basis for intervention.
	Self-report inventories	Allows for quantitative and qualitative evaluation of specific components of fears/anxieties. Provides treatment targets.
Relaxation	Progressive muscle relaxation	Decreases muscle tension and somatic complaints.
	Controlled breathing	Decreases tension and regulates breathing.
Countercondi-tioning	Systematic desensitization	Breaks association between anxiety-producing cues and fear response.
Social skills training	Puppet role plays	Provides practice of social skills in a graduated fun manner.
	Fogging	Gives children a verbal skill to defuse teasing.
	Ignoring	Provides simple way to "escape" teasing circumstances.
	Observation	Gives children data on social skills options and provides models.
Cognitive self-control techniques	Talking Back to Fear	Facilitates acquisition and application of more adaptive internal dialogues. Good with younger children (ages 8–11).
	Dreadful Iffy	Decreases catastrophic thinking patterns (good with younger children ages 8–11).
	Real versus False Alarms	Provides way for youngsters to check whether their worries are accurate or not (good for younger children ages 8–11).
	Just Because	Offers a way to separate others' opinion from fact.
	Behavioral experimentation	Gives children opportunities to test out their predictions through practice.
	Test of evidence	Allows for consideration of acts supporting or disconfirming their anxious beliefs.
Performance-based procedures	Exposure	Provides genuine data on performance, helps children habituate to fear and test out beliefs.
	Red Light/Green Light	Fun way to practice exposure: child "freezes in place" to simulate exposure
Self-reward	Badge of Courage	Reward that records success.

SELF-MONITORING

Self-Monitoring with Children

Subjective Units of Distress (SUDS) ratings are conventional ways to self-monitor (Masters et al., 1987). SUDS ratings titrate the level of each fear or worry. The child judges the intensity of each fear and gives the item a numerical value. The more intense the fear/worry, the higher the level of subjective distress. Friedberg et al. (2001) modified the SUDS rating process in a *Bubble-Up* procedure. The rating scale consists of a series of bubbles and the child simply colors the number of bubbles that corresponds to each fear.

Tracks of My Fears (see Figure 12.2) is a fun self-monitoring task for youngsters in which they learn to recognize the relationship between various situations, thoughts, feelings, and actions. The task is a relatively simple and straightforward one that utilizes train, track, and station metaphors. Tracks of My Fears gives you more specific data regarding children's fears since youngsters identify the individual components associated with their fears.

Tracks of My Fears begins with the child drawing a train; this engages the youngster in the task. The next step requires the child to track his/her fears. As Figure 12.2 reveals, there are six stations the train visits (Who Station, Mind Station, Where Station, Action Station, Body Station, and Feeling Station). It is important that the child visit each station. However, the order in which the train visits the various stations is irrelevant.

When the train stops at a station, the child colors in the building. Then the youngster responds to the question at the station. The therapist should help the child to answer each question or prompt as specifically as possible. The child records his/her responses in the spaces provided in the station. You could use the completed sample worksheet contained in Figure 12.3 as an example.

You are encouraged to introduce Tracks of My Fears in a lively and engaging manner. The following transcript offers an introduction that has proved to be successful with children.

THERAPIST: Paying attention to places, people, and things around you also is an important way to help you track your fear. The Tracks of My Fears worksheet is another way to be in charge of your fears. Do you like trains or roller coasters?

HOLLY: Yes.

THERAPIST: What do you like about them?

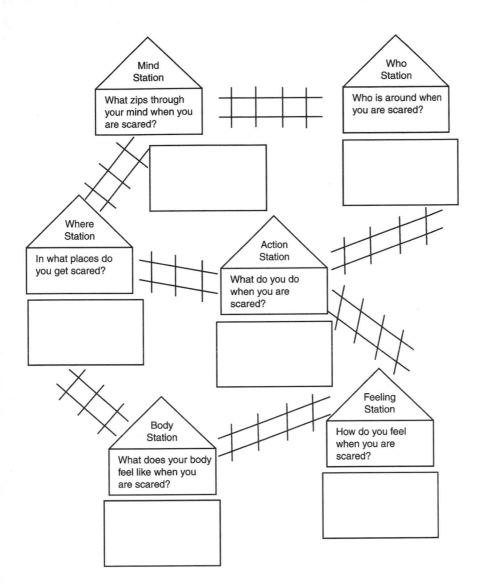

FIGURE 12.2. Tracks of My Fears Worksheet. From Friedberg and McClure (2002). Copyright by The Guilford Press. Permission to photocopy this figure is granted to purchasers of this book for personal use only (see copyright page for details).

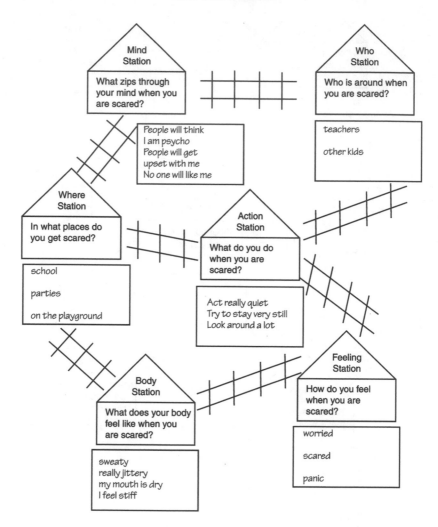

FIGURE 12.3. Completed Tracks of My Fears Worksheet.

HOLLY: They're fun.

THERAPIST: I like them because they stop at different places. How do you think your fears and worries are like a train?

HOLLY: I don't know.

THERAPIST: They're like trains or roller coasters because when boys and girls worry, their minds race around like a train engine. Their hearts beat fast and they sweat. Finally, when you worry a lot, your worry train goes off the track and it's harder to get where you want to go.

The train metaphor is an especially productive one for many children. You might use the train metaphor to represent railroads, subways, or even roller-coaster cars. For instance, the notion of a train careening out of control may match the child's phenomenological experience of his/her anxiety. Moreover, using the train metaphor to talk about being derailed or going off-track may click for many youngsters. Finally, the stations emphasize the different components of anxiety. For example, children may readily recognize the physiological components (Body Station) and behavioral aspects (Action Station) of their fear, but be relatively unaware of their anxiety-producing thoughts (Mind Station). You can apply the tracks, stations, and trains metaphor to illustrate this process to children. The following dialogue provides some pointers on augmenting the train metaphor and maintaining a playful attitude.

THERAPIST: Have you ever been on a train or roller coaster?

RAY: Yes, I go to an amusement park where there is a roller coaster. Sometimes I get scared when I ride it. My dad gets dizzy.

THERAPIST: The roller coaster goes fast around lots of curves.

RAY: It races up and down hills too.

THERAPIST: The train kind of goes out of control, doesn't it?

RAY: That's what makes it scary.

THERAPIST: Exactly, your fears and worries are kind of like a roller coaster. They take you on a scary ride that is full of surprises. Do you think if you knew in advance where the roller coaster stops or picks up speed you would be as scared as you are?

RAY: I don't know.

THERAPIST: How would it be to find out?

RAY: OK, I guess.

THERAPIST: Let's give it a try. First, let's read the worksheet together. (*Reads together with Ray.*) Go ahead and draw the type of train your fear would look like.

RAY: Can I use whatever colors I want?

THERAPIST: It's your fear, so it's all up to you.

RAY: OK. I'm going to make it really bright red. (*Draws the train.*)

THERAPIST: Let's pretend your worries and fears are passengers or riders on this train. Which ones would be riding on your bright red train?

RAY: The worries about other kids not liking me or my teacher being mean to me.

THERAPIST: OK. Let's see where this train goes. You move the train along the tracks to each station. Each station has its own name. Go ahead and read each station's name.

Self-Monitoring with Adolescents

Self-monitoring with older children and adolescents is generally straightforward. Silverman and Kurtines (1996) designed the *Fear Thermometer* as a useful self-monitoring tool. The Fear Thermometer is a drawing of a thermometer with different gradients of fear. Teens could draw their own Fear Thermometers or you could supply them with blank illustrations. Regardless of how these Fear Thermometers are drawn, we think it is important that the adolescent determines the rating scale or fear degrees. Thus, for some teens, a 1–5 scale will meet their needs; others may want to design a 1–100 scale. Adolescents should be encouraged to complete the Fear Thermometer in any way they like. For instance, some young people prefer to simply circle the degrees of fear on the Fear Thermometer. Others may want to shade in the mercury in the Fear Thermometer to reflect their fear level.

Self-report instruments such as the RCMAS or the MASC are also useful self-monitoring tools for adolescents. Teens can take the inventories on a regular basis (we generally recommend once per week for 4 weeks). Scores should then be graphed and given to the adolescent as a way to self-monitor. The scores could then be used as cues for coping and problem solving (e.g., "What do you do when you feel shy at a 3?").

RELAXATION TRAINING

Relaxation training seems best suited for anxious children with somatic complaints (Eisen & Silverman, 1993). Relaxation training requires youngsters to focus on their breathing and muscle tension. Ruminative children will have difficulty focusing attention on their bodily cues. In these instances, we work on the ruminative cognitions first or concurrently with the relaxation. Relaxation training also involves somewhat elaborate instructions. Care should be directed at making instructions concrete and understandable, especially for younger children.

Highly restless anxious children will be a challenge for a therapist teaching relaxation techniques. It is hard to get the child to relax if he/she can't sit still! Sports metaphors might be helpful for these children (Sommers-Flannagan & Sommers-Flannagan, 1995). For instance, you could prep the child by showing him/her an athlete on videotape engaging in relaxation. The child and therapist could watch basketball, baseball, or tennis players as they ready themselves for a foul shot, important pitch, or big point. Videotape is a good idea because you can match the child's interest, gender, and ethnicity with an appropriate model. You can also stop and review each tape with the child (e.g., "What is the player doing to relax? How still is he/she?").

Simplifying the procedure will also help. Relaxation can become a graduated task. For instance, you may start progressive muscle relaxation with just one or two muscle groups (Kendall et al., 1992). Then, with the child's increasing skill, you could add other muscle groups. Often, youngsters have difficulty grasping the tension–relaxation phase of muscle relaxation. Squeeze toys, whistles, and other toys can be helpful and add to the fun (Cautela & Groden, 1978, as cited by Morris & Kratochwill, 1998). When a youngster properly tenses a muscle group, he/she gets a response (e.g., the squeezy duck quacks) that tells him/her that he/she is doing the skill properly. Similarly, blowing through a whistle or blowing bubbles teaches a child the fundamentals of controlled breathing (Warfield, 1999).

For some youngsters, the act of focusing on their bodily sensations is itself anxiety producing. Anxiety-sensitive children scan their bodies for any signal of distress and catastrophically misinterpret normal bodily reactions (Kendall et al., 1991; Vasey, 1993). Accordingly, progressive muscle relaxation and controlled breathing might be perceived as quite threatening by such children. In these cases, setting up the relaxation as an experiment might help (e.g., "What do you predict might happen?"). Children may also fear losing control. Using cognitive techniques to test out children's expectations is also productive. The following transcript illustrates how to work with a child's fear of sensations related to the relaxation procedure.

THERAPIST: You look uncomfortable, Irma.

IRMA: I'm worried that I'm not going to catch my breath. It feels like I might go out of control.

THERAPIST: I see. Do you think we could test it out and practice the breathing to see what happens?

IRMA: I don't know. If I start to lose control and can't catch my breath, can we stop?

THERAPIST: Of course. You're in charge of how long we do the relaxation. How long do you think we can try it before you start to worry about losing control?

IRMA: Maybe 2 minutes.

THERAPIST: Let's shoot for that. We'll stop before that if you want to, and if you don't get worried we can go for a little longer. How does that sound?

What does this exchange demonstrate? The relaxation procedure and Irma's fears were set up as a graduated experiment. If Irma tolerated the relaxation for 2 minutes or more, the relaxation procedure could be extended the next time. If 2 minutes was too long for her, the therapist would need to shorten the procedure and attend to any additional fears and beliefs she has about the procedure and focusing on her bodily sensations.

SYSTEMATIC DESENSITIZATION

In this section, we present an example of a 14-year-old boy who is highly fearful of his ninth-grade state proficiency test. The example illustrates many of the pivotal steps in constructing an impactful systematic desensitization. Let's call our young client Herman. Herman completed the hierarchy by assigning SUDS to 10 situations (see Figure 12.4). As you can see, the items reflect a temporal–spatial hierarchy with each circumstance reflecting how close in time and physical space Herman is to the testing.

The next step is to ask Herman to write out in as much detail as possible the physiological, mood, behavioral, cognitive, and interpersonal aspects of his fear. Let's say Herman, like most other 14-year-olds, does not fully report all these elements. You will need to help him flesh out the relevant details in order to construct a vibrant image. You might ask him questions such as "Who is around you?"; "How do they look?"; "What do you imagine they are thinking about you?"; "What does the room look like?"; "What does your body feel like?"; and so on until you are confident you have a robust image. Further, we recommend that the images be multisensorial (Padesky, 1988). Therefore, you might try to have Herman imagine the sights, sounds, smells, and tactile sensations embedded in the situation. By doing so, both Herman and you can get a "feel" for the situation. Figure 12.5 presents an example of a robust scene.

Herman needs to be skilled in relaxation imagery before he can formally begin the desensitization procedure. This imagery training should be paired with the bodily relaxation procedures we described in the previ-

SUDS	SCENE
10	Day of proficiency test, sitting in class with booklet being passed out. Starting to panic in class.
9	Walking to school on day of test worried about passing. Other kids talking about test while waiting to enter school.
8	Night before proficiency test, laying in bed worrying about failing.
7	Three days before test. Teachers seeming stressed. Lots of last-minute reviews. Think I am coming down with a cold.
6	Five or six days before test. Worrying, I can't remember what I studied. Teachers getting critical. Parents getting worried.
5	Week before test. Lots of practice tests. Parents talking about it a lot.
4	Month before test. Talking to other kids about test. Comparing scores on practice test. Sitting in review sessions.
3	Couple of months before the test. Sitting in auditorium being oriented to test. Hearing "horror" stories from teachers about students who don't prepare.
2	Six months or so. Study sessions start. Wonder what group I will be in.
1	Summer before school. Read newspaper article about tests. Talk to friends about it.

FIGURE 12.4. Herman's hierarchy.

It's the day of the proficiency test. My palms are really sweaty. My heart is beating really fast and I think I can feel it pounding. I think I am getting a slight headache and won't be able to concentrate. I feel light-headed. The noises seem really distracting. The other kids' voices sound almost like buzzing. People are squirming around, kind of shuffling at their desks. They are so nervous. They are fidgety and dropping stuff. There is a line of kids by the pencil sharpener. I check and double check my pencils and my pencil sharpener. My hands are sweating so much sweat is on my desk and on my pencil sharpener. Tests are being passed out and I hear moans from the other kids. The papers are rustling. The chair feels hard on my back and my shirt collar feels rough and tight around my neck. Almost like a noose. The room smells kind of like wet books. I grab my test and the paper sticks to my hands. I feel a little faint and nauseous as I look at the instructions. I worry my mind will go blank. I almost see myself running out of the room screaming and all the kids are shocked and laughing. All this work is wasted, I think.

FIGURE 12.5. Example of one of Herman's scenes. SUDS: 10.

ous section and in Chapter 8. When I (RDF) think about introducing the positive imagery technique to youngsters, I am reminded of the movie *Happy Gilmore*. In the movie, Happy, an aspiring golfer who is betrayed by his unbridled rage, is taught to imagine his "happy place." This simple phrase can be used to describe pleasant imagery to youngsters. You can instruct them to create a happy, safe psychological space in their mind. In this space, they can imagine themselves as calm, relaxed, satisfied, and in control as they do some of their favorite activities. Once the youngsters have created their happy place they are ready to begin to juxtapose their anxiety-producing situations with the happy place's images and bodily relaxation techniques.

As noted in Chapter 8, you begin with the lowest item on the hierarchy and then move up toward the highest rated items. If the child reports anxiety during the presentation of the scene, end the scene and instruct the youngster to return to his happy place. The following exchange picks up at a point where Herman and his therapist are working on Item 8 and Herman has just completed his relaxation and positive imagery induction.

THERAPIST: Herman, lift your finger when you feel in a calm, relaxed, and confident state.

HERMAN: (*Lifts his finger.*)

THERAPIST: Now gently lower your finger. You are in a deep relaxed state. You are feeling calm and confident. I am now going to ask you to imagine in your mind's eye the scene where you are walking to school on the day of the proficiency test. You leave your house hearing the door slamming behind you, crashing like a drum roll. Your head starts to pound and your stomach is churning. You seem to be walking in slow motion and your legs feel heavy. Worries about passing the test and having to take it over and over go through your head. Lift your finger if you are able to picture this scene.

HERMAN: (*Slowly lifts his finger.*)

THERAPIST: Now, gently lower your finger.

HERMAN: (*Lowers his finger.*)

THERAPIST: Hold onto this scene and picture it as if it is happening to you. Bring it into focus just like you were fine-tuning a TV show. When your image is really clear, scan your body for signs of anxiety. Then use your breathing to rid yourself of the fears.

HERMAN: (*After a brief pause, uses the breathing technique.*)

THERAPIST: When you feel relaxed, lift your finger.

HERMAN: (*Lifts his finger.*)

THERAPIST: Now we are going to change the scene a little more. As you are walking to school, you meet up with a group of other kids. You see the fear and anxiety in their faces. It sounds like their voices are going really fast. You heard them talking about possible questions and you feel panicky. Your heart is pounding and you feel out of breath. You worry that you can't think of any answers. When you have this scene clearly in your mind's eye, slowly raise your finger.

HERMAN: (*Raises his finger.*)

THERAPIST: If you are feeling anxious, raise your finger.

HERMAN: (*Raises his finger.*)

THERAPIST: Hold onto this image for a bit. Now, with the power of your breathing and imagery skills, see if you can reduce your anxiety when you see this picture of yourself.

What does this exchange teach us? First, the imagery includes various sensory modalities. Second, the therapist was careful not to reinforce Herman's relaxation by saying "Good" or "Good job" when he did not report anxiety. Third, the therapist worked slowly and deliberately, making sure Herman was seeing the scene in his mind's eye and experiencing the accompanying anxiety.

SOCIAL SKILLS TRAINING

In this section, we illustrate several social skills intervention components with Dannica, an 11-year-old girl who is being teased by her classmates. Dannica is a bright yet socially awkward girl who does not know what to say or do when her classmates taunt her. She becomes very posturally stiff, verbally inexpressive, and cognitively rigid in these interactions.

The first social skill we taught her was ignoring and walking away. We taught her to relax; take a deep breath; say to herself, "Just because they call me a slob does not make me one"; say nothing to her tormentors; and calmly walk away. These strategies were written down and recorded on index cards. Additionally, Dannica was taught to engage in another task (e.g., do a math exercise) to distract herself from the teasing.

The ignoring technique was initially successful, but over time it became annoying and burdensome for Dannica. Since ignoring is a passive solution, her anxiety and frustration built up, compromising her concentration in school. Dannica needed to see herself as more in control. The ignoring did not change her perception of herself as a victim.

Subsequently, we taught Dannica "fogging." *Fogging* is an assertiveness technique that disarms teasers (Feindler & Guttman, 1994). When you "fog" a teaser, you agree with the tease. By acting nonplussed and responding with humor, the teased child disappoints his/her teasers, who are looking for a strong negative reaction. Dannica was initially taught the fogging technique via puppet play in the following exchange.

THERAPIST: OK, Danni, let's use these puppets to learn what to do when the other kids tease you.

DANNICA: How can we do that?

THERAPIST: Well, you decide what puppets we will use. We'll pretend the puppets are the other kids teasing you. What do you want to play?

DANNICA: I'll play myself.

THERAPIST: What will your plan be if the kids tease you?

DANNICA: Ignore them.

THERAPIST: How about trying to use fogging?

DANNICA: Oh yeah.

THERAPIST: Let's start playing. What puppet is going to be you?

DANNICA: I'll be the giraffe because I'm so tall. Elly will be the tiger because I think she is fierce.

THERAPIST: So I'll play Elly. Remember, try to use fogging when I tease you.

DANNICA: OK, I'll try.

THERAPIST: Now, what is your giraffe's name and what is my tiger's name.

DANNICA: Umm. Let's see. My name is Rosy and your name is Rory.

THERAPIST: OK. I'll start. Oh, Rosy, you are so geeky looking with your long neck.

DANNICA: I'm not going to listen to you.

THERAPIST: What a big baby you are. Baby, baby, baaa-by! What are you going to do, tell the teacher? What a real dweeb you are.

DANNICA: (*Pretending to talk to another animal.*)

THERAPIST: (*Coming out of role.*) Danni, what was it like to do this?

DANNICA: I felt nervous—like I didn't know what to do.

THERAPIST: How much is that like what happens at school?

DANNICA: Pretty much.

THERAPIST: What went through your mind?

DANNICA: She's going to get over on me. Everyone will see how nervous I am.

THERAPIST: OK. So you have to take charge in a way. Do you think fogging might help?

DANNICA: I don't know.

THERAPIST: Let's try. How could you use fogging with Rory?

DANNICA: I don't know.

THERAPIST: Let me see if I can help you. I'll share my ideas about fogging with you. Let's see. I'll play Rosy and try to do fogging. You tease Rosy with your tiger.

DANNICA: OK. That will be fun. Rosy, you are so gawky. Why don't you ever wash your hair, it's so yellow.

THERAPIST: Thanks for the advice. My hair is really yellow.

DANNICA: Yellow. Yellow. You really need my advice. Your fur is so matted down. You are afraid of the ball in class. You are a scaredy-cat too. So afraid of the ball.

THERAPIST: Wow! You really pay attention to me. I know you think I'm scared of the ball.

DANNICA: You are. Scaredy-cat. Yellow scaredy-cat.

THERAPIST: You sure do think you know me. (*Coming out of role.*) Danni, what was it like for you when I was fogging.

DANNICA: It made it hard to keep teasing. I don't know if I can think of things to say.

THERAPIST: We'll write some things on cards for you to practice and remember. Are you willing to try it?

What does this dialogue teach us? First, the practice puppet play revealed that Dannica did not have the skills to cope with continued teasing. She had not sufficiently acquired the fogging technique. Accordingly, the therapist switched roles to model the fogging tactic for her. Second, the therapist and Dannica will write down effective fogging statements so Dannica will have a script. Third, the therapist and Dannica will switch roles once again so Dannica can practice more with fogging.

Observation is another way to build social skills. In addition to directly teaching Dannica ignoring, fogging, and assertiveness skills, we worked with her to observe how the other children in her class handled teasing. She noted how many other kids were teased and how they coped.

She also identified the positive and negative consequences of each strategy. Then she drew conclusions about which were the best options based on her observations.

Finally, Dannica needed to experiment with her newly acquired skills. Thus, we had her complete a modified tease diary when she was mocked (see Figure 12.6). We asked her to write down each situation in which she was teased. Then she recorded her feelings, thoughts, coping behaviors, and their success. By doing so, she practiced applying her coping skills and registered their degree of success.

COGNITIVE SELF-CONTROL

Talking Back to Fear is a self-control/self-instructional technique to help youngsters construct coping thoughts that challenge beliefs associated with their anxious feelings. The Talking Back to Fear skill is a relatively simple approach that may be a good initial step with anxious children. The Talking Back to Fear Worksheet is presented in Figure 12.7. The following transcript offers an example of the way you might present the task to the child.

> "We've really heard your fear talking today. When you were worried, you thought your teacher will think you are stupid and your parents will feel really badly if you don't do well. You worried that everyone will notice how much you messed up. Your fear talked you out of what you knew you could do. The fear kind of bullied you. So I'm going to teach you how to talk back to your fear."

How I was teased	How I felt	What went through my mind	What I did to handle it	How it worked (t = terrible g = great)

FIGURE 12.6. Dannica's tease diary.

My fear says: _____

Here are some things you could say to yourself that can help you **talk back** to your scared feelings:

- Scared feelings are like the wind. They blow over you and then they are gone.
- Everybody feels scared sometimes. These feelings just make me human.
- These feelings are just signals to use my new skills.
- I know I can do this. The main reason I think I can't is because I feel scared. I just have to remember it's my fear talking.
- Keep cool. I can talk back to my fear.

Write down five more things you can say to yourself to **TALK BACK TO YOUR FEAR:**

1. _____
2. _____
3. _____
4. _____
5. _____

Write down all these ways to talk back to your fear on index cards. Read them over twice a day.

FIGURE 12.7. Talking Back to Fear Worksheet. From Friedberg and McClure (2002). Copyright by The Guilford Press. Permission to photocopy this figure is granted to purchasers of this book for personal use only (see copyright page for details).

The Talking Back to Fear skill includes several phases. In the first phase, the therapist teaches and models coping statements. In the second phase, the children craft their own coping statements. In the third phase, youngsters write down their personalized coping statements on an index card. Youngsters can put the statements in their pocket, wallet, or purse, and carry them to situations where they might become anxious. The Talking Back to Fear Worksheet systematizes this process for youngsters (see Figure 12.7).

Figure 12.8 shows a completed Talking Back to Fear Worksheet. The youngster's fearful inner voice told him he would "mess up" his oral book report. He then circled several prepared coping statements he believed would quiet the fear. Next, he wrote down five more ways he could talk back to his fear. Finally, he transposed these coping statements onto index cards. Thus, he was able to access a relatively full deck of coping skills.

My fear says: <u>I will mess up my oral book report.</u>

Here are some things you could say to yourself that can help you **talk back** to your scared feelings:

- Scared feelings are like the wind. They blow over you and then they are gone.
- Everybody feels scared sometimes. These feelings just make me human.
- These feelings are just signals to use my new skills.
- I know I can do this. The main reason I think I can't is because I feel scared. I just have to remember it's my fear talking.
- Keep cool. I can talk back to my fear.

Write down five more things you can say to yourself to **TALK BACK TO YOUR FEAR:**

1. <u>I am bigger than my fear.</u>
2. <u>This is just my fear talking. I don't have to listen to it.</u>
3. <u>My fear doesn't know what is going to happen. I can handle this.</u>
4. <u>Every time I face my fear I get stronger. I can stand up to my fear.</u>
5. <u>My fear is bullying me. I need to talk back to it. My fear will break down.</u>

Write down all these ways to talk back to your fear on index cards. Read them over twice a day.

FIGURE 12.8. Sample Talking Back to Fear Worksheet.

The Talking Back to Fear skill set can be a springboard to other experiential/play exercises. For example, puppet play is a natural extension of the exercise. You can set up the exercise by having the child pick two puppets. One puppet will represent the child's adaptive self-talk while the other puppet will represent his/her fear talking. The child can be asked which role he/she wants to play. Children who are well skilled in talking back to their fear may be encouraged to play the adaptive self-talk role first. For children who are not as well skilled, you should play the adaptive self-talk puppet role. In this way, you could model how to talk back to fear for the child.

When children first play this game, they may have trouble accessing the coping statements. Therefore, we recommend that you remind your clients that they can use their coping card deck. Readily available coping materials boost children's confidence. Moreover, this strategy reinforces the notion that carrying the cards with you is a good idea.

As children become better practiced with the skills, you can increase the task difficulty. For example, when you play the fear's voice, you could increase the frequency and intensity of the catastrophic predictions. The anxiety-producing cognitions are well-practiced beliefs and consequently will not relent easily. Thus, you should encourage youngsters to be persistent with their coping self-talk.

Often young children's excessive worry is punctuated by "What if" questions (Lerner et al., 1999). For example, "What if I have a test and forget everything I studied" may pop into their heads. *Dreadful Iffy* is an exercise that simplifies the decatastrophizing process and teaches youngsters to challenge their dire predictions. The Defeating Dreadful Iffy Worksheet (see Figure 12.9) includes a self-monitoring component and a change technique embedded within its content. First, children record their worrisome "What if" question. Then they work themselves through five successive questions and derive a conclusion that helps them "Talk Back to Dreadful Iffy."

You may elect to introduce the Dreadful Iffy exercise in the following manner:

> "Many times when boys and girls worry, they wonder 'What if?' For example, one time a boy was on his way to a party and worried, 'What if the other boys and girls make fun of me?' Another example is when a girl worried the night before the first day of school, 'What if I don't do well in my new grade?' This is called 'Dreadful Iffy Thinking.' When you do Dreadful Iffy Thinking, you start to stay away from the things you fear. You guess that the worst is going to happen and you will not be able to handle things. Listening to Dreadful Iffy Thinking just makes you feel worse. So we are going to learn to talk back to Dreadful Iffy so we can defeat him."

Many times when you worry, you wonder, "What if something bad happens?" You sometimes guess that the worst is going to happen and you won't be able to handle it. This is called **Dreadful Iffy thinking**. Let's use this worksheet to **Defeat Dreadful Iffy**.

When I worry what if . . .

_____

_____

_____ I feel really scared and worried.

Ask yourself questions:
How sure am I that what I am worrying about will really happen? Circle one.

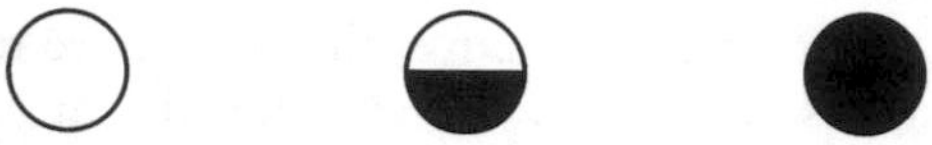

Not sure   Pretty sure   Very sure

Has it ever happened before? Circle one.

YES   NO

If it has not happened in the past, what makes me think it will happen now?

_____

_____

If I have handled it in the past, how dreadful is it really? Circle one.

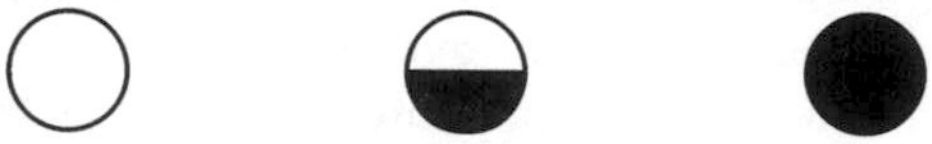

Very dreadful   Kind of dreadful   Not dreadful

Now that you have answered these questions, what is a new way to talk back to Dreadful Iffy?

_____

_____

_____

_____

FIGURE 12.9. Defeating Dreadful Iffy Worksheet. From Friedberg and McClure (2002). Copyright by The Guilford Press. Permission to photocopy this figure is granted to purchasers of this book for personal use only (see copyright page for details).

The first prompt on the worksheet asks the child to write down his/her anxious prediction. You should help the child write as specific a question, worry, or prediction as possible. Further, you should check that the material recorded is psychologically meaningful and associated with appropriate levels of emotional intensity.

The questioning or testing process is introduced with two basic questions: "How sure am I that what I am worrying about will really happen?" and "Has it every happened before?" The child chooses between three choices (Not sure, Pretty sure, and Very sure) for the first question and two choices (Yes/No) for the second question. Question 3 follows from Question 2 and asks the child to list his/her previous coping efforts. If the circumstance the child worries about has never happened before, the child skips Question 3 and proceeds to Question 4. Question 4 asks for the basis of the worry: "What makes me think it will happen now?" Responses to this question will help the therapist and the child evaluate whether the worry is well founded.

Question 5 follows from Question 3. Question 5—"If you have handled it in the past, how dreadful is it really?"—is a Socratic question designed to create some dissonance by juxtaposing previous coping with predicted disaster. This question helps the child access heretofore neglected coping resources and apply them to current circumstances.

Question 6, the summary question, asks the child to consider his/her responses to the previous questions. After reviewing his/her responses, the child derives a conclusion. This conclusion can then be recorded on an index card and used as a coping statement. A sample of a completed Defeating Dreadful Iffy Worksheet is included in Figure 12.10.

There are several ways you can increase the fun level associated with Dreadful Iffy. First, a sample Dreadful Iffy cartoon is included with this worksheet exercise. The child can color in this cartoon as he/she talks about his/her dreadful thoughts. Second, since the skill set is entitled "Defeating Dreadful Iffy," the child can be instructed to put an X through the cartoon whenever he/she talks back to his/her disastrous predictions. Third, the child can make a Dreadful Iffy hand puppet by pasting the cartoon on a brown paper sandwich bag. Therapist and child can role-play talking back to Dreadful Iffy in a manner similar to the puppet play suggested in the Talking Back to Fear skill set. For example, the puppet play may include a sandwich bag puppet and another puppet with a child's self-portrait drawn on it. If the child prefers, he/she can draw or paste a picture of a hero or coping model instead of a self-portrait. The child's puppet and the Dreadful Iffy puppet might engage in an animated discussion where the hero talks back to Dreadful Iffy. The following transcript illustrates the way children might talk back to Dreadful Iffy.

Many times when you worry, you wonder, "What if something bad happens?" You sometimes guess that the worst is going to happen and you won't be able to handle it. This is called **Dreadful Iffy thinking**. Let's use this worksheet to **Defeat Dreadful Iffy**.

When I worry what if . . .

<u>Something bad happens to me or my mom or dad or brother</u>

_____

_____ I feel really scared and worried.

Ask yourself questions:
How sure am I that what I am worrying about will really happen? Circle one.

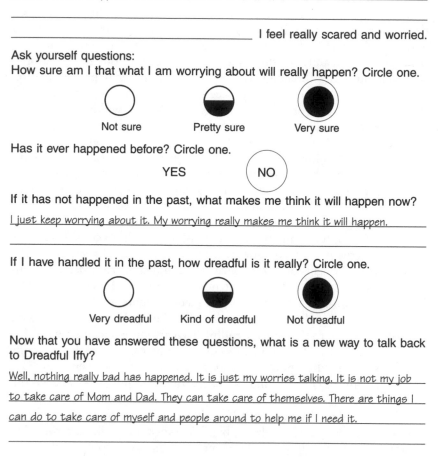

Not sure   Pretty sure   Very sure

Has it ever happened before? Circle one.

YES   (NO)

If it has not happened in the past, what makes me think it will happen now?

<u>I just keep worrying about it. My worrying really makes me think it will happen.</u>

_____

If I have handled it in the past, how dreadful is it really? Circle one.

Very dreadful   Kind of dreadful   Not dreadful

Now that you have answered these questions, what is a new way to talk back to Dreadful Iffy?

<u>Well, nothing really bad has happened. It is just my worries talking. It is not my job</u>
<u>to take care of Mom and Dad. They can take care of themselves. There are things I</u>
<u>can do to take care of myself and people around to help me if I need it.</u>

_____

FIGURE 12.10. Sample Defeating Dreadful Iffy Worksheet.

THERAPIST: You did a good job making these puppets. Do you want to have a puppet show where you talk back to Dreadful Iffy?

RUBIN: Sure.

THERAPIST: Who do you want to play?

RUBIN: I'll play myself.

THERAPIST: Then I'll be Dreadful Iffy. Now I'll start to say lots of things Dreadful Iffy might say to you when you get nervous. You have to use your puppet to talk back to Dreadful Iffy.

RUBIN: I'll get you, Dreadful Iffy puppet!

THERAPIST: That's right but also use your Dreadful Iffy skills and your Talking Back to Fear skills.

RUBIN: OK.

THERAPIST: Are you ready to play?

RUBIN: Yes, let's play.

THERAPIST: Oh no. I have to go up in front of the class to do long division. The kids are going to laugh at me and the teacher is going to yell at me. Everybody's going to think I'm stupid.

RUBIN: No, they won't.

THERAPIST: You don't know that. I know that everyone will laugh at me. They'll not want to play with me. I'll get so scared that I'll throw up right in front of the class.

RUBIN: Shut up Dreadful Iffy! You're stupid! I'm strong!

THERAPIST: Let's stop here for a second. When Dreadful Iffy is saying these things, how do you feel?

RUBIN: Bad!

THERAPIST: What is making you feel badly?

RUBIN: Dreadful Iffy is mean.

THERAPIST: When you get really worried, how easy is it for you to think up things to say to yourself to help you feel less worried?

RUBIN: Not very easy.

THERAPIST: This is what this puppet play is all about. It's a chance for you to practice the things you can say to yourself that will help you feel better. What do you think about looking over your Dreadful Iffy worksheets and Talking Back to Fear worksheets and writing helpful statements down on your index cards so you will already have some things to say.

RUBIN: Can I keep the cards and read them?

THERAPIST: Of course.

> (*Rubin and the therapist review the worksheets and transcribe some coping statements onto index cards. Then they engage in more role-playing practice.*)

Anticipatory anxiety is likely related to children's catastrophizing. Anxious children subjectively imagine dangers where no objective danger exists. They predict disaster and they act as if their predictions are totally reliable. Several cognitive-behavioral clinicians refer to inaccurate catastrophic predictions as "false alarms" (Craske & Barlow, 2001; A. T. Beck et al., 1985). Thus, as therapists, we need to help youngsters view their "alarming" predictions with greater skepticism.

For older children and adolescents, behavioral experiments are good tools. Behavioral experiments are designed to test the reliability of the child's predictions. For instance, 16-year-old Nia believed that unless she worried about things, something bad would happen. The following transcript illustrates the way you may set up a behavioral experiment to test this belief.

THERAPIST: Nia, what belief should we test?

NIA: I guess the one where I think if I don't worry something bad will happen.

THERAPIST: Well, what do you suppose the worrying prevents?

NIA: Something bad happening.

THERAPIST: So what do we need to keep track of?

NIA: Whether something bad happens.

THERAPIST: Do we need to connect it to anything?

NIA: How much I worry.

THERAPIST: Good. Let's make a couple of columns. [see Figure 12.11]. We'll call the first one "How much I worry." What should we put in this column?

NIA: Maybe I could grade my worries from like 1 to 10. Just like we do on the thought diaries.

THERAPIST: Exactly. Which is high and which is low?

NIA: 1 is just a few worries and 10 is the most worries.

THERAPIST: OK. We'll rate your worries on a scale from 1 to 10. We'll call the next column "The bad thing that happened." In this column, you

DATE	HOW MUCH I WORRY (level of worry)	THE BAD THING THAT HAPPENED	HOW BAD WAS IT?
Mon.	5	Nothing	0
Tues.	6	Nothing	0
Wed.	7	Nothing	0
Thurs.	5	Pop quiz that I was not expecting	3
Fri.	8	Nothing	0

FIGURE 12.11. Nia's experiment.

write down any bad thing that happened over the week. The last column we'll call "How bad was it?" because not all bad things are the same. Some could be disasters and some could just be a hassle. How should we keep track of this?

NIA: On another grading scale. Maybe 1 to 10?

THERAPIST: OK, let's do that. Now, we can check out several things about this. First, does your worrying prevent bad things from happening? Second, does the amount you worry have any influence on how bad things go? If you worry less, will things turn out worse?

NIA: I'm not sure.

THERAPIST: I know. That's why we're going to check it out.

What can we take from this exchange? First, the therapist worked with Nia to concretely test her perceived correlation between worrying and preventing something bad from happening. Second, the therapist also designed the task so it would address the severity of the worry. By doing so, Nia could discern whether the amount of worrying would ward off dreaded outcomes. Finally, by recording the amount of worrying and any negative outcomes side by side, Nia could see that worrying and the nonoccurrence of bad things happening were unrelated.

Many anxious children in general and most socially phobic children in particular fear others' ridicule or criticism. Their social behavior is severely limited by their fears. Their emotional, cognitive, and behavioral responses are stiff and rigid. Next, we will present ways for therapists to teach children how to lessen their fears of negative evaluation and cope with potential criticism or embarrassment.

Children who fear others' judgments and appraisals possess several blind spots in their thinking. First, like socially anxious adults, they confuse fact with opinion (Burns, 1980). Anxious youngsters generally are quite approval seeking and see others' opinions as indisputable gospel. In short, they unwittingly question their own competence and their identity is based on frequently ill-founded criticisms or other comments by peers.

We have found the *Just because* technique to be a productive intervention (Elliott, 1991). The technique does not require much rational analysis and it can provide the child with much needed perspective. In this task, the youngster debunks the myth that opinions equal fact (e.g., "Just because Ernie thinks I'm stupid does not mean that I am."). The child first captures the negative thought (e.g., "Jill and Susan will think I'm immature."). Then, he/she simply inserts the "just because" phrase prefacing the negative automatic thought (e.g., "Just because Jill and Susan think I am immature does not mean I am.").

The "Just because" technique can be followed by more sophisticated rational analysis. While others' evaluations naturally have greater or less relative degrees of importance, rarely does another's opinion *absolutely* define oneself. In the following transcript, examine the way the therapist and 15-year-old Marla Socratically evaluate fears of negative evaluation.

MARLA: The girls in my class really annoy me. I worry all the time about what they think.

THERAPIST: What is it that they say that you worry about?

MARLA: I worry that they will make fun of the way I talk and what I wear.

THERAPIST: You really feel uncomfortable around these girls. What goes through your mind?

MARLA: They think I'm not with it. You know, that I'm not as good as them. They think that they know how to wear their hair and how to act. They seem to think I'm so 5 minutes ago.

THERAPIST: How will they criticize you?

MARLA: They'll think my clothes are bad or I act weird or something like that.

THERAPIST: I see. How well do you know these girls?

MARLA: They're in my class.

THERAPIST: Do you hang around with them?

MARLA: No, not really.

THERAPIST: Have you ever gone to their houses?

MARLA: No, never.

THERAPIST: Have they ever gone to your house?

MARLA: No.

THERAPIST: Ever been to a party or a movie with them?

MARLA: Never.

THERAPIST: So how well do they know you?

MARLA: Not well at all.

THERAPIST: Hmm. That's curious. So they don't know you well? And yet you seem to give them a lot of power over defining who you are. What do you make of that?

MARLA: I don't know.

THERAPIST: Well, that might be something for us to consider. The other thing I was wondering is, who made them the experts on fashion and behavior?

MARLA: I don't know. I guess I made them the experts.

THERAPIST: I see. But how can they be experts on your "coolness" and your fashions when they don't really even know you?

In this example, Marla clearly defined herself through the eyes of these other girls. The therapist helped her recognize that these youngsters held a very narrow view of her. In fact, they did not know her at all! Second, the therapist worked at evaluating the foundation for the "experts' " opinion (e.g., "Who made them the experts on fashion and behavior?"). Finally, the therapist juxtaposed all the information with a Socratic question (e.g., "How can they be experts on your 'coolness' when they don't really even know you?").

Being stung by teasing mockery and criticism is made doubly painful by children's expectation that they should be liked by everyone. They often feel that if a child or a group of children ridicule them, then they are unpopular or rejected by all children. Simply, they overgeneralize and engage in all-or-none thinking. Therapy should guide the child toward the recognition that some children will like them, others will dislike them, and still others won't have strong feelings either way.

There are various ways to help youngsters cope with negative peer reactions. For the child who becomes dismayed by the mistaken belief "Nobody likes me" when other children make fun of him/her, we create a type of test of evidence. For instance, we invite the child to make three lists. The first one includes all the children who make fun of him/her, the second has the names of children he/she considers nice who are his/her friends, and the third holds the names of children who are kind of in between and don't have strong feelings either way. The child then compares the three lists and constructs a conclusion. The following exchange illustrates the process.

ANDY: Nobody likes me. They say I throw like a girl and I'm a dweeb. They laugh at me when I play sports. I don't have any friends.

THERAPIST: Andy, would you like to check that out using a new tool.

ANDY: OK, Dr. Bob.

THERAPIST: Let's take this sheet and make three columns. The first is the kids who make fun of you. Write down all their names.

ANDY: What color pencil should I use?

THERAPIST: Whichever one you like.

ANDY: I hate the color green so I'll use that one.

THERAPIST: OK, next list all the children who are nice to you and you think are your friends.

ANDY: OK. I'll use my favorite color for that one.

THERAPIST: Now list the kids who you know but you don't hang out with and who don't pick on you.

ANDY: Kind of like the kids who can take or leave me?

THERAPIST: Exactly.

ANDY: OK.

THERAPIST: Good job! Now, lay these lists down side by side. Which lists have the most names?

ANDY: My friends.

THERAPIST: Which has the least names?

ANDY: The mean kids.

THERAPIST: I see. Now, how is it possible that nobody likes you if your friends outnumber the kids who pick on you?

ANDY: It isn't. It just feels that way sometimes.

THERAPIST: I know it does. So when it feels that way sometimes, what can you say to yourself?

ANDY: This may feel bad but most other kids like me.

THERAPIST: What about this third column?

ANDY: Well, most kids like me, some don't care either way, and only two kids pick on me.

THERAPIST: What does that mean?

ANDY: Most kids like me.

THERAPIST: Let's write these new thoughts down on index cards.

Younger children will need more concrete stimuli when working through this belief. I (RDF) learned an inventive way from Dr. Christine Padesky to do a similar test of evidence with a young child. In an exercise called the *Friend Game*, we drew faces on strips of paper. A happy face represented a friend, a sad or angry face represented someone who is not a friend, and a blank slip of paper represented a child who was neutral. You want to create more friend slips than not friend or neutral slips. The game begins with each player taking a turn by picking a slip of paper. Each player puts a friend slip, not a friend slip, and a neutral slip in a pile. At the end of the game, each player counts the numbers in each pile and then the child is asked to make a conclusion comparing the different amounts in each pile (e.g., "Can I still have lots of friends even if some boys and girls don't like me?"). As you can see, this playfully simplifies the kind of work presented in the Andy transcript.

EXPOSURE

Exposure- or performance-based treatments provide children with opportunities for greater self-control and self-determination. It is important that they see themselves as collaborating and participating in the experience rather than seeing exposure as something that is done to them. Adam is a 9-year-old, highly intelligent, athletic, socially skilled boy who fears elevators. He fears that the elevator will crash or become stuck between floors. If the elevator becomes stuck, Adam predicts he will suffocate.

Graduated performance-based treatment for Adam began with relaxation and self-instructional skills. Adam learned to modulate his physiological arousal and develop coping thoughts. Treatment then progressed to graduated exposure opportunities and rational analysis skills. He recorded his anxiety level and his thoughts and feelings about riding elevators. He also gathered information about elevator operation and crashes. After collecting data, Adam concluded that while elevator crashes and injuries were possible, they were highly improbable.

Adam was now ready for greater exposure to his fear: the elevator.

We began with Adam determining how close he would stand to an elevator and how long he could tolerate the anxiety. As the first step in the hierarchy of approaching the elevator, Adam stood about 12 feet away from and around the corner from an elevator. As he stood there, I (RDF) verbalized his anxiety-producing thoughts (e.g., "Oh no. I'm going to have to go in the elevator. It will get stuck and there won't be enough air to breathe. I'll turn blue and die."). Adam successfully mastered several more steps in the hierarchy, each time moving closer to the elevator. Soon, he was at the elevator door, looking in. To my amazement, he then volunteered to step inside. At first, he entered timidly. Then we examined the elevator car together. Adam quickly identified the "rescue" factors in the elevator (e.g., the telephone and emergency bell). Then he proclaimed, "I'm ready to ride."

Next, we developed a hierarchy for riding. Riding just with me was the easiest for Adam (e.g., "There is more air for me, you could calm me down or know what to do if we got stuck."); riding in a half-full car was more difficult for him; and riding with a full car of people was most anxiety producing. Naturally, we began with the lowest rung on the hierarchy.

What does Adam's example teach us? First, Adam stayed in charge of his exposure by collaboratively designing tasks with his therapist. Second, the use of facilitative skills enabled him to profit from the exposure tasks. Third, imaginal "exposures" such as collecting information about elevators and watching a documentary on elevators paved the way for his fuller exposures.

Creating exposure opportunities for children can be challenging. First, remember that most exposures should be carried out in a graduated manner. Second, try to make the exposures as realistic as possible. There is often a theatrical element in creating initial exposures. You may elect to bring in props or do some role playing (Hope & Heimberg, 1993). Third, flexibility and ingenuity are necessary.

Socially anxious children dread acting silly. Thus, in our work with these youngsters, we encourage them to act silly. We may invite the child to do a silly dance or to sing a silly song in front of his/her peers. Naturally, we urge the youngster to explore his/her own reactions as well as the reactions of his/her peers. We elicit the child's expectations before doing the exercise and then compare them with his/her actual experience. Often, this is an experience that can disconfirm his/her expectations. The following transcript of part of a group session illustrates the process.

NICK: I don't want to jump around and dance. It's not cool and popular.

THERAPIST: What do you suppose will happen?

NICK: People will think I'm a maniac.

THERAPIST: Are you willing to test this out?

NICK: No.

THERAPIST: How about the rest of you boys and girls? (*The rest of the children agree to try.*) What do you make of that, Nick?

NICK: I don't know.

THERAPIST: Do you think Nancy, Chloe, Matt, and Jeremy want to be unpopular?

NICK: No.

THERAPIST: Do you think they want to call you a dweeb?

NICK: I don't know. Probably not.

THERAPIST: So if they don't want to be unpopular and don't want to call you a dweeb, how safe is it to act silly right now?

NICK: Pretty safe.

THERAPIST: Are you willing to give it a try? I'm going to act silly too.

NICK: OK.

(*Therapist and children dance around acting silly and singing.*)

THERAPIST: What was that like for you, Nick?

NICK: Pretty weird.

THERAPIST: Tell us about it.

NICK: I don't know. Umm. I think I looked like a jerk.

THERAPIST: Do you want to check that out with the others?

NICK: They think I'm weird.

THERAPIST: Can we ask them?

NICK: Do you think I'm weird?

NANCY: No, we all did it.

JEREMY: I wasn't looking at you.

CHLOE: I didn't think you looked weird. We all were laughing. It was kind of fun.

THERAPIST: What do you make of that?

NICK: I guess nobody thought I was a dweeb.

THERAPIST: What was it like for you to ask the other boys and girls?

NICK: Scary.

THERAPIST: Let's all talk about the scary feelings we have when we talk and check things out.

This example illustrates several important issues. As you review the transcript, you can see that the exchange includes several different phases. In Phase 1, the therapist worked with Nick's reluctance to act silly. In Phase 2, the experiment was attempted. Phase 3 was built around processing the experiment. Finally, in Phase 4, Nick's fears of negative evaluation were challenged.

For many of the socially anxious children we treat, reading aloud in front of the class is an excruciating experience. The group format is a handy way to do graduated exposures to reading aloud. We simply encourage the child to read in front of the group. When we do school-based groups, we usually hold our sessions in a classroom. The classroom atmosphere adds to the realism. The child is reading aloud to same-age peers in a situation that closely approximates a classroom experience. The sights, sounds, and smells of the educational institution are present.

Consider the following example. Marc is an 10-year-old child who is so painfully socially anxious that reading aloud in class is torture for him. His social anxiety disguised his considerable academic skills, contributed to his teacher's doubts about his abilities, fueled his own fears of negative evaluation, and decreased his self-confidence.

During group therapy, we taught Marc how to make better eye contact and project his voice. Then we put these skills to the test. As Kendall et al. (1992) would say, we wanted Marc to "show that I can." Marc was repeatedly invited to read in front of a group. Initially, Marc physically shook and his voice trembled as he reluctantly read. It was hard for the therapists and even the group members to resist the urge to rescue this obviously distressed child. However, rescue would only reinforce his view of himself as fragile. With repeated practice, Marc learned to identify the thoughts associated with his anxiety. He then tested out these beliefs with the audience (e.g., "Did you think I was foolish?"). Subsequently, the other children reassured him that they did not see him as foolish.

But this was not enough. We felt we needed to prepare Marc for the possibility of negative feedback. Therefore, we asked him, "What if someone thought you were stupid?" He then needed to apply his coping skills to this possibility. Moreover, we went so far as to point out the slight errors in his performance. From this, he learned to cope with our evaluation without subjecting himself to self-debilitating criticism. He learned to think, "I can't always be perfect. Even really good students make mistakes. Two mistakes don't mean I'm stupid," instead of thinking, "I must be perfect and in control or else I'm stupid."

Another interesting exposure trial is based on an idea borrowed from the literature on family variables and anxiety disorders (Chorpita & Barlow, 1998; Kendall et al., 1992; Morris, 1999). For children who get anxious doing a new task or performing in front of others, and/or who have perfectionistic parents who become overinvolved in their projects, completing a project in session is a nice graduated exposure. Craft kits in which children make beaded necklaces or key chains are ideal projects. Arts-and-crafts supply kits that are found in any toy store (e.g., bottle-painting kits, jewelry-making kits, models) are also good for this exposure exercise.

The child is presented with the project and he/she has to complete it in session. If you find that the child has fears about performing the task, we suggest you ask the child to make predictions about what is going to happen. Remember to bring thought diaries to the session so you will have them handy. When the child experiences the anxiety associated with doing a novel task or making a mistake, you can capture the moment on a thought diary. As the child works him/herself through the project, you should process his/her thoughts and feelings with him/her. The following transcript illustrates the process.

THERAPIST: Gary, I want you to try to make this beaded key chain. You'll have to follow the directions yourself and figure out how to make it. I'll watch you and ask you how you are feeling and what is going through your mind. Are you ready?

GARY: Sure. I like this shark key chain.

THERAPIST: Yes, it's a nice one. OK, go ahead.

GARY: (*Opens the box and begins reading the directions. Starts making the project and begins to have some difficulty.*)

THERAPIST: What's going through your mind right now?

GARY: I can't do this. I'm going to mess up. Will you help me? I'm confused.

THERAPIST: How are you feeling?

GARY: Nervous.

THERAPIST: On a scale of 1 to 10, how nervous?

GARY: Maybe an 8. Can you figure this out for me?

THERAPIST: I want you to try it yourself. Hang in there and see what you can come up with.

GARY: (*Continues working on his own.*) I'm getting it. Look. I did the fin. This was tricky.

THERAPIST: How are you feeling now?

GARY: Proud.

THERAPIST: What is going through your mind?

GARY: I did it myself. It was hard.

THERAPIST: How close was this to what happens in school?

GARY: Pretty close.

THERAPIST: On a scale of 1 to 10, 1 being completely different and 10 being identical, how close was it?

GARY: About an 8.

THERAPIST: So it was very close. What did this tell you about handling new assignments?

GARY: I can do it, if I stay calm.

THERAPIST: What was it like for me not to help you?

GARY: It bothered me at first.

THERAPIST: What about it bothered you?

GARY: I thought it was mean.

THERAPIST: If I helped you, would you have felt as proud?

GARY: Probably not.

THERAPIST: So what does that tell you about trying new things on your own?

GARY: Even though it freaks me out at first, if I stay with it I can do it, even on my own.

What can we learn from this exchange? The therapist helped Gary persist in the task even though he became anxious and requested more direction from the therapist. Second, the therapist processed the experience (e.g., identified thoughts and feelings after completing the task, drew similarities between the experiment and Gary's school situation). Finally, the therapist helped Gary form a new conclusion about himself in these situations based on the experiment.

The arts-and-crafts project also provides a graduated exposure to the parenting variables that contribute to children's anxiety. Parents who are perfectionistic and overcontrolling will probably not stand back and let their child do the task on his/her own. Rather, they will more likely direct the child, correct his/her mistakes, or possibly even take over the task. It is excruciatingly difficult for these parents to let go and allow their child to "mess up." The child, in turn, begins to see any failure as disastrous.

Because he/she is consistently rescued, his/her confidence in his/her coping capacity is weakened.

The craft should be presented as a task to be performed. Giving ambiguous instructions is proper here (e.g., "Go ahead and make this."). The ambiguity will allow the typical familial interaction patterns to emerge. When these interaction patterns pop up in session, be ready to process the thoughts and feelings associated with them.

Exposure trials can be introduced and simplified for young children. *Red Light, Green Light* is a therapeutic variation of the children's game of the same name. As children line up next to one another, as far away from the leader as space permits, the leader calls out either "Red light" or "Green light." When the leader calls out "Green light," the children are free to move forward, toward the leader. Conversely, when the leader calls out "Red light," the children must freeze in place. In this psychological version of the game, the "Red light" command serves several purposes. When children freeze in their tracks at "Red light," you can use this experience to teach them about the effects of anxiety. Figuratively, the freezing reflects being scared stiff and represents the emotional paralysis that often accompanies anxiety. Children can be asked to scan their bodies for signs of tension. Their increasing ability to identify these pockets of tension can serve as a foundation for relaxation training.

Freezing at "Red light" is also a graduated exposure opportunity. When children freeze at the "Red light" instruction, you induce anxiety-producing imagery. For a child who fears ridicule, negative evaluation, and embarrassment, you might construct an image where the child is exposed to criticism. You might have the child imagine him/herself raising his/her hand in class, being called on by the teacher, and then forgetting the answer. The child then has to apply a coping skill when the therapist induces the anxiety-producing imagery.

When Red Light, Green Light is done in a group setting, the other children could serve as consultants to a child if he/she is unable to develop coping skills. For instance, they might be asked if they could think of something Johnny could say to himself that could unfreeze him. For many socially anxious children, simply being "put on the spot" in a group exercise such as Red Light, Green Light may be anxiety producing. In this way, you could use a here-and-now approach to processing the anxiety. Examine the following transcript to gain a sense of the process.

THERAPIST: Green light . . . OK, everybody, go. Red light, everybody stop. (*Notices that Johnny is blushing and appears quite self-conscious.*) Johnny, let's see how you might talk back to your fear. Johnny, what's going through your mind right now?

JOHNNY: Nothing really.

THERAPIST: How does your body feel?

JOHNNY: All tight.

THERAPIST: Concentrate on the tightness and see if you can hear your fear talking. What's going through your mind right now?

JOHNNY: I hope this ends soon.

THERAPIST: I bet you do. As you look around and see all the other boys and girls watching you, what are you saying to yourself?

JOHNNY: This is embarrassing.

THERAPIST: When you feel embarrassed, what goes through your mind?

JOHNNY: This is stupid. I look like a geek.

THERAPIST: Great job, now your fear is talking. Let's see if we can use one of your skills. What skill could you choose?

JOHNNY: I don't know.

THERAPIST: Who can help Johnny?

BILLY: Maybe he could try Talking Back to Fear.

THERAPIST: What do you think of that idea?

JOHNNY: Good.

THERAPIST: How can you talk back to the thought "The boys and girls will think I'm a geek."

JOHNNY: I'm not sure.

THERAPIST: Who can help him?

SALLY: He could say, "I'm not a geek, this game is stupid." (*The boys and girls laugh.*)

THERAPIST: That's one possibility. How about another?

JENNY: He could say, "Who cares whether they think I'm a geek? They may think I'm a geek now but maybe later they won't."

THERAPIST: Another good idea. Let me ask you a question, Johnny. What do you think of the other children helping you out?

JOHNNY: I don't know.

THERAPIST: How many boys and girls tried to help you out?

JOHNNY: Pretty much everybody.

THERAPIST: How many laughed at you or teased you?

JOHNNY: None.

THERAPIST: So, did what you actually fear happen?

JOHNNY: I guess not.

You are well advised to keep the game moving. You should not stay with one child for too long a period. The other youngsters may become bored and the game will lose its reinforcement value. The child should become sufficiently anxious rather quickly and then the therapist can use the other children's input to help moderate the youngster's distress.

While we are enthusiastic advocates of exposure treatment, there are some special considerations to mull over before attempting exposure-based approaches. First, when a child has coexisting anxiety and depression, we generally prefer to treat or target the depression first. Lifting the depression before attempting exposure makes the exposure training somewhat easier. Depressed children likely lack the necessary self-confidence to encounter even the most minimal anxiety-producing cue. Second, depressed children's inactivity, passivity, and pessimism makes exposure difficult.

Needless to say, exposure is an intense experience. Therefore, you should be careful that the child has medical clearance for the procedure. Thus, we recommend a thorough physical and medical evaluation before beginning exposure treatment. Medical clearance will give the child (and you!) peace of mind when conducting the exposure.

Rewarding Exposure Efforts

We find that rewarding children's efforts at exposure is key. In fact, we make a big deal out of their accomplishments! For younger children, we create a "Badge of Courage" that summarizes and amplifies the gains they achieve. The badge is a way to remind children about their ability to cope and master their insecurities.

When we make a Badge of Courage, four questions are included. The first question asks, "What was the fear I faced?" Therapists can coach children to specifically record the fear they faced (e.g., "Asking a group of children if I could play."). Specificity is very important because the goal is for children to look at the "badge" and recall their exact successes.

The second and third questions require children to record how long and how often they faced their fears. These questions provide concrete feedback on children's capacity to confront and endure their dreaded events. In our experience, change is rarely linear. Often, past avoidance exerts a strong magnetic pull, forcing the child into old behavior patterns. When this happens, the Badge of Courage might stimulate positive memories associated with previous coping successes.

The fourth question asks children to list the ways they cope with their fear. In their examples, the children may include the specific strategies and skills that propelled approach behavior. After the exposure trials, the child can review his/her successful strategies. A sample Badge of Courage is show in Figure 12.12 and a completed badge is illustrated in Figure 12.13.

There are several ways you can augment the Badge of Courage. For instance, the badge could be placed in a plastic sleeve and presented as a certificate. Further, the badge could be laminated so that it serves as a lasting reminder and reward to the child. The child could also create a small badge. A pin could be attached to the back and the child could wear the small badge.

Another innovative idea is providing feedback on children's coping via photographs (Kearney & Albano, 2000). Children could be photographed when they attempt the feared activity and successfully master it. The pictures could then be attached to or accompany the badge. By attaching the photographs to their Badges of Courage, children can literally "picture" themselves coping.

CONCLUSION

Helping anxious children calm and control their fears and worries will take patience and ingenuity. Coaching children and adolescents to step toward their anxiety rather than back away from it requires a systematic plan that includes a variety of clinical tools. In this chapter, we have recommended multiple ways for you to reach anxious youngsters. We encourage you to remember that anxious children need to face their worries and fears rather than just talk about them. Use the ideas and strategies in this chapter to invite youngsters to directly cope with their fears and develop genuine self-efficacy.

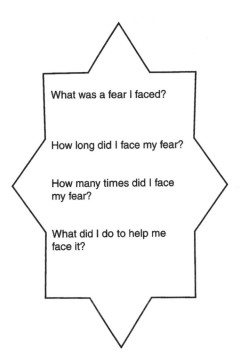

What was a fear I faced?

How long did I face my fear?

How many times did I face my fear?

What did I do to help me face it?

FIGURE 12.12. My Badge of Courage Worksheet. From Friedberg and McClure (2002). Copyright by The Guilford Press. Permission to photocopy this figure is granted to purchasers of this book for personal use only (see copyright page for details).

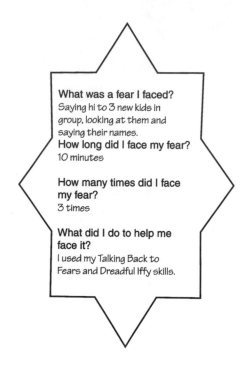

FIGURE 12.13. Sample My Badge of Courage Worksheet.

13

❖

Working with Disruptive Children and Adolescents

COMMON SYMPTOMS OF THE DISRUPTIVE DISORDERS

Disruptive children impact us in different ways than anxious or depressed children. I (RDF) can never forget the time early in my training when an 11-year-old boy with severe behavior problems locked me in the time-out room! These youngsters can elicit strong feelings of anger, frustration, and anxiety in us.

A recent report by the U.S. Surgeon General (1999) notes that disruptive disorders are marked by antisocial acts such as aggression, noncompliance, oppositionality, rebelliousness, and disregard for people and property rights. Conduct disorder generally includes a persistent pattern where the child violates the rights of others and age-appropriate social rules and norms (American Psychiatric Association, 1994; Kazdin, 1997). These violations fall into four broad categories: aggression, destruction of property, deceitfulness and/or theft, and serious violations of rules. More specifically, bullying, fighting, physical cruelty to people and/or animals, fire setting, stealing, running away, lying, and truancy are representative behaviors (American Psychiatric Association, 1994; Kazdin, 1997). Vandalism, precocious sexual activity, substance use, and school expulsion are also frequent occurrences with these youngsters (U.S. Surgeon General, 1999). Not surprisingly, these children are described as resentful, boisterous, hyperactive, and suspicious (Kazdin, 1997). Kazdin (1993,

1997) reported that children with conduct disorder also demonstrate lower achievement levels, failure to complete homework, poor reading skills, diminished social skills, and higher levels of peer rejection.

Sam is a 15-year-old whom his parents describe as incorrigible. He has been suspended repeatedly from school due to his aggressive and unruly behavior. Most recently, he chased several other boys around the school wielding a broken tree branch. He claims he was set off by others' rude comments and looks. Sam is of average intelligence but does not apply himself to his studies. In fact, at times, he has ripped up assignments in class because they were "bogus." His parents reported that Sam repeatedly steals money and completely ignores house rules and curfews. Sam has a record of joyriding. He believes that "rules are meant to be broken" and he works hard at maintaining a "Don't mess with me" attitude. His parents confess that Sam runs the house; they also admit they are afraid of him. His teachers claim he can be cooperative when they make no demands upon him but in general they see him as a bully, a liar, and a troublemaker.

Oppositional defiant disorder is characterized by a persistent pattern of defiance, disobedience, and hostility toward authority figures such as parents and teachers (American Psychiatric Association, 1994; U.S. Surgeon General, 1999). Specific signs of oppositional defiant disorder include chronic arguing and fighting, temper tantrums, high levels of irritability/annoyance, vindictiveness/spitefulness, noncompliance, stubbornness, and blaming others for one's own mistakes. These children are "Teflon kids": responsibility just does not stick to them. Younger children with oppositional defiant disorder often show high levels of intolerance for frustration, have difficulty delaying gratification, and kick and thrash (Kronenberger & Meyer, 1996). Kronenberger and Meyer noted that older children with oppositional defiant disorder talk back to parents, reveal passive–aggressive behavior problems, and are described by their parents as touchy, stubborn, and argumentative.

Lou is a 10-year-old boy who is pushing his parents to their limits. While at school, he is compliant, cooperative, and studious. However, at home, he curses at his mother's commands, "flips the bird" at his sister and parents, and generally dominates his family members through various power struggles. Lou sees rules as being unfair and unreasonably imposed on him (e.g., "Why do I have to do this?"). Finally, he distances himself from responsibility by externalizing blame (e.g., "How can this be my fault?").

The core clinical criteria for attention-deficit/hyperactivity disorder are inattention, impulsivity, and hyperactivity (American Psychiatric Association, 1994; Cantwell, 1996). An early age of onset (before age 7), 6-month duration, and presence of problems in more than one context is required for diagnosis (American Psychiatric Association, 1994). A child may be identified with a primarily inattentive type of the disorder, a hyperactive–impulsive type, or a combined type. Inattention is marked by symptoms such as careless mistakes in schoolwork, difficulty maintaining attention in play or school, difficulty organizing tasks, and frequently losing things. Hyperactivity is characterized by fidgeting, squirminess, excessive talking, and acting as if driven by a motor. Blurting out answers in class, difficulty waiting turns, and intruding on others in a conversation reflect impulsivity.

Alice is a 10-year-old girl who teachers and parents report "can't sit still." She is frequently out of her seat in school and can't stop herself from chatting with her neighboring classmates. Alice's schoolwork is careless and messy; her desk looks like a tornado hit it. She frequently forgets to do or misplaces her homework assignments. During the intake session, Alice crawled under the couch to investigate a buzzing sound. Her mother describes her as similar to the cartoon character "The Tazmanian Devil." Alice feels sad and lonely because she thinks her peers reject her. She believes they think she is "weird."

CULTURAL CONTEXT AND GENDER ISSUES

Elevated rates of antisocial behavior are reported for Hispanic American, African American, and Native American youth (Dishion, French, & Patterson, 1995). Dishion et al. recommend that we carefully assess the unique contributions ethnicity, economic hardship, limited employment, peer relationships, parenting, and living in a high-risk neighborhood make to behavior problems. Additionally, the psychological effects of oppression, discrimination, prejudice, and stereotyping are also salient. Dishion et al. aptly wrote, for example, "perceived ethnic stigmatization among children would likely contribute to social information processing, in particular, the likelihood of making hostile attributions in ambiguous situations" (p. 455).

Cartledge and Feng (1996a) wrote that Southeast Asian youth in the United States encounter unique obstacles such as language problems, poverty, prejudice, pervasive uncertainty, and loss of country, friends, family, and social status (Rumbault, 1985, as cited by Cartledge & Feng, 1996a). Southeast Asian American children appear to be at-risk for school attrition (Dao, 1991, as cited by Cartledge & Feng, 1996a). Chin (1990, as cited by Cartledge & Feng, 1996a) reported that the initial emergence of Chinese gangs was associated with high racial tensions in neighborhood schools. "Attempting to escape the pressures of an alien society, many of these youngsters indulge in self-destructive behaviors such as violent action and substance abuse" (Cartledge & Feng, 1996a, p. 106).

Gibbs (1998) writes that "while the prevalence of conduct disorders among African-American adolescents is not known, it can be safely said that they have disproportionately high rates of conduct problems in school settings" (p. 179). Teachers judged students' academic potential on the basis of their appearance, gender, and language ability and these determinations persisted over time (Irvine, 1990, as cited by Cartledge & Middleton, 1996). Citing a number of other studies, Cartledge and Middleton (1996) wrote that African American males are overrepresented in referrals for learning and behavior problems. Alarmingly, African American students are two to five times more likely to be suspended than their white peers (Irvine, 1990, as cited by Cartledge & Middleton, 1996). Carmen (1990, as cited by Cartledge and Middleton, 1996) reported that in a school where African Americans accounted for 24% of the school population, the behavioral disorder program included 52% African Americans. Cartledge and Middleton aptly write, "From the outset of their formal schooling, many of these youngsters learn that school personnel often devalue the way they look, talk, think, share experiences, and live. Failing to be affirmed in the schools, they often turn to other environments to verify their self-worth" (p. 149).

Cochran and Cartledge (1996) describe various factors that put Hispanic youth at risk for disruptive behavior problems. They argue that "for a significant minority of Hispanic-American youth, the negative influences of poverty, inadequate schooling, urban living conditions, and psychological alienation contribute to a focus on aggression and violence" (p. 261). Ramirez (1998) found that oppositional defiant disorder was the second most frequent diagnosis given to Mexican American youngsters at his clinic.

Gender differences are also salient in the disruptive disorders. Before puberty, the rates for oppositional defiant disorder are higher for boys than for girls but the rates become equal after puberty (U.S. Surgeon General, 1999). Most studies report much higher rates of attention-deficit/hyperactivity disorder in boys than in girls. However, Biederman et al. (1999) state that one million girls may suffer with attention-deficit/hyperactivity disorder even if a conservative 5:1 gender ratio is chosen. Further, they suggest that although the basic clinical picture for attention-deficit/hyperactivity disorder is the same for boys and girls, there were some specific differences in symptom expression. Girls in their study tended to have more inattention, mood, and anxious features in their symptom picture than did boys. Biederman et al. also argue that girls with attention-deficit/hyperactivity disorder may be at a somewhat greater risk for developing a substance abuse disorder. Finally, Biederman et al. conclude that we may be underestimating the prevalence of attention-deficit/hyperactivity disorder in girls.

Gender somewhat shapes symptom expression in conduct disorder. Girls tend to be more likely to engage in prostitution and runaway behavior (U.S. Surgeon General, 1999). Further, Woodward and Ferguson (1999) found that women whose conduct problems at age 8 were in the highest 10% suffered a 2.6 times greater risk of becoming pregnant at 18 years of age than their peers in the lowest 50% of disturbance. Finally, the majority of teens who have comorbid depression and conduct disorder are male whereas more than three-quarters of teens with comorbid anxiety and conduct disorder are female (Lewinsohn, Ruhde, & Seeley, 1995, as cited by Stahl & Clarizio, 1999).

In their review, Johnson, Cartledge, and Milburn (1996) noted that boys demonstrate more aggression than girls; they argue that guilt and fear inhibit girls' aggressive behavior. Crick and Grotpeter (1995) described relational aggression in girls. Specifically, relational aggression refers to "behaviors that are intended to significantly damage another child's friendships or feelings of inclusion by the peer group" (Crick & Grotpeter, 1995, p. 711). Children who are relationally aggressive dump their peers from their play group, withdraw their friendship as a way to control other children, and "diss" other children by spreading rumors about them so they will be rejected by their peers. Crick and Grotpeter found that girls engage in more relational aggression than boys. They concluded that rejected girls may disrupt peers' relationship with each other.

ASSESSMENT OF DISRUPTIVE BEHAVIOR PROBLEMS

The Achenbach Child Behavior Checklist (CBCL) is a widely used measure in clinical child psychology (Kronenberger & Meyer, 1996). There are separate scales for parents (Achenbach, 1991a), teachers (Teacher Report Form [TRF]; Achenbach, 1991b), and children (Achenbach, 1991c) to complete. Items are rated on a 0–2 scale to assess the extent to which the behavior is representative of the child. The scales are appropriate for children ages 4 to 18. Comparing the reports from different data sources is an excellent clinical strategy (Kronenberger & Meyer, 1996). For example, Kronenberger and Meyer wrote that "a problem-ridden TRF coupled with a relatively normal CBCL profile suggests that the child may behave adequately in the less structured, more individualized home environment while becoming disorganized and misbehaving at school" (p. 27).

The Eyberg Child Behavior Inventory (Eyberg, 1974, 1992; Eyberg & Ross, 1978) is another checklist that assesses children's disruptive behavior patterns. Parents report their children's behavior problems at home on a 7-point Likert scale. The scale is appropriate for children ages 2 through 16. However, the scale does focus more on annoying behavior problems than on the more severe conduct problems (Kazdin, 1993). There is a variation of the ECBI for teachers. The Sutter–Eyberg Student Behavior Inventory (SESBI; Sutter & Eyberg, 1984) contains some items identical to those on the ECBI and items particular to the school setting. Similarly to Achenbach scale interpretation, it is commonly useful to compare reports from different sources.

The Conners Parent Rating Scales (CPRS) and Conners Teacher Rating Scales (CTRS; Conners, 1990) are extensively researched and widely used in the assessment of ADHD (Kronenberger & Meyer, 1996). There are different forms that vary in length. Since the Conners Scales emphasizes attention-deficit/hyperactivity disorder symptoms, they are particularly useful if you need an in-depth and closer look at specific attention-deficit/hyperactivity disorder symptoms (Kronenberger & Meyer, 1996).

TREATMENT APPROACH

Since disruptive behavior disorders are characterized by multiple behavior problems, a multimodal treatment package works best. Figure 13.1 illustrates the different conceptual components and a proposed sequence. We begin with education about the treatment model. Disruptive children and adolescents do not generally enter treatment with motivation to change themselves. Rather, they generally want others to change (DiGiuseppe, Tafrate, & Eckhardt, 1994). Thus, engaging them in the treatment rationale is crucial.

The second tier involves teaching the youngster and his/her caregivers basic behavioral skills. Depending on the nature of the child's disruptive problems, different behavioral skills will be delivered. Depending on the circumstances, techniques such as social skills training or relaxation training may be in order. Parents usually are taught basic child management strategies to quiet down the youngster's aggressive and disruptive behavior. The techniques for parent training described in Chapter 14 are well suited to this phase of treatment. Family problem-solving training and individual problem-solving approaches for the disruptive youngster are also included in this second tier.

The third tier reflects increasingly sophisticated techniques. In this tier, we teach self-instructional skills to help disruptive children rethink situations and replace provocative internal dialogues with soothing self-talk. Further, since disruptive youngsters who behave aggressively often lack empathy, we add an empathy training component.

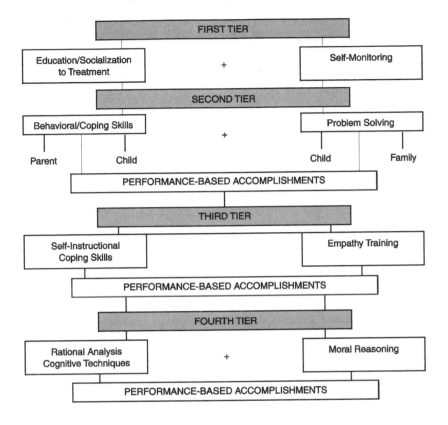

FIGURE 13.1. Treatment approach with disruptive youngsters.

The techniques included in the fourth tier represent the most complex cognitive procedures. Rational analysis procedures such as reattribution focus on exploration of various alternatives and decreasing youngsters' hostile attributional biases. Due to the finding that aggressive youth often lack a moral link to others (Goldstein, Glick, Reiner, Zimmerman, & Coultry, 1987), efforts at increasing their moral reasoning capacities are indicated. In this phase of treatment, children are presented with moral dilemmas and discuss the moral rationale for their decisions.

In each tier, performance-based accomplishments follow the specific skill acquisition. As with the treatments for depression and anxiety, cognitive-behavioral techniques need to be applied in the context of negative affective arousal (Robins & Hayes, 1993). Performance-based exercises, activities, and assignments allow youngsters to practice what we are preaching to them.

BUILDING RELATIONSHIPS WITH DISRUPTIVE
CHILDREN AND ADOLESCENTS

Establishing a good relationship with the disruptive youth is crucial. Therapeutic relationships must be based on trust, understanding, respect, and a sense of genuineness. How do we get to that place with these disruptive children? For us, limit setting is key. By knowing what is expected, children feel safe. However, in our experience, we have found that it is relatively easy to fall into a rigid authoritarian style or to lapse into an overly permissive style with these young clients. Isn't it interesting that this seems to parallel the dysfunctional parenting strategies that accompany these youngsters' disruptive behaviors?

In order to establish therapeutic limits and boundaries, we all must know our own limits. What is acceptable and unacceptable behavior? For instance, can a child swear in session? If he/she can use foul language, can he/she use any "bad" word he/she wants or are some words outlawed? Can he/she put his/her feet on a chair? Can he/she have a session if he/she is high? In order to be clear with these children, we have to have clear limits in our own heads.

After we clearly state our limits, we must be consistent about enforcing them. Consistency promotes trust. If you set a limit and follow through with it, you are saying that your words and actions are meaningful. We believe that if you have to say "Trust me" to a child, you probably are not following through with limits. Limits also communicate that you care about the child. Thus, when you demonstrate caring and trust through flexible limit setting, therapy becomes a safe place.

Consider the following example. I (RDF) was doing therapy with a group of inpatient adolescents with disruptive behavior disorders. One of the group rules was that no one was allowed to hurt him/herself or anyone else. During the group, I noticed that a young girl had something shiny in her hand and seemed to be picking herself with it. I asked her what was in her hand and she showed me a bloody paper clip. At this point, I reassured her (and the rest of the group!) by enforcing a limit. I said, "I need to make sure you don't hurt yourself. I'm going to take care of you now by asking you to go to the nurse's station to get your wrist cleaned and bandaged. After you do that, come back to group and we'll talk about what's going on with you. I won't let you hurt yourself in group." By authoritatively limiting the child, I communicated my concern.

Flexibility is also important in limit setting with disruptive youngsters. Without flexibility, you can enter into unwanted power struggles and escalate conflict. In another example on the same unit, I (RDF) was in group with several very disruptive and unruly teens. A new group member referred from juvenile hall came into session. He had a gang background and an assaultive history. Like most aggressive children, he was quite territorial and controlling. Early in session, he challenged my leadership by proclaiming, "We're going to have a problem because I'm in charge here. I'm real close to messing you up." He was clearly trying to frighten me—quite honestly, he was succeeding! I asked myself, "How could I set the limit without escalating the situation?" I elected to say, "I'm in a tough spot, now. You're scaring me but I still have to do my job." Fortunately, the group members responded by saying, "Don't scare the doc." The teen backed down and the group proceeded. Why did this limit work? First, I think the youngster needed to know he could scare me; once he did, that was enough for him. Second, he needed to clearly know I would not let go of the reins of the group. Thus, he could frighten me, but I nevertheless had to do my job. Third, the group helped me out by reinforcing my limit.

TEACHING PARENTS ABOUT BEHAVIOR MANAGEMENT AND FAMILY PROBLEM SOLVING

In this section, we first describe the familial interaction patterns that contribute to disruptive behavior disorders in children and then suggest strategies that may repair these interactions. It is important to begin with a discussion of the impaired processes because they form a rationale for the interventions.

Barkley et al. (1999) cogently describe the processes that impair families. First, there is a low level of reinforcement for any existing compliance. Put simply, parents neglect the positive behaviors and almost exclusively attend to the negative behaviors. Indeed, always attending to the negative is tiresome. Not surprisingly, then, parents become frustrated and agitated around noncompliance and defiance. Barkley and his colleagues note that, depending on their individual circumstances, parents/caretakers enter into a cycle of either inconsistent punishment or inappropriate acquiescence. In other words, consequences for defiance are not delivered well. Parents then will likely resort to angry threats. The parent–child relationship deteriorates into one bruised by insults, putdowns, and destructive name calling. Coercive family processes ensue, interpersonal conflict increases, and everybody's self-esteem suffers (Barkley et al., 1999).

Barkley et al. (1999) aptly note that parents and children doggedly hold onto grudges toward each other. We think these grudges form an information-processing wall that blocks each family member's capacity to see any positive behavior in the other. For example, if a teenage girl has built a grudge against her mom and sees her as a "controlling bitch," she will be relatively unable to see her mom's nurturant and responsive behaviors. On the other hand, if the mom sees her daughter as a "defiant, uncontrollable slut," she will be equally unable to see her daughter's "good" behavior. This may explain the "war bunker" mentality we see in many families with disruptive behavior.

As a function of all these factors, parents begin to abdicate their parental role (Barkley et al., 1999). They give up keeping track of their youngsters' behavior and adopt a "whatever" attitude. Barkley notes that this parental acquiescence is correlated with increases in a variety of more severe forms of disruptive behavior.

There are several compelling reasons to begin the family behavior management by increasing the level of positive reinforcement (Barkley et al., 1999). First, increasing the level of positive reinforcement combats this tense and hostile family tone. Second, due to the parents' overuse of punishment and response cost techniques, their youngster probably has habituated to these interventions. Third, positive reinforcement techniques serve as a counterweight to what the parents are already doing. Finally, due to the overuse of punishment techniques, coercion, and name calling, parents have become aversive stimuli to their child, and therefore it is unlikely that the child will listen to his/her parents' messages.

To modify this critical and hostile climate as well as to reestablish parental authority, Barkley et al. suggest a simple yet sophisticated intervention. They recommend teaching parents to give the child a command to do something he/she likes and then to reward his/her compliance. For example, if a child likes chocolate cake, the parent/caretaker may tell the child, "Andy, go get yourself a big piece of cake for dessert." Then when Andy complies, he is rewarded (e.g., "Thanks for doing what I asked you to do.").

The beauty of this technique is that it not only improves the family climate, but it also provides parents with an opportunity to practice giving commands and reinforcing compliance. Additionally, successful use of this technique reestablishes the proper executive functioning for parents. They can reaffirm that they are the legitimate authority in the house without resorting to coercion and punishments.

Despite the simplicity and straightforwardness of this task, we need to add several cautions. First, you will likely need to teach the parent how to give these commands. Remember, parents are coming into your office with a history of giving vague and indirect instructions. Thus, you will need to model how to give the instruction, role play with the parents to help them practice, give them corrective feedback on the practice, include the child in the session, practice again with the parent giving the child the command, and provide additional feedback.

For instance, suppose one parent began the exercise with the command, "Josie, you like going to the mall. Go ahead and go with your friends." Think about what is problematic about this command! First, the parent did not stipulate when Josie could go. Was it right now? After dinner tonight? Tomorrow? Second, how long should Josie go? An hour? Six hours? The whole day? What were the expectations once she was there? Do anything she wants?

Another caution is making sure that the parent is genuine with the command. Parents may give the command snidely or in a sarcastic manner. Pay attention not only to what parents say but to how they say it. Watch their body posture and facial expressions. Disingenuous commands sabotage their effectiveness.

Praising the child for spontaneous compliance is another way to increase his/her level of positive behavior and reward in the family (Barkley et al., 1999). You can teach the parent to look for times when the misbehavior or defiance does not occur. By trying to catch the child when he/she is on his/her better behavior, parents are shifting their attentional set. This technique can decrease families' all-or-none thinking (i.e., parents think child is always sullen and disrespectful; child thinks parents only see him/her in a bad light). In this way, each member gains a broader perspective of each other.

Barkley et al. (1999) also recommend family problem-solving training with disruptive and defiant youngsters. In distressed families, the problem-solving processes become very rigid. The goal in family problem solving is to loosen up these rigid patterns. You will want to help family members distinguish between negotiable and nonnegotiable issues. Like giving commands, this sounds simpler than it really is. Parents may unwittingly give mixed messages to their youngsters. Take, for example, the mother who caught her 16-year-old daughter kissing her boyfriend in her bedroom. She proclaimed, "Take it outside. I won't have you having sex in my house." The mother really wanted to communicate that sex was a nonnegotiable issue. However, what her daughter heard was that it was OK for her to have sex so long as it wasn't in her mother's house. Thus, you will have to work diligently to help parents and children separate negotiable from nonnegotiable items.

Blos (1979, p. 147) noted that troubled adolescents often "do all the wrong things for the right reasons." In their effort to become their own person and form their identities, teens rebel. Parents cannot gratify most adolescents' demands and consequently teens become frustrated. Family problem solving helps manage conflicts surrounding these frustrations.

We have found one of Barkley et al.'s modifications quite compelling. In their approach, therapists help parents and children hear problems from each other's perspective. This process can soften rigid patterns and pave the way for more productive problem solving. Being able to hear the problem from another perspective will not be easy for many distressed parents and children. Therefore, we suggest that you adopt a relatively directive stance.

Clementine is a 16-year-old girl who is in conflict with her mother over her clothes. According to her mother, Clementine is wearing revealing clothes and giving off the "wrong type of messages." Mother has been watching Clementine "like a hawk," closely monitoring her choice of school clothes. The problem came to a head when mother discovered that Clementine kept a change of clothes in her locker at school. See if you can determine how the following dialogue loosens up the mother and daughter's problem-solving processes.

THERAPIST: Mom, tell Clementine what worries you about the way she dresses.

MOTHER: She looks trashy. She's going to get herself a reputation or worse.

CLEMENTINE: I know what I'm doing. You don't have to worry about me. You're just doing this for yourself . . .

THERAPIST: I'm going to stop you here for now, Clementine. I am asking you to just listen and then you'll get a chance to have your own voice next. Are you willing to do that with me?

CLEMENTINE: (*Reluctantly.*) OK.

THERAPIST: Good. Now, Mom, what about Clementine getting a bad reputation bothers you?

MOTHER: I just don't want that to happen. She's so young. I want to protect her.

THERAPIST: I see. What's the reason you want to protect her so much?

MOTHER: She's my daughter.

THERAPIST: Help us understand. What about her being your daughter makes you care so much?

MOTHER: I love her.

THERAPIST: I see. You really worry about Clementine's outfits giving off the wrong impression and getting her into dangerous situations, so you work to protect her because you love her and don't want bad things to happen to her.

MOTHER: That's right.

THERAPIST: Clementine, what did you hear Mom say?

CLEMENTINE: She thinks I can't handle myself so she has to take over. It makes me sick.

THERAPIST: Hold on a second. Think back to what you heard her say. What's the reason Mom tries to take over?

CLEMENTINE: She says it's because she loves me.

THERAPIST: Now you sound like you don't believe her right now and you don't have to but I'm asking if you could look at Mom and repeat what you heard her say.

CLEMENTINE: You said you want to protect me because you love me and don't want anything bad to happen to me.

THERAPIST: Now, Clementine, what is your take on the reason Mom likes to take over.

CLEMENTINE: She doesn't trust me. She thinks just because I dress this way I'm going to do something stupid. I just want to look like this. It's me and she can't see me if I don't look like her.

THERAPIST: What bugs you about Mom not trusting you?

CLEMENTINE: She thinks I'm stupid and I'm a little kid.

THERAPIST: What do you want from her?

CLEMENTINE: I want her to respect me and understand that I'm not an idiot. I want her to see me as someone who can be in charge.

THERAPIST: And if she saw you in that way, what would that mean?

CLEMENTINE: That she'd like and approve of me.

THERAPIST: You really want Mom to see you as you are and approve of you. Mom, can you repeat what you heard Clementine say?

MOTHER: I know she wants me to see her but what I see sometimes scares me.

THERAPIST: Mom, I want you just to see if you can tell Clementine what you hear her say.

MOTHER: She wants me to back off and let her know that I like and approve of her.

In this dialogue, the therapist helped make mother's and Clementine's motivations more visible (e.g., Mom loves her, Clementine wants Mom to approve of her). Second, once the authentic motivations emerge, each family member profits from the broader perspective. By doing so, they became less entrenched in their own argument and able to engage in the problem-solving process.

EDUCATION AND SELF-MONITORING

Explaining the treatment rationale and focus is an especially key issue in working with children who have disruptive and aggressive behavior problems. Frequently, these youngsters see us as adversaries rather than allies. DiGiuseppe et al. (1994) commented that engaging these youngsters in treatment is made difficult by their tendency to blame others for their problems. For example, 14-year-old Romy's goal for treatment was for her mom to stop acting bitchy. Changing her own rebellious and defiant behavior was far more secondary.

Presenting the *ABC model of behavior* is a typical first educational step with these youngsters (Barkley et al., 1999; Feindler & Guttman, 1994). In the ABC model, "A" stands for the antecedents or triggers to behavior, "B" denotes the behavior, and "C" represents the consequences that either increase or decrease the behavior's frequency. We like the ABC model because it is so simple. Almost everyone understands that "A" comes before "B" and "C" follows "B." We rarely use technical words such as "antecedents" or "consequences." Rather, we prefer phrases such as "the things that come before" and "the things that come after."

For example, consider Romy's view of the problem. As a first step, you might ask her to define the bitchy behavior (B). For her, it was her mom's nagging, yelling, grounding her, and so on. Then, ask what happens after Mom's behavior (e.g., Romy does not comply, which increases the intensity/frequency of unpleasant consequences). Next, you should address the "A's," or things Romy does to elicit Mom's "bitchy behavior" (e.g., violating curfew, not listening). The model then simply illustrates how Romy's behavior contributes to her own definition of the problem. By doing so, you can help her see how by changing her own behavior patterns she can decrease Mom's problematic behavior.

Brondolo, DiGiuseppe, and Tafrate (1997) offer several interesting ways to present treatment to disruptive youngsters. Disruptive and aggressive youngsters often have a vested interest in acting tough and mean. In fact, aggression may be a competency in some violent neighborhoods (Howard, Barton, Walsh, & Lerner, 1999). Dishion et al. (1995) wrote that "aggressive children . . . live in a world in which they are frequently attacked and consequently their biases may be an accurate reflection of their high base rates for such behavior" (p. 437). Thus, Brondolo et al. (1997) recommended framing treatment as a way to maintain greater control rather than as a way to tolerate maltreatment. Using martial arts training or other sports analogies can be helpful in illustrating these points (Brondolo et al., 1997; Sommers-Flannagan & Sommers-Flannagan, 1995).

We often find simple experiential exercises useful in educating these youngsters. For example, suppose Drake is a 13-year-old boy who is impulsive, disruptive, and aggressive. Drake believes he has no choice but to act in this way. Others make him lash out and fight. As his therapist, you can wad up a piece of paper into a ball. Then ask Drake, "Do you know how to catch a ball?" Following his response, you ask, "Can I toss you this ball?" You then toss Drake the paper ball. After he attempts to catch it, ask him, "Did I make you catch the ball?" This little exercise demonstrates that although the situation may typically call for a particular response, the circumstance does not absolutely determine the individual's action. Simply put, he could have done something else.

Vernon (1989a) offers a creative exercise that I (RDF) have adopted with inpatient youngsters. I begin this activity by telling the clients that we are going to conduct an experiment. I hold up an egg and ask them, "What is this?" In the second step I announce that I am going to tap the egg on the side of a bowl and ask, "What is going to happen now?" In the third step, I crack the egg and ask, "Take a look at the bowl. Who knows what happened?" Inevitably, the youngsters report that the egg has cracked. Finally, I ask Vernon's key question, "But did the egg choose to crack?"

We like this exercise because it so simply demonstrates the notion of choice. After doing this exercise, you can ask youngsters what are the differences between themselves and an egg. The discussion frequently yields a better understanding of the ways impulsivity overrides reason. Commonly, I refer back to this exercise when a youngster mindlessly reacts and ask, "Are you being an egg?"

Self-monitoring techniques may include rulers, thermometers, traffic signals, and/or volume dials. You might want to pick the scaling technique based on the child's interests and preferences. For example, a child who enjoys NASCAR racing may embrace an angry gas tank gage (see Figure 13.2). The child can draw the gage on a piece of cardboard and cut out an indicator arrow from another piece with scissors. He/she then attaches the arrow to the cardboard with a small clasp. In this way, the arrow can move up and down the dial.

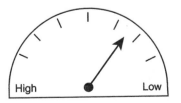

FIGURE 13.2. Angry gas tank gage.

Youngsters also need to track the antecedents and consequences to their disruptive behavior. Most adolescents have the skills to complete a chart in which they list the antecedents and consequences of their behavior (Feindler & Ecton, 1986; Feindler & Guttman, 1994). For younger children, you may have to "jazz up" this process. For example, you could equate the antecedents to buzzers that jolt the youngster, propelling him/her toward acting-out behaviors. A worksheet with buzzers drawn on it could be easily developed (see Figure 13.3).

We like the buzzer metaphor because it can lead in multiple directions. You could bring in a buzzer from a board game like Taboo to augment the worksheet. The sound effects may be quite engaging to children! Additionally, the buzzer metaphor may cue subsequent coping and you can ask, "How can you beat the buzzer?" Third, we find the buzzer a more neutral word than "trigger" with angry children. Finally, we often use action verbs in our questions to help children identify their buzzers (e.g., "What sparks your anger?"; "What fuels your anger?").

Youngsters could be asked to complete a thought diary whenever they feel angry or have an argument with a parent. Feindler and her colleagues (Feindler & Ecton, 1986; Feindler & Guttman, 1994) developed very handy self-monitoring devices they call *Hassle Logs*. In their Hassle Logs, youngsters monitor their thoughts, feelings, and behaviors by completing a checklist. Prototypical situations and reactions are listed and the youngsters need only check what happened. Thus, there is little demand for written responding.

A key for us in doing anger management work is helping children distinguish between feeling angry and acting aggressively or disruptively. You want to let the child know it is OK to feel angry, but it is not OK to hurt yourself or someone else when you are feeling angry. For younger children, we use a very specific and concrete way to help them learn the difference between being angry and behaving aggressively.

Casey was a 9-year-old boy who was referred to us for his aggressive and disruptive behavior. Early in treatment, Casey was taught to tell the difference between the emotion and the behavior. Casey drew a picture of himself when he was mad. Then he was asked to draw a picture of himself doing something when he was mad. Casey drew a picture of himself kicking another boy. I (RDF) then asked Casey which of these pictures were OK things. At first, he thought both the angry feelings and the angry behavior were not OK. Later, after we talked about the feelings being acceptable, but the behavior not being acceptable, Casey was able to distinguish between feelings and actions. He wrote "OK" beneath the mad face and "Not OK" beneath the kicking drawing.

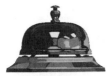 Angry buzzers with parents.

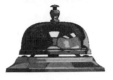 Angry buzzers with teachers.

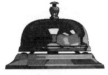 Angry buzzers with friends/peers.

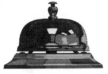 Angry buzzers with brothers or sisters.

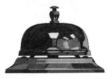 Other angry buzzers.

FIGURE 13.3. Angry Buzzers. From Friedberg and McClure (2002). Copyright by The Guilford Press. Permission to photocopy this figure is granted to purchasers of this book for personal use only (see copyright page for details).

INDIVIDUAL PROBLEM SOLVING

Problem solving is often another difficult "sell" to disruptive children and adolescents. Thus, priming them for problem solving becomes even more critical. I (RDF) originally developed this idea with inpatient adolescents (Friedberg, 1993). In the first phase, the therapist tosses a foam Nerf ball to the youngster. (Be sure the ball is a *foam* ball!) After the client catches the ball, the therapist asks, "How common is it for you to catch it when a ball is tossed to you?" Then the therapist instructs the child to do any-thing else he/she can think of other than catch the ball (e.g., duck, bat the ball back with his/her hand, etc.) After children do something different, the therapist processes the experience with them (e.g., "What was it like to do something different?").

So what's the point? This exercise serves several purposes. First, the game is fun! Second, the youngster is likely to be surprised by the activity and won't be exactly sure what to make of it. Third, the exercise offers experiential practice in generating options, thereby paving the way for problem solving.

Problem solving with disruptive children requires considerable flexi-bility. The youngsters' maladaptive problem solving can be quite reinforc-ing. For example, when discussing alternative problem-solving strategies, a teen replied, "Hey, Doc, Why should I give up selling drugs where I make $500 a week to work at McDonald's? The car you drive is a joke." In order to help an adolescent like this to develop more productive alter-natives, you have to consider each option's reinforcement value. Clearly, for this youngster, the immediate cash benefits of drug dealing out-weighed the consequences of criminal activity.

When we explain this issue to supervisees, we construct a simple analogy. Imagine you have to go on a diet. As part of this diet, you have to give up doughnuts—which you love! Instead of having a doughnut, you have to eat a carrot (P.S. nothing against carrots!). More likely than not, you are thinking, "Yuk, a carrot for a doughnut? You've got to be kidding." The carrot simply does not come close to the satisfying proper-ties of the doughnut. Thus, when we try to replace maladaptive strategies with more productive ones, substituting carrots for doughnuts dooms us.

Another sinkhole for problem solving with these youngsters is work-ing too abstractly. These individuals live in the now and often espouse a "live hard, die young" philosophy. I (RDF) am reminded of one young teen client who, when asked to think about the future consequences of his behavior, responded, "Why should I worry about my future? I'm going to be dead by 18 or 19. Most of the boys I know are going to be dead or in jail." In these circumstances, you have to help teens see how better prob-lem solving can serve their immediate needs.

Consider the following example. Wesley is a 16-year-old determined to be the meanest, baddest, toughest guy in school. He sees no advantage in changing his stance. Here is a way problem solving may help.

THERAPIST: So, Wesley, is there something you want that you don't have right now?

WESLEY: No, not really.

THERAPIST: Nothing? Really?

WESLEY: Well, I would like to go out with this girl named Caty.

THERAPIST: I see. How much are you dating now?

WESLEY: Not much.

THERAPIST: What, maybe two dates a month?

WESLEY: OK. I'm not dating at all.

THERAPIST: Hmm. How do you suppose the girls you like in your school see you?

WESLEY: I don't know. I can't see inside their heads.

THERAPIST: How do they act when you are around?

WESLEY: Like they are scared of me.

THERAPIST: That sure does make sense—if you are the meanest guy in school, you'd scare off lots of people. You've taught them well. So remind me again, how does this behavior get you everything you want?

In this example, the therapist tied Wesley's behavior to direct consequences. He wanted girls in his class to be attracted to him, but, in fact, he scared them off with his behavior. This example is a good one because Wesley selected a meaningful topic to him (i.e., dating). The therapist was able to help Wesley see how his behavior was causing him problems in this area.

Problem solving has five basic steps. Specifying these five steps in some sort of acronym is a handy tool for youngsters. In *Switching Channels* (Friedberg et al., 1992), we spelled out the problem-solving steps in a COPE acronym. "C" stands for *catching* the problem, "O" refers to listing the *options*, "P" denotes *predicting* long- and short-term consequences, and "E" stands for *evaluating* the anticipated outcomes and then taking action based on this review. We commonly add an "R" to this model to make the youngster a "COPER." The "R" is for *self-reward* for following the steps and attempting productive action. These problem-solving steps can be placed on a card and laminated for future reference (Castro-Blanco, 1999).

Kazdin (1996) uses five verbal prompts to facilitate prosocial problem solving. Each prompt is a form of self-instruction. The five cues include: (1) "What am I supposed to do?"; (2) "I have to look at all of my possibilities"; (3) "I had better concentrate and focus in"; (4) "I need to make a choice"; (5) "I did a good job" or "Oh, I made a mistake" (Kazdin, 1996, p. 383). As you can see, these steps closely resemble the COPER model described above. Kazdin also recommends priming and experiential activities to prime problem solving such as teaching sequential reasoning by playing Connect Four. We especially like Kazdin's concept of "super-solvers" (p. 384) where parents and children are given *in vivo* assignments for problem solving.

TIME PROJECTION

We have found time projection to be particularly useful in helping youngsters to see the consequences of their actions and to put their impulses in perspective. Imagine you are working with Tom, an 11-year-old boy, who has just been suspended for 3 days for fighting in the cafeteria. You have seen him about six times prior to this incident. During the session, you elect to use time projection to help him gain perspective on the incident.

THERAPIST: Tom, when Steve cut in front of you in the cafeteria, how mad were you on a scale of 1–10?

TOM: I was about a nine. That's why I shoved him.

THERAPIST: Ok. About an hour later, how mad were you?

TOM: Maybe a 7 or 8.

THERAPIST: Would you have shoved him and hit him if you were that mad?

TOM: Probably. I hate to be that mad. I have to do something.

THERAPIST: How mad did you feel 6 hours later at dinner?

TOM: I don't know. Maybe a 5.

THERAPIST: Would you have shoved and hit him at a 5?

TOM: Maybe, I'm not sure.

THERAPIST: I see. So 6 hours later you're not sure you'd do the same thing. How about a day later? How angry do you feel today about it?

TOM: Maybe a 3. I am still pissed though.

THERAPIST: Do you feel like hitting him right now?

TOM: No, but I did at the time.

THERAPIST: I know you did. But let me ask you this. Your angry feelings and your urge to hit him lasted about a day. Right?

TOM: I guess.

THERAPIST: How long does your suspension last?

TOM: Three days.

THERAPIST: Let me get this right. So you are paying for 1 day of feeling angry with 3 days of suspension?

TOM: Yep.

THERAPIST: How does that work out for you?

What does this exchange illustrate? First, Tom and his therapist tracked his anger over time. Second, they connected his level of anger to his actions. Third, the therapist Socratically guided Tom's discovery that although his anger lasted only a short time, he will be paying the penalty for his impulsive actions for a longer time.

SOCIAL SKILLS TRAINING

In this section, we suggest several additional ways to enhance social skills with disruptive children. We tend to use social skills approaches with these youngsters to decrease their aggressive and antagonistic behavior, decrease inappropriate intrusions/interruptions, increase prosocial behaviors, and increase friend-making skills. Hands-on activities will help make abstract social skills principles come to life for youngsters.

Cochran and Cartledge (1996) invite therapists to use "jigsawing" as a social skills exercise. *Jigsawing* (Aronson, 1978, as cited by Cochran & Cartledge, 1996) is an exercise in which a group of youngsters is given a project and the project is divided into it constituent parts. Each individual child is responsible for being the expert on his/her part and is required to teach this part to the other youngsters. Planting a garden, building a sand castle, and acting out stories are just some of the examples of jigsawing that Cochran and Carledge offer.

In our minds, jigsawing offers therapists multiple opportunities. For example, youngsters could be given a project to build a model. Each child is given a portion of the directions and becomes an expert on their portion. They have to interact and cooperate to get tasks done. In essence, the way they interact with each other is a genuine sample of behavior. You can intervene to highlight appropriate interactions and provide corrective feedback on inappropriate social interactions.

The *Joining Jar* is another fun way to promote better social skills (Cartledge & Feng, 1996a). A jar is placed in a group therapy room. If the therapist observes any member of the group engaging in a prosocial behavior such as being empathic, listening, or responding nonaggressively to confrontation, he/she places a marble in the jar. The therapist gives special rewards to the group members when the marble total tops a certain amount. You could also invite the group members to reinforce each other by placing marbles in the jar, thereby delivering a reinforcement whenever they see a peer interacting well.

We agree with several authors who advocate the use of popular literature and movies as ways to teach social skills (Cartledge & Feng, 1996a, 1996b; Cartledge & Middleton, 1996; Cochran & Cartledge, 1996). Books, movies, and music can facilitate greater cultural responsivity. Biographies of Jackie Robinson, Malcolm X, Thurgood Marshall, Harriet Tubman, Cesar Chavez, Henry Cisneros, and others provide good role models for children of color. Specific titles we recommend include *Hoops* (Myers, 1981), *Fast Sam, Cook Clyde, and Stuff* (Myers, 1975), *Scorpions* (Myers, 1988), *Famous All Over Town* (Santiago, 1983), *In the Year of the Boar and Jackie Robinson* (Lord, 1984), *New Kids on the Block: Oral Histories of Immigrant Teens* (Bode, 1989), *Hawk, I Am Your Brother* (Baylor, 1976), *Racing the Sun* (Pitts, 1988), and *I Speak English for My Mom* (Stanek, 1989) (Cartledge & Feng, 1996a, 1996b; Cartledge & Middleton, 1996; Cochran & Cartledge, 1996; Lee & Cartledge, 1996). For teens and children who do not read well, movies or documentaries may fit the bill as teaching tools.

Positive Adolescent Choices Training (PACT) is an innovative violence-prevention program specifically tailored to African American adolescents ages 12–15-years-old (Hammond & Yung, 1991). PACT is especially sensitive to racial, ethnic, and cultural issues. Communication, negotiation, and problem-solving skills are taught to youngsters via direct instruction and videotaped modeling. In general, the training is done in groups of 10–12 adolescents. They learn six skills: giving positive feedback, giving negative feedback, accepting negative feedback, resisting peer pressure, solving problems, and negotiating. Role plays and psychodramas are presented in videotaped vignettes to facilitate peer and self-modeling. As Hammond and Yung (1991) argue, "Models which capture the distinct style of minority teen subcultures are more credible and convincing to them" (p. 365).

The PACT skills and videotapes featuring African American teen role models are available in a video series and leader's manual (Hammond, 1991). The videotapes, which run from 14 to 20 minutes, emphasize three basic skill sets. In *Givin' It*, youngsters learn to express criticism, disappointment, anger, and/or displeasure in a calm and self-controlled manner. Further, this readies the youngster for better conflict resolution. *Takin' It* helps teens listen, understand, and react to others' criticism and anger in a productive manner. Negotiation is taught with the *Workin' It Out* skill. Here, youngsters learn listening, problem identification, generation of alternative solutions, and compromising skills.

EMPATHY TRAINING

Aggressive and violent children lack empathy for others (Goldstein et al., 1987). If they truly had empathy for the target of their aggression, they would be less likely to attack. I (RDF) am reminded of an incident I witnessed when I was consulting at a preschool. The teachers were having difficulty with a child who was hitting, biting, kicking, and otherwise making the school routine difficult for other youngsters. When I observed the classroom, the child wanted a crayon that another student was using. When the other child did not give him the crayon, the child bit him hard on the arm. The teacher rushed up to the child and firmly stated "Biting hurts!" The child looked incredulously at the teacher and then wandered away to another part of the classroom.

Why was this teacher's intervention ineffective? The misbehaving child already knew "biting hurts." In fact, that was the reason he bit the other child! The problem was that he did not care that he hurt the other child. His need for the crayon superseded his concern for others. The teacher would have been more successful if she had applied a negative consequence for the behavior and worked on building his empathy skills.

We believe empathy training has to be active. We do not take for granted that aggressive youngsters have empathy. Therefore, we generally adopt a graduated approach to empathy training. For the most unempathic children, we might begin training by watching a movie or reading a book with characters who experience different feelings and stressors (e.g., being bullied, being teased). Unempathic children may have difficulty responding to real characters. Using fictional characters is one step removed from real characters. Thus, we practice the skills with these characters first to build empathic capacity. Many therapists elect to use pets (dogs, cats) as a first step. Certainly, we think this is also a good first step unless the child is cruel to animals.

Group therapy is especially well suited to empathy training. The peer group exercise allows opportunities for real-life practice. Consider this example. Eddy, a 9-year-old boy, saw Josh cry in group. Eddy automatically called him a "little crybaby." Naturally, the group focus shifted to the interaction between Josh and Eddy. How would you use this as a therapeutic teaching moment?

We suggest you work with Eddy so that he gains a sense of how Josh feels. For instance, you might ask him, "When you called Josh a crybaby, how did he look?"; "What might he say to himself?"; "What did he do?"; and "How do you suppose he felt?" Additionally, you might elect to focus on Eddy's motivations: "How did you want Josh to feel when you called him the name?"; "What does Josh feeling that way get you?"; "If someone called you a name, how would you feel?"; "How are your feelings like and not like Josh?" Finally, once Eddy gains a bit of empathy for Josh, we recommend that Eddy communicate his understanding (e.g., "What can you say to Josh that will show him you understand?").

SELF-INSTRUCTIONAL APPROACHES

We find that angry children need to be prepared for self-instructional approaches. *On Purpose or By Accident* is a priming self-instructional-type technique tailored to decrease an aggressive child's hostile perceptual bias. The tool includes 10 events; the child's task is to determine whether they happen "on purpose" or "by accident." These items are followed by two questions (see Figure 13.4). The first asks the youngster to list five ways he/she can tell if someone does something on purpose or by accident. This question helps the youngster develop different ways of interpreting interpersonal situations. The last question, "What is important about learning to decide whether somebody does something on purpose or by accident?," reinforces the rationale for the technique.

A useful way to use the tool is to have the child read each item and then decide whether the event happened on purpose or by accident. You can then engage the youngster in a discussion regarding what went into his/her decision. By doing so, you can begin to help the youngster more accurately determine whether someone's behavior was deliberate. After the child works through the exercise, he/she can be instructed to write the question on an index card. You can coach him/her to ask this question of him/herself before he/she automatically leaps to conclusions about others' intentions.

We have found that metaphors improve our self-instructional techniques. One metaphor that may be helpful in your work with angry youngsters is "Putting Fights on Ice." When children put fights on ice, they use imagery and self-control skills to cool off their anger. The procedure begins with a discussion of the tool and its rationale. Then children imagine or draw themselves sitting on a block of ice. They practice developing "cool down" statements and record these statements on a worksheet or index card. Figure 13.5 shows a sample worksheet.

Circle whether each thing listed below happens to you on purpose or by accident.

A classmate does not say hello.	On purpose	By accident
Your mother asks you to wash the dishes.	On purpose	By accident
Your teacher calls you by the wrong name.	On purpose	By accident
At lunch, your friend spills milk on your tray.	On purpose	By accident
Your friend did not get you a birthday present.	On purpose	By accident
Someone cuts ahead of you in line.	On purpose	By accident
Someone bumps into your desk when he/she is not looking where he/she is going.	On purpose	By accident
Someone takes your pencil and won't give it back.	On purpose	By accident
A classmate makes fun of you and calls you names.	On purpose	By accident
Someone gives you a strange look.	On purpose	By accident

List five ways you can tell if someone does something on purpose or by accident.

1. _____
2. _____
3. _____
4. _____
5. _____

What is important about learning to decide whether somebody does something on purpose or by accident?

_____
_____
_____

FIGURE 13.4. On Purpose or By Accident. From Friedberg and McClure (2002). Copyright by The Guilford Press. Permission to photocopy this figure is granted to purchasers of this book for personal use only (see copyright page for details).

The following dialogue illustrates how you might use Putting Fights on Ice with a 12-year-old boy.

THERAPIST: OK, Eric. When you get angry and are ready to fight, how do you feel?

ERIC: Really hot, like I'm burning up inside.

THERAPIST: I see. Would it help you if you found a way to cool down?

ERIC: I suppose so.

THERAPIST: I agree. When you get in fights, it's almost as if you are having a meltdown. Let's see if together we can find a way for you to put your fights on ice. Here is this worksheet (*presents sheet*). I want you to draw yourself sitting on this ice. Have fun with it.

ERIC: (*Draws on the sheet.*)

THERAPIST: What could you say to yourself to cool off?

ERIC: Maybe "Freeze!" "Stop!" "Think about what you're doing!"

THERAPIST: Good. Do you think you could come up with five more statements that you could try?

ERIC: I think so.

THERAPIST: I also want you to try imagining sitting on this block of ice when you get really angry and are ready to fight. Do you think you can get that picture you drew in your mind's eye?

What does this dialogue teach us? First, the therapist used metaphors to illustrate anger (e.g., having a meltdown; putting fights on ice). Second, self-instructions (e.g., "What could you say to yourself to cool off?"; "I also want you to try imagining sitting on this block of ice. . . . ") were applied. Third, the therapist integrated the imagery technique into the exercise.

Disruptive children simply do not stop and think! *Picture This* (Friedberg, 1993) is a game-like technique developed with inpatient adolescents to help them become less impulsive. The game is usually played in groups of youngsters with pictures out of popular magazines. Preferably, the pictures are packed with stimuli and there is plenty going on in the photographs. There are two rounds. In the first round, the picture is presented for about 5 seconds and participants have 10 seconds to record everything they recall seeing. Players share their lists and earn points for each unique answer. If two or more players have the same response, they each receive 0 points. Additionally, depth of processing is rewarded. When players synthesize, integrate, or combine stimuli, they receive addi-

Draw yourself sitting on this block of ice.

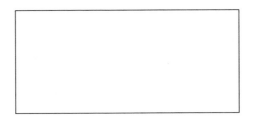

Color the ice a nice *cool* color.

Write down five cool-down statements.

1. _____

2. _____

3. _____

4. _____

5. _____

Next time you feel really angry and you are ready to melt down, imagine yourself sitting on this cool block of ice thinking your five cool-down statements.

FIGURE 13.5. Putting Fights on Ice. From Friedberg and McClure (2002). Copyright by The Guilford Press. Permission to photocopy this figure is granted to purchasers of this book for personal use only (see copyright page for details).

tional bonus points. For example, "A girl is worth 1 point, a girl sitting on a porch is worth 2 points, and a girl sitting on a porch petting a puppy dog is worth 3 points."

In the second round, the display time is increased to 15 seconds and children have 10 seconds to record their recall. After playing the second round, you help the youngsters connect the game to the stop-and-think process. For instance, you can ask, "In which round did you see more things?"; "What was it like to stop and think?"; and "When was it easier to solve the problem, when you stopped and thought things over or when you just acted?" Then you could connect stopping and thinking to their presenting problems: "When do you stop and think?"; "Do you suppose stopping and thinking might help you get a fuller take on your problems?"

"Simon Says" is another nonthreatening game that can teach younger children the benefit of stopping and thinking. As you remember, Simon Says requires players to attend, listen, and inhibit their behaviors due to simple commands. You cannot do well in the game if you are inattentive and noncompliant. Simon Says is a playful way to teach children to respond to commands. When playing the game, you can process different types of instructions. For instance, you might ask, "What was it like to do what Simon said?"; "What made you successful in doing what Simon said?"; and/or "What did you have to do to do well in Simon Says?" Further, you might ask, "How were you able to stop yourself from doing things?"; "What did you need to do so you were not out of the game?"; and "Which of the skills in Simon Says can you do in school and at home?"

There are several other ways to teach youngsters stopping and thinking skills. Whistles are handy tools for reminding children to stop. For example, you might elect to use a sports analogy, such as "Parents and teachers often act like referees! When a foul is called, a referee blows the whistle and play has to stop." You and the child might create a list of common situations and then decide whether the situation is a "foul" and deserves a whistle. Penalty flags could also be used instead of a whistle. Additionally, children could draw or paint the penalty flags.

RATIONAL ANALYSIS TECHNIQUES

The rational analysis techniques for anger management are best applied to work with adolescents rather than younger children. Similarly to the work with anxious and depressed youngsters, rational analysis should be done when children are moderately rather than severely agitated.

The first set of techniques are reattribution procedures. Remember that angry children's cognitions involve hostile attributions of malevolent intent (Dodge, 1985). Thus, you will want them to ask themselves, "What's another explanation for the trigger situation?" Let's consider the following example. Imagine you are working in a school setting. Jake, a 14-year-old boy with whom you have been working, comes into your office. He is agitated because Omar called him a name. He believes Omar is testing him, playing him for a fool, and that his manhood is being called into question. He believes he must retaliate and teach Omar a lesson.

JAKE: I gotta go get him during lunch. I've got to show him he can't disrespect me.

THERAPIST: You are so pissed off that you really want to attack him to show Omar you are the man?

JAKE: You've got that right!

THERAPIST: What is going through your mind right now?

JAKE: He's showing me up. Everybody is waiting to see what will happen. If I don't fight, they will think I'm afraid of him. I'll be out of control.

THERAPIST: How in control will you be if you fight him?

JAKE: A lot. If I hit him hard enough.

THERAPIST: He really gets you going. The volume on your anger really gets turned up.

JAKE: You've got that right, too.

THERAPIST: Now, it sounds like Omar is in charge of the volume knob.

JAKE: How is that?

THERAPIST: By getting Omar, how in control are you?

JAKE: I'm out of control. I'm a maniac. That's why nobody messes with me.

THERAPIST: So is it possible that fighting and paying the penalty for all this fighting makes you more out of control?

JAKE: Maybe. But I am still the man.

THERAPIST: Can you be the man without fighting?

JAKE: Why?

THERAPIST: When you think you are the man, how cool do you think you are?

JAKE: Really cool.

THERAPIST: And if it is so easy to pump up your anger volume, how cool are you?

JAKE: (*Pauses.*)

THERAPIST: You look a little confused.

What does this exchange teach us? First, the therapist used the analogy of a volume knob on a disc player to help Jake see that Omar was pumping up his anger volume. Second, the therapist attempted to shake Jake's belief that fighting made him a man. Third, the therapist tried to create doubt and confusion regarding Jake's belief that fighting was cool and meant he was in control.

Many aggressive youngsters are certain that there is only one way to explain things that happen to them. For example, during an inpatient group session, an angry adolescent I'll call Simon spied a peer looking at him with his head slightly cocked and with his arms crossed. Immediately he thought, "This guy is testing me. He's disrespecting me." The youngster was certain he was being baited. At this point, Simon needed to develop alternate attributions. Check out the following dialogue to gain a sense of how to help a youngster form reattributions.

SIMON: Look at him. He's just waiting to see what I'm going to do!

THERAPIST: What makes you think he is disrespecting you?

SIMON: I've been around. He's giving me the signals.

THERAPIST: What signals?

SIMON: Disrespect!

THERAPIST: I see. So you see his head being cocked as a sort of test of your manhood?

SIMON: You've got that straight.

THERAPIST: What if it meant something else?

SIMON: Like what?

THERAPIST: I don't know. Maybe he's just tired. If he's just tired, you may be getting yourself all worked up for nothing. Are you willing to be courageous enough to look for other reasons?

The therapist reframed reattribution as an act of courage (e.g., "Are you willing to be courageous enough to look for other reasons?").

All-or-none thinking characterizes many disruptive adolescents. They think in dichotomous categories and label others in either "good" or "bad" ways. Indeed, if you see someone as a "total a-hole," defying him/

her becomes a more acceptable response. Therefore, we often use a continuum technique to help adolescents challenge their all-or-none thinking.

Let's take the example of Mitch who is in frequent conflict with Mr. Robinson, his homeroom teacher. Mitch is belligerent and defiant with Mr. Robinson's commands. He sees Mr. Robinson as a "total a-hole." Clearly, Mitch does not want to obey someone he sees so poorly. Therefore, by using the continuum technique, the therapist is trying to find a way for Mitch to see Mr. Robinson in less of an all-or-none way.

The basic procedure begins by placing the youngster's categorical labels on each end of the dimension (see Figure 13.6). Thus, Mitch places "total a-hole" on one end and its opposite, "totally cool," on the other end of the continuum. Then Mitch needs to define the two ends of the continuum. The following transcript illustrates the process.

THERAPIST: So, Mitch, what makes someone a total and complete a-hole?

MITCH: They're a jerk. They write you up for every mistake you make. They look for you to mess up.

THERAPIST: How about the way they would treat your car? Like if they backed into it and drove away?

MITCH: That would be a real a-hole thing to do.

THERAPIST: What about stealing some of your favorite stuff?

MITCH: Yeh. That would be a-hole.

THERAPIST: Anything else make somebody an a-hole in your mind?

MITCH: Being nasty to my family. Maybe being cruel to my dog.

THERAPIST: Now how about the other end? What does someone do who is totally not an a-hole?

MITCH: They're cool.

THERAPIST: Tell me more. How do you know when someone is cool?

MITCH: They never hassle me. They let me be me. They play music loud and drive fast.

THERAPIST: How do they act in school? Do they study? Do they talk back to teachers?

MITCH: They're cool. They don't always talk back. They study the stuff they think is important.

THERAPIST: I see. Let's see who we can place on this line. Where would your best friend be? How close to the end would he be? How about your brother? . . . Father? . . . Mother? . . . The guy who hit your car? . . . Mr. Robinson? [See Figure 13.6.]

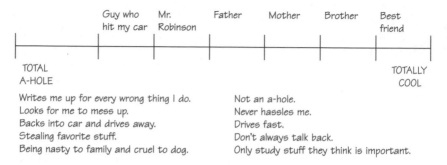

FIGURE 13.6. Mitch's continuum.

MITCH: (*Completes the diagram.*)

THERAPIST: When you look at the line, does it seem to say "Mr. Robinson is a total, 100% a-hole"?

MITCH: No, but he's on the end.

THERAPIST: Do you think your mom and dad are total a-holes?

MITCH: (*Pause*) No.

THERAPIST: How close on the line is he to them?

MITCH: Pretty close.

THERAPIST: So what does that mean?

MITCH: Maybe he's kind of an a-hole but not total.

THERAPIST: What does that do to your anger toward him?

MITCH: (*Pause*) Makes it lower.

Mitch's anger decreased due to his softened view of Mr. Robinson. The harsh label of a total a-hole was lessened. Obviously, Mitch did not develop a positive view of Mr. Robinson. However, thanks to this exercise, in the future he will be more likely to respect and comply with someone he does not see as a total a-hole.

MORAL REASONING

Goldstein et al. (1987) recommended adding a moral reasoning component to an anger management package. In their innovative approach, therapists lead discussion groups that focus on moral dilemmas. Goldstein and colleagues (1987) said change is accomplished by creating cognitive conflict or dissonance. For Goldstein, when youngsters try to resolve their dissonance, they will experiment with different forms of moral reasoning. The general idea is to move the youngster from low-level immature reasoning to higher, more sophisticated reasoning.

In their text, Goldstein et al. present numerous moral dilemmas for youngsters to discuss. Sommers-Flannagan and Sommers-Flannagan (1995) also suggest creating moral dilemmas around alcohol and drug use, abstaining/engaging in sexual intercourse, cheating on exams, stealing, and violating curfew. Finally, the board game Scruples also offers many moral or ethical dilemmas. The advantage of a board game may be that it adds a playful tone to the discussion. Regardless of the type of dilemma you use, Goldstein et al. (1987) alert us to several salient considerations. Dilemmas should generate significant cognitive conflict. You want to unbalance youngsters' heretofore moral equilibrium. While the dilemmas should create dissonance, they also need to be interesting, relevant, and productive.

Setting the stage for the discussion is an important preparatory step. Overall, there are four goals in this phase (Goldstein et al., 1987). First, you should explain the rationale and purpose of the dilemma discussion group to the youngsters (e.g., to develop and experiment with new perspectives). Second, you should discuss the group format, making sure you communicate to the youngsters that there are no right answers, everyone will have a turn, and the group members have the responsibility for generating discussion. Third, you should explain the facilitator's role to the youngsters. Here, you might tell them that you will not evaluate their responses but rather help them focus the discussion and ensure that everyone follows group rules and has a chance to talk. Goldstein et al. encourage therapists to periodically play the Devil's advocate. Finally, you should outline the ethical rules for group behavior. Goldstein et al. (1987) stress that youngsters should be informed that disagreement is a way to learn from each other.

In guiding the discussion, you assess the stages of moral reasoning youngsters demonstrate. Then you create a debate between the lowest level reasoners and the members whose reasoning is one stage higher. The idea is to unbalance reasoning patterns by pointing out injustice and contradictions. You can change the scenario and add in hypothetical information.

Goldstein et al. (1987) also suggest various ways to manage insensitive participation, overactive participation, and underactive participation. Aggressive youngsters may resort to put-downs and insults during the discussion. In these instances, Goldstein et al. suggest a directive approach where you intervene quickly, point out why you are stopping the discussion, and coach the group members to focus on the topic rather than on personal qualities. Overactive participation, which reflects egocentrism, also needs to be discouraged. In these circumstances, youngsters want the discussion to focus entirely on their own ideas. To decrease the egocentrism over participation, you will need to summarize the participants' viewpoints and also set some limits on their participation. Underactive participation is a third dilemma for leaders. Goldstein et al. recommend that you discuss the reasons for the relative inactivity (e.g., anxiety, difficulty grasping the material, boredom). In these instances, empathy, gentle prompts, and providing greater structure are indicated.

EXPOSURE/PERFORMANCE ATTAINMENT

Like anxious children, angry, aggressive youngsters need experiences to *show* them that they can manage their emotions. In fact, DiGiuseppe et al. (1994) assert that anger and anxiety both have high levels of autonomic nervous system arousal and both ready the individual for action. We agree with many other cognitive-behavioral clinicians who advocate constructing experiential learning opportunities for angry youngsters (Brondolo et al., 1997; DiGiuseppe et al., 1994; Feindler, 1991; Feindler & Ecton, 1986; Feindler & Guttman, 1994). Brondolo et al. (1997) write that "as individuals learn to tolerate the experience of anger, they become more flexible in their responses to provocation" (p. 86).

In our experiences, most aggressive youngsters readily acquire the skills presented in the previous sections. Nowhere was this more apparent than on an inpatient unit where I (RDF) worked. The adolescents would seemingly grasp the tools of anger management in a 1:00 P.M. skills group yet not uncommonly get into an altercation with staff or peers by 4:00 P.M. It wasn't that these young people could not learn the skills; it was more that they could not apply the skills when they were angered.

For safety and efficacy reasons, we strongly recommend that exposure training follow the acquisition and application of self-control skills. You want to be sure the youngsters have learned the self-control skills before you put them in a situation where they have to perform them. Additionally, we also recommend graduated exposure trials. Brondolo et al. (1997) recommends that "with very disruptive or impulsive children, it may be necessary to work slowly with few people and distractions in the room and starting with the least offensive rather than the most offensive words or use imaginal rather than in-vivo provocations" (p. 88). Brondolo and her colleagues comment that regarding extremely disruptive youngsters, establishing the proper rules of conduct for exposure could take up to a year. Finally, we agree with Brondolo et al. that you should carefully sift through worst case scenarios before you begin performance attainment strategies.

Feindler and Guttman (1994) offer several structured, graduated, exposure-based activities and exercises. In *Circle of Criticism* (p. 184), youngsters sit in a circle and are instructed to criticize the person sitting to their right. If you adopt a graduated approach to the task, you could supply the criticisms so you can control the intensity of the remarks. The criticism could be placed in a box and randomly picked. By doing so, many criticisms may not be personally relevant or intensely provocative at first. The target of the criticism is instructed to use fogging (see Chapter 8) as a response. Group members would receive rewards or tokens for participating appropriately. As the group members learn to tolerate greater criticisms, you could write more provocative remarks on the slips of paper in the box. In the beginning phase of this training, you might want to provide the youngsters with scripted fogging remarks. With greater practice, the scripts could be removed and the youngsters would then have to come up with their own responses.

Feindler and Guttman (1994) also make use of the *Barb technique* (p. 195). Adolescents are taught that a barb is a provocation or stressor. Essentially, somebody is trying to push your anger buttons. Similarly to the Circle of Criticism exercise, the youngsters are "barbed" with certain provocative statements (e.g., "Why aren't you respecting me?"). These barbs can be designed to resemble provocative statements made by their parents, caregivers, teachers, or other authority figures. You should prepare the youngster for this activity by warning him or her: "I'm going to barb you." The barbs are generally delivered by the therapist. The youngsters should respond with self-control strategies (e.g., self-instructional statements such as "Calm down, stay in charge of myself.") or social skills (e.g., empathic assertiveness, fogging). As in the Circle of Criticism exercise, youngsters could have prepared scripts or lists of coping skills to rely on. Gradually, these prepared scripts could be faded out as the youngsters progress through training.

In running inpatient groups with angry youngsters, I (RDF) have generally used the group process as an *in vivo* learning experience. During group sessions, we had group rules and anger management skills posted for handy review. For instance, one angry young man was extremely upset when anyone disagreed with him. In one session, the group therapists told him we were going to disagree with him. The other group members were instructed to either say nothing or to disagree with what the young man said. At first, this was extremely difficult for him and he became agitated. We had to take a time-out, help him write down skills on paper, and remember to refer to the posted skills and rules. Over time, with repeated practice, he was able to better tolerate the disagreement by relying on his self-control skills.

Brondolo et al. (1997) give us some useful tips for doing these graduated exposures. For instance, when the youngsters are practicing delivering criticisms, disagreements, or other provocative statements, begin by teaching them to remove the emotional inflection from their words. As Brondolo et al. aptly note, flat tones allow people time to reflect about what is bothering them rather than to react immediately. Additionally, we like their suggestion to sit next to the youngster who is practicing anger management and conflict resolution. This subtly communicates our support and makes it easier to help youngsters through the process. Brondolo et al. also recommended that you ask permission to push or provoke the youngsters. We heartily endorse this idea. In fact, when I (RDF) was working in a psychiatric hospital, the staff and inpatients nicknamed me "Dr. can I push you on this?" because I commonly prefaced emotionally intense moments with this remark. Finally, adding gentle self-instruction to foster conflict resolution is encouraging to young clients. Brondolo et al. offer statements such as "I am going to sit right next to you like this and put my hand on your arm to remind you to stay relaxed. What do you think about that? Keep breathing, calm yourself, you don't need to respond to this attack" (p. 91).

CONCLUSION

As you can see from these previous sections, working with children and adolescents suffering from disruptive behavior disorders is often a long, slow, deliberate process. Communicating to the youngster that you are "in it for the long haul" is important. We encourage you to make use of multiple treatment strategies and to creatively apply the tools we have described.

14

❖

Working with Parents

Doing child psychotherapy is impossible without working with adults. Children's problems occur far more often outside of the therapy office than in-session. To effectively impact a child's environment, parents must become cocaptains with therapists. If parents and therapists are not working on the same "game plan," children receive confusing signals and the effectiveness of the intervention is lessened. We have included a "playbook" of interventions that we have found useful in helping parents shape their children's behavior.

The first strategy in working with parents is education. You must ensure that parents have basic general information, such as knowledge of developmentally appropriate behavior and recognition of the antecedents and consequences of behavior. We educate them through discussions, readings, and modeling. Providing parents with resources such as brochures or reading lists of books on cognitive therapy and child development may also be helpful. For example, we often recommend Seligman et al.'s (1995) *The Optimistic Child* to parents of depressed youth. In addition, handouts with guidelines for behavioral interventions and homework assignments will assist parents in implementing behavioral strategies at home.

ESTABLISHING REALISTIC
EXPECTATIONS FOR BEHAVIOR

Often, parents expect too much or too little from their children, which leads to conflict. We find that some parents' complaints about their children's behavior are in part related to unrealistic expectations for the child. Five-year-old Linda's mother complained that Linda did not "make her bed and clean her room, even though she knows she is supposed to." Working with Linda's mother on what are realistic expectations regarding chores for a 5-year-old, as well as educating her on how to effectively give directions, is a good strategy in this case. Micky's father was an "emotional perfectionist." He believed people, including Micky, should never feel sad, so whenever Micky showed a blue mood, his dad became overly alarmed.

Many parents mistakenly confuse *desirable* behavior with *expected* behavior. For example, it is desirable for siblings to play together for hours without arguing. However, we do not expect (certainly, it is not reasonable to expect) siblings to do so. When parents hold these unrealistic expectations, they will become frustrated with constantly trying to enforce them and failing. Fifteen-year-old Sean's father reported, "There is no reason he should ever pick on his little sister." Reminding Sean's father that in the real world no one is right or behaves perfectly 100% of the time may help him to develop more realistic expectations for his son's behavior.

In discussing with parents what is reasonable behavior for their child, we must consider several issues. We must consider the child's skill level and previous performance in the target area. For example, Bradley had been given limited responsibilities prior to age 10 years. His mother accurately stated that it is reasonable to expect a 10-year-old boy to assist in packing his lunch for school. However, Bradley had never been expected to do such tasks independently. Therefore, we pointed out that Bradley's parents first had to teach him the steps to packing his own lunch, and then they had to explain to Bradley the consequences of completing or not completing this task, before their expectation could actually be considered "reasonable."

Unique issues regarding realistic expectations are relevant when working with adolescents. Too often parents (and sometimes therapists) confuse adolescence with adulthood, forgetting that adolescence is a transitional phase preparing teenagers for adulthood. For example, some parents expect adolescents to *never* make mistakes in judgment or to *always* do what the parent desires (Barkley et al., 1999). Fifteen-year-old Darlene's father complained, "She knows homework must be done first before watching TV or talking on the phone." Sixteen-year-old Derek's mother stated, "I can't believe he got a traffic ticket! He knows better than to speed." Adolescents are learning to be autonomous, and inevitably will sometimes make poor choices. Although parents need to enforce consequences for these poor choices, they should expect their teens to make some imperfect and improper decisions.

A different type of expectational error is also common with parents of teens. When teens exhibit problematic or defiant behaviors, parents understandably may begin to expect such undesirable behavior from their teens all the time, as well as to presume that their teens are intentionally trying to anger them (Barkley et al., 1999). After Andre repeatedly violated his curfew, his mother reported, "I know he is doing this just to get to me." Confronting the issue in therapy revealed that most of Andre's friends had curfews an hour later than his, and that his disobedience sprang from wanting to hang out with them versus wanting to aggravate his mother.

Understanding cultural practices and expectations will also aid in parent training and intervention. While there are more similarities than differences in parenting practices across cultures, some parenting practices vary among cultural groups. For example, when you work with African American families, you may discover that extended family networks (e.g., grandparents, aunts and uncles, older brothers and sisters, other family members, neighbors, church members) are often very involved in "parenting" the child (Forehand & Kotchick, 1996). By recognizing these supports, and drawing on their strengths, you can incorporate these individuals in the treatment. Latino parenting also traditionally involves a greater reliance on extended family and other supports (Forehand & Kotchick, 1996). Note, however, that Latino culture generally includes more permissive parenting styles. Therefore, the expectations of parents in Latino culture may differ from those in cultures that put more emphasis on strict rules and obedience. Native American parenting styles vary according to the practices of many distinct tribal groups. But many Native American groups emphasize a shared responsibility for raising children and employ a cooperative and noncompetitive approach (Forehand & Kotchick, 1996). Thus, minimal punishment is used, with practices generally including the use of persuasion and inducing emotions such as fear, embarrassment, or shame (Forehand & Kotchick, 1996). Asian American cultural beliefs about parenting emphasize academic achievement, hard work, and parental authority (Forehand & Kotchick, 1996). Thus, all parents act as teachers, promoting the child's focus on goals for success.

Although none of these cultural practices necessarily precludes the use of certain parenting techniques presented here, they may impact the parents' views of therapeutic strategies and their motivation to use various disciplinary practices (Forehand & Kotchick, 1996). Therefore, part of your job as therapist is to assess the cultural values and standards of each client and to carefully consider how those values interact with expectations for behavior.

HELPING PARENTS DEFINE PROBLEMS

By assessing the frequency, intensity, and duration of the presenting problem, you will be able to gain insight into whether parental expectations are realistic. For example, many behaviors typically occur at a low to moderate frequency, but are only considered problematic when the frequency is high. Consider 7-year-old Taylor, whose mother reports that she "cries all the time." If Taylor cries four or five times a week when she doesn't get her way, this problem is much different than if she cries four or five times a day. To help the mother to assess the severity of Taylor's crying, the therapist had her complete a frequency chart similar to the one in Figure 14.1. The data she collected objectively showed her that Taylor's tantrums were really occurring much less frequently than she had estimated. Charts can also help identify patterns in behaviors. Eight-year-old Craig's parents used a frequency chart and discovered more frequent tantrums an hour after his afternoon snack and favorite TV show. Simply by changing his schedule, they reduced his tantrums.

Intensity of behavior is another potentially subjective aspect of defining problems. The therapist and parents can collaboratively design a scale for rating intensity to assess how atypical a behavior is. Nine-year-old Brian's parents were distressed by his fighting with his 6-year-old brother (e.g., "They can't be in the same room without fighting. He is so aggressive."). Therefore, we wanted to assess the severity of the aggression to determine appropriate interventions, as well as to provide a baseline to

	Monday	Tuesday	Wednesday	Thursday	Friday	Saturday	Sunday
7:00 A.M.	√		√√√√				
8:00 A.M.		√√		√√			
9:00 A.M.							
10:00 A.M.			√				√
11:00 A.M.							
12:00 P.M.							
1:00 P.M.							
2:00 P.M.							
3:00 P.M.		√√√√	√				√√√
4:00 P.M.							
5:00 P.M.							
6:00 P.M.			√				

FIGURE 14.1. Taylor's frequency chart.

help detect changes in behavior in the future. One of our jobs as therapists is to see how the parents' subjective perceptions match the objective data. With Brian's family, a 5-point scale was developed for measuring the intensity of the behavior: 1 point indicated arguing, 2 points indicated yelling, and so on, up to 5 points for punching and kicking. Identifying intensity is also beneficial for establishing guidelines for parental intervention (at 3 points or above), and independent problem solving (1 to 2 points).

Duration of the problem behaviors is also an important consideration. Two-minute tantrums should be addressed differently than 30-minute tantrums. Likewise, 15-year-old Katlyn's parents would be advised to respond differently if she delayed her chore of taking out the trash 10 minutes versus 10 days. Specific strategies for increasing desirable and decreasing undesirable behaviors are discussed in detail later in this chapter.

Anastopoulos (1998) discussed the importance of teaching parents of children with attention-deficit/hyperactivity disorder general behavior management principles to prepare them for later training in more specific behavioral techniques. We recommend using handouts, discussions, modeling, and examples from the family's presenting problem to help educate parents about basic behavioral principles. The ABC model is used to illustrate how children's Behaviors can be modified by "altering" Antecedent events and Consequences (Anastopoulos, 1998). Remember, children's behavior is purposeful for receiving/gaining positive consequences or to avoid undesirable situations (Anastopoulos, 1998).

The ABC model can be explained to parents in a manner similar to the example presented below. Verbal and visual presentation will make the information you present more memorable for parents. The following transcript can be used as a guide.

THERAPIST: You said that you see Megan's tantrums as your biggest problem, so we agreed to start by focusing on those. When we talk about Megan's temper tantrums, it will be helpful to do so using what is called an ABC model. "A" stands for what happens before the behavior ("B") occurs. "A's" kind of set the stage for "B's." Typically, antecedents are the triggers that "set off" the behavior. Sometimes they are the instructions and commands that alert your youngster. During the intake interview, you gave several examples of antecedents when you described times that Megan has tantrums. What types of antecedents can you think of now?

MS. MATERNAL: So antecedents would be like when I tell her to do something, or when she has to share.

THERAPIST: Those are all antecedents. (*Writes them on the ABC work-sheet, in the "A" column.*) You are one step ahead because you have already identified the triggers for "B"—the behavior. Sometimes the antecedents can be hard to identify and the behavior seems to just "come out of nowhere." However, you have already identified some triggers to the tantrums. You also gave several examples of tantrums where you did not know what the trigger was. Figuring that out will help us to understand and therefore change the behavior. As I said, the "B" in the "ABC" stands for behavior. We have said temper tantrums are the behavior, but what specific behaviors do the tantrums include.

MS. MATERNAL: Yelling, crying, laying on the ground and refusing to walk. (*Writes in "B" column of worksheet.*)

THERAPIST: OK. "C" is for consequences. That means the thing that happens after the behavior that either makes it happen more or happen less.

MS. MATERNAL: (*Laughs.*) Like Megan getting her way?

THERAPIST: That has been one consequence. Can you think of others?

MS. MATERNAL: Well, she doesn't always get her way. Sometimes she is punished. I send her to her room, take away her bike, or spank her. (*Writes on worksheet in the "C" column.*)

THERAPIST: So the consequences can vary. What do you think happens when Megan does not know what consequences to expect for her behavior?

MS. MATERNAL: Sometimes I think she gets even madder and throws a bigger fit if I don't let her get away with it. She probably thinks she'll get away with things and then she gets even madder if she doesn't get her way.

THERAPIST: What we want to do is have a clear consequence to follow the behavior so that Megan knows what the consequence will be when she does the behaviors. Understanding the ABC's of her behavior will help us make the changes necessary for the behavior to improve.

The therapist in this dialogue worked with Ms. Maternal to explicitly outline the ABC's related to Megan's behavior. Doing so not only helped Ms. Maternal understand the behavioral principles involved in the ABC model, but also helped her "tune in" to her own responses related to the consequences of Megan's behavior, as well as predicting potential triggers (antecedents).

HELPING PARENTS INCREASE
THEIR CHILD'S DESIRABLE BEHAVIORS:
"I JUST WANT HIM TO BEHAVE"

Parents commonly present for treatment stating that they would like to see more "good" behaviors in their children. Techniques for increasing specific behaviors represent the offensive playbook in parenting. Through using the techniques we describe in this chapter, you can work with parents on ways to increase desirable behaviors by being "proactive." Techniques for increasing desirable behaviors are generally applied before a negative behavior has occurred. You are teaching the parents to catch children behaving appropriately.

Reinforcement

Beginning parent training by teaching parents to reinforce their child's "good" behavior is an idea shared by most parent trainers (Barkley et al., 1999; Becker, 1971; Forehand & McMahon, 1981). *Reinforcement* is somewhat of a "catchall" term for anything that occurs following a behavior in order to increase the frequency of that behavior. Reinforcement is a basic behavioral strategy that generally produces quick results in increasing target behaviors. Thus, reinforcement is the primary way of increasing behavior and is implemented in many ways. The reinforcement, or reward, may involve giving something positive, such as praise, hugs, a toy, or playtime, or removing something negative, such as having to do chores.

Many parents neglect reinforcement with their children. The child's behavior is only noticed when it is disruptive or undesirable. Parents need to understand that by consistently leaving the child alone when they are behaving appropriately, they are essentially ignoring positive behavior. Some parents report that they do not want to reinforce the child during good behavior because they do not want to interrupt the behavior for fear that it will stop. Other parents believe that if they "disturb" the child, the youth will then demand continual attention (Forehand & McMahon, 1981). Still other parents believe that children should not be praised for appropriate behavior, and that praise and other forms of reinforcement should be used only when the child engages in extraordinarily good behavior (Webster-Stratton & Hancock, 1998).

Reinforcement comes in two types: positive and negative. Positive and negative reinforcement can be confusing to first-year doctoral students, let alone lay parents! Thus, we employ a simple teaching strategy. First, we emphasize that all reinforcement *increases* the desired behavior. The terms positive (+) and negative (−) reinforcement refer to whether *something good is added* to increase the rate of desired behavior (positive reinforcement) or *something bad is subtracted or removed* to increase the rate of desired behavior. The (+) and (–) signs are good cues for this explanation. Most people recognize that a (+) stands for both adding and something positive and that a (–) refers to both subtracting and something negative. We find it helpful to emphasize that the descriptors refer to the reward aspect, but the end result is always an increase in desirable behavior. Thus, if Karen cleans her room, she *gets* a hug, verbal praise, 15 extra minutes of TV time, or a special snack. This is an example of positive reinforcement. Karen could also be rewarded for cleaning her room with a negative reinforcer: her father *stops* yelling at her for being messy, lazy, and so on.

What parent has not heard his/her child say, "Hey Mommy, Daddy, look at me!" Indeed, attention is one of the most overlooked reinforcers by parents. Yet most children crave it. Therefore, giving children attention is an effective way for parents to increase desirable behavior. Smiles, hugs, verbal praise, and pats on the back are all ways to positively attend to the child. Simply watching 9-year-old Teri build with blocks and commenting on her good work provides attention, and thus is reinforcing to Teri.

Play Time (Noncontingent)

The Greenspans offers some wonderful ideas in their parenting books (Greenspan & Greenspan, 1985, 1989). These books, aimed mainly at parents of young children, emphasize the value of floor time. *Floor time* is simply a time parents or caregivers devote to playing with their child on the floor and following the child's lead. We encourage parents to have floor time with their young children everyday for 10 minutes or so.

When parents do make time to spend with their children, the child is reinforced and the bond between child and parent is strengthened. Play interactions also provide rich environments for reinforcing children's positive behavior and for increasing the child's self-esteem by focusing on the youth's skills and strengths. The child feels valued by the parent, which frequently leads to increased compliance, which generalizes to other situations. Playtime can also serve as an opportunity to practice and model problem solving for the child. Ten-year-old Joel became very self-critical when he made mistakes. While playing a board game with Joel, his father consistently modeled positive coping, as when he drew a card requiring him to move back five spaces on the board (e.g., "Oh well, maybe I'll get a better card next time.").

Play is the fabric of a child's world. By following the child's lead in his/her play, parents enjoy opportunities to see positive behavior in their child and attend to those behaviors; they can also ignore mildly inappropriate behaviors (Anastopoulos, 1998). A common pitfall for parents is trying to control the play, being too directive, and taking over the task. Teaching parents to narrate rather than instruct is a helpful strategy ("You are building a tower of blue blocks," vs. "Let's make a house."). Parents should be taught to be more descriptive and less interrogative in their comments regarding the child's play (Webster-Stratton & Hancock, 1998). Eight-year-old Connie's mother was taught to change questions (e.g., "What are the dolls doing in the house?"; "Where is the girl doll going in the car?"; "What are they going to do after the picnic?") into descriptive statements (e.g., "The dolls are sitting in the house."; "The little girl is going for a drive."; "They are all having a picnic."). Another frequent mistake made by parents is being too disengaged in the play, such that they are essentially watching the youth play. Consider 7-year-old Mary Lou, who became quickly bored and attention seeking while playing with her dollhouse when her mom just watched while sitting beside her. In another example, 11-year-old Vince's father became overly directive while assembling a model airplane with him. Vince quickly lost interest and became oppositional.

Regarding play with their children, parents should be encouraged to describe events and behaviors, praise appropriate behavior, and ignore negative behaviors as long as they are not dangerous or destructive (Eyberg & Boggs, 1998). Allowing the child to take the lead minimizes the opportunities for noncompliance. At times when parents need to direct the activity, they should offer specific commands (e.g., "Put the cars on the shelf" instead of "Why don't we clean up?"). Parents should be more directive when behaviors cannot be ignored, the behaviors are reinforced by something other than parents, or the behaviors do not extinguish easily (Eyberg & Boggs, 1998).

Inviting the parent and child to play during session will allow you to observe the parent and shape the use of techniques. Eight-year-old Blake's father reported that every time they tried to play a game together, it ended in a fight. In session, the two were observed interacting while playing Candy Land. When Blake stated, "I'm losing again. I'm such a loser," his father responded by telling him not to talk like that. Then the father gave Blake a lengthy lecture on why Blake should not put himself down. The father had a good intention: he did not want Blake to be so hard on himself. But his approach led to frustration and irritation for both of them. After the therapist worked with the father and reviewed ways to reinforce, attend, and model, the father and Blake had greater success and the game was more enjoyable. The following week, the two again were playing the game. Blake's father lost the game. He responded with a smile and stated, "It was fun playing that game with you. Maybe next time I will win," thus modeling positive coping, rather than lecturing.

Spending noncontingent time with teens is also highly recommended (Barkley et al., 1999). Allow the adolescent to choose something he/she enjoys. Parents should then participate with positive observations, but should not ask questions, give directions, or make corrections. The main goal is to be interactive, but nonjudgmental! Computer games, art projects, cooking, sports, card games, or board games are all potential activities. Fourteen-year-old Nicholas wanted to make brownies with his mom. His mother got out the recipe and the ingredients. Initially, she took control of the activity, saying, "Here, let me." Then she caught herself and thereafter said things like "Nicholas, what does it say to do first?" and "You are doing a nice job mixing."

Providing Choices

Providing children with choices is another form of parental reward. Choosing is a very rich experience for most children and adolescents. Joe was a 5-year-old boy who often dawdled behind and darted away from his mother. His mother learned to use choice as a simple reward (e.g., "Joey, since you came when I called you and you stayed by my side when we walked, you can choose whether we go in the front door or the back door."). Eight-year-old Tabitha became easily frustrated, distracted, and impatient at restaurants. Her father used choices effectively as a way to increase her positive behavior (e.g., "Tabby, because you waited without jumping on me and whining, you get to pick the table we sit at."). Finally, 16-year-old Moe often fought with his 10-year-old sister during car rides. His mom and dad "caught him" behaving well with his sister. Accordingly, they said, "Moe, since you are talking to your sister without yelling and teasing, you can pick the radio station we will listen to until we get to Grandma's house."

Helping Parents Increase Reinforcement

Increasing the frequency of reinforcement will produce quick and effective behavioral results. Therapists and parents should begin by identifying two or three behaviors to target. For example, if a child frequently fights with her younger brother, the parents could reinforce her nonfighting interactions with her brother. Once target behaviors are identified, a list of potential reinforcers can be generated. Parents are then required to increase the frequency with which they reinforce that behavior. It is important to emphasize that simply by reinforcing a child one time for a particular behavior will not necessarily ensure the child will do the desired behavior again. Rather, parents must reinforce the behavior on numerous occasions before it is likely to change (Patterson, 1976). In addition, the praise must occur immediately following the behavior in order to be most effective (Webster-Stratton & Hancock, 1998). When tucking him into bed at night, Dalton's mother always praised him for the good things he had done that day. However, her lack of immediate reinforcement during the day made it difficult for Dalton to connect the "end of the day" praise to his actual good behaviors.

One challenge for therapists involves parents who report that their children never do anything worthy of praise. This typically reflects frustration on the parent's part, and may result in a lack of attention to positive behaviors. We find it helpful to remind parents that children are not "bad" 100% of the time, and that it is important to find times that they are exhibiting desirable behaviors and reward them. Putting forth the effort now will decrease the need for more punishment, as well as make future interactions smoother and less conflictual. In general, increasing positive feedback to at least the frequency of negative feedback is recommended (Barkley et al., 1999). Indeed, this is commonsensical. If parents increase the amount they reinforce positive behavior, they are spending less time and effort on punishment. If they are reinforcing positive behavior, negative/disruptive behavior should become less frequent until it is crowded out by the new positive behavior. More specifically, when the child is present, his/her parents should aim to initially give him/her some form of reinforcement several times an hour at the minimum. Reminding parents that reinforcement may be as simple as a look and a smile will help them to keep this task in perspective. However, for parents who find this assignment too overwhelming, a more graduated approach may be needed. You can help parents select a specific time period (e.g., the 15 minutes after dinner) to begin attending to the child's behavior. Once the parent has developed basic skills through practice, they can be generalized.

For instance, Grace's parents wanted to reduce her oppositional behavior. It seemed that Grace responded to all their requests with a definitive "No!" When asked what things they praised in Grace, her parents responded with several sporadic examples: "Well, last week I told her she did good work on her spelling worksheet. And, when her cousin was over last weekend, I told Grace I liked how she shared." These were both very appropriate times to reinforce Grace. However, the difficulty the parents had in generating examples of their use of reinforcement, and its seemingly rare occurrence, was a clue that a dramatic increase in reinforcement was needed. Thus, we praised the parents' efforts and use of positive statements, but emphasized the importance of praising Grace at least several times a day. A homework assignment recording their own use of reinforcement was used to provide a structure under which the parents could practice.

Teaching Parents Different Ways to Reinforce a Child

Shaping involves reinforcing graduated steps toward the desired behavior. Each step is like a subgoal toward the overall desired behavior. Initially, a small step is reinforced (e.g., taking clean laundry from the laundry room to the bedroom) until it is consistently demonstrated. Then, more advanced steps must be completed for the reinforcement to be received (e.g., folding clean clothes, putting clean clothes in dresser drawers). "Homework" assignments are given to parents instructing them to initially reinforce early steps. As the child begins to demonstrate those behaviors, more advanced steps must occur for reinforcement to be given. Applying differential reinforcement is also taught. Thus, more complex behaviors, or "higher" levels in the sequence, receive more reinforcement than the simpler, lower level behaviors.

Teaching parents to use a variety of specific reinforcers will increase their effectiveness and prevent habituation to any one reinforcer by the youth. Verbal praise, physical reinforcement, enjoyable activities, and tangible rewards can all be utilized by parents. The specificity of the verbal praise is just as important as providing tangible positive reinforcement. Merely telling 11-year-old Lynn "Good job!" provides little information regarding what behavior the parent is pleased with. Lynn may not be able to figure out which behavior the parent is reinforcing. Rather, statements such as "I like the way you hung up your coat" will lead to increased future compliance.

Reviewing potential reinforcers with parents is recommended. Parents should make a list of things they can say and do to reinforce their child.

Verbal rewards must also be nonjudgmental and immediate. Reinforcement should be a reward, and should not be coupled with criticism. Thus, no "but" should follow the reward (e.g., "I like how you cleared your dishes, *but* you did not put them in the dishwasher."). The verbal praise should describe the behavior the parent likes, not judge the child. When the parent praises without judging, the child does not then misinterpret praise or its lack as accepting or rejecting of him/herself, but rather of the behavior. (e.g., "Good job raking up all the leaves" vs. "You are such a good boy for raking the leaves").

Working to Overcome Parents' Reluctance to Give Positive Reinforcement

Some parents who are having trouble managing their children's behavior are initially reluctant and perhaps even skeptical about the value of positive reinforcement. These parents have come to you for help in designing new and harsher penalties for misbehavior. In our opinion, it is important not to collude with the parents' agenda to first develop stiffer penalties for misbehavior. So, how do we work with parents who do not share our view that increasing the level of positive reinforcement is an effective intervention?

Here's what we try. First, we might ask the parent what it is he/she really wants. The bottom line for him/her is for the child to listen to him/her and do what he/she says. This prompts questions such as "How effective are you in getting the child to hear you now?"; "How easy is it for a kid to listen to someone who is nagging, scolding, and punishing?"; and "Do you really listen to people who do these things?" A second pass through this issue involves teaching parents that positive reinforcement lightens the family tone (Barkley et al., 1999; Becker, 1971; Forehand & McMahon, 1981). As mentioned in Chapter 13, many of these families' homes are characterized by tense, hostile, and conflictual emotional climates. Adding positive reinforcement combats this overbearing atmosphere. Finally, you can increase the parents' motivation to try positive reinforcement by helping them see that punishment is not working and their child has likely habituated to the negative consequences. It is this habituation that leads the parents to seek even more punitive methods.

Socratic questioning is quite useful in these circumstances. Consider the following brief example where Mr. Punish thinks positive reinforcement is a load of baloney and wonders why he has to "bribe" his child.

MR. PUNISH: You know, I don't get why I have to bribe my own kid. Why does he need a carrot out in front of him? He should just do what we ask without any payoff. Hell, if I acted like that my father would have kicked my a _____ out!

THERAPIST: I understand Mr. Punish. Tommy is not following your rules for his behavior or even how a son should react to his father. It is really frustrating.

MR. PUNISH: That's right. The idea of every day being Christmas for good behavior just doesn't sit right.

THERAPIST: I can see that. Remind me just for a minute. How have your punishments been working?

MR. PUNISH: They don't. The kid doesn't seem to care. They don't make a dent in his behavior.

THERAPIST: I see. You really want things to change, don't you?

MR. PUNISH: Something's got to give.

THERAPIST: I agree. Let me ask you something. Have you ever tried this positive reinforcement stuff in the way I described before?

MR. PUNISH: No. You know that.

THERAPIST: Help me understand. You want things to give or change. What you are doing now is not working. You have never tried the positive reinforcement. So, how can you be certain it won't help?

The important part of this dialogue is that the therapist actively dealt with Mr. Punish's reluctance to use positive reinforcement. Rather than lecturing him, the therapist constructed a Socratic dialogue so Mr. Punish could examine his own position.

TEACHING PARENTS TO GIVE COMMANDS/DIRECTIONS

Many parents spend a large amount of time telling their children what to do and what not to do. Yet giving directions is a basic parenting task that is frequently overlooked (Barkley, 1997). Teaching parents more effective strategies for giving commands will decrease the number and frequency of commands, as well as increase their children's compliance rates (Barkley, 1997). Barkley (1997) recommends that parents first attend to the instructions they are giving and only give directions they are willing to enforce. He notes that a series of unreinforced commands will only lead to more noncompliance by teaching children that the consequence of not following directions is that they will "get out of" the requested behavior! Five-year-old Abby frequently played with her food at the dinner table rather than eating. Her parents threatened numerous times, "Once more and you are going to your room." Abby responded with "No! No!" Her parents warned, "Then you better settle down." A few minutes later the cycle continued. When her parents finally sent her to her room, Abby would throw a temper tantrum. This is a cycle many parents fall into, but luckily you can teach parents techniques to stop it.

You need to teach parents that giving a command means giving the child directions, rather than making requests (Barkley, 1997). A request or question leaves room for choice (e.g., "Will you please clean up your room?"—"No!"). Thus, children should never be asked to do something unless parents are willing to accept "No" for an answer ("Clean up your trucks and cars now" will be more effective than "Can you clean up your cares and trucks?"). Forehand and McMahon (1981) suggest that many parents have trouble with this aspect of giving directions, because as adults we do not often make this distinction. How often have we said "Would you mind getting the phone?" when it is ringing? When doing so, we are asking a question, but our intent is really for the person to answer the phone.

Similarly, parents should avoid pleading with their child. Mary Ann and Kathy's father often pleaded, "Please stop fighting, just for me?" Again, pleading sends the message that the child has the power to choose not to follow the direction. Although children can even refuse commands, these guidelines reduce the opportunity to do so. Noncompliance must then be met with specific consequences addressed later in this chapter.

Finally, parents should avoid using "Let's . . . " with commands unless they truly intend to complete the task with the child (Forehand & McMahon, 1981). Thus, when the parent says, "Let's clean up the blocks," he should intend to help the child clean up all the blocks, not just start the task and then walk away, expecting the child to complete it independently. Not only has this statement misled the child, the parent is also modeling incomplete follow-through.

Commands should be specific and include a time frame for expected completion (e.g., "Eric, you need to put your clothes away before dinner."). Making only one command at a time will increase the chance of compliance. Multiple tasks presented at one time, or chain commands, are likely to be forgotten; moreover, they leave little room for success as all the commands must be fulfilled for success to occur (Forehand & McMahon, 1981). Further, a child may be overwhelmed when presented with a list of instructions. One command will seem more manageable, will invoke less discomfort, and will more likely be followed. Following a command with a lengthy rationale is also a common error parents make. This may lead to noncompliance because by the time the parent is done, the initial instruction has been lost (Forehand & McMahon, 1981). Compliance should be followed immediately with specific praise. With a child who has particular difficulty attending to and following directions, parents should have him/her repeat back the directions to ensure his/her understanding (Anastopoulos, 1998).

As mentioned in Chapter 13, vague and weak parental commands sabotage compliance. Think about this example. Stan is a 12-year-old boy who suffers from attention-deficit/hyperactivity disorder. His room looked like a bomb hit it. Stuff was everywhere! His mom ordered him to "clean his room!" Stan spent about an hour tidying his floor so you could see the carpet. He transferred all the stuff from his floor to his desk, so all the stuff was piled high covering the desk. Mom returned and reacted lividly. "How could you do this?" she screamed. Mom and Stan got into a huge shouting match. Mom resented Stan's apparent noncompliance and Stan was perplexed about what was annoying Mom.

So, what happened? The vague command gave rise to differing expectations. For Stan, cleaning his room meant getting everything off his floor. Mom, however, had a different expectation. She expected that his room would be completely in order and tidy. But her expectation was not communicated via her command.

What could Mom do differently? First, she needs to make her request clear and specific (e.g., "Stan, I want you to pick up the dirty clothes on the floor and put them in the laundry basket."). Second, she needs to be sure to break the task down into small accomplishable tasks. Rather than giving the ambiguous directive, "Clean your room," Mom should divide the tasks into subgoals (e.g., "Pick up the clothes, put away the toys, stack the books."). Finally, as with any child with attention or behavior problems, Mom has to give one direction at a time and reinforce efforts at compliance. Therefore, Mom should tell Stan to first pick up the clothes and put them in the laundry basket. Next, he is to check in with her for a reward and a new assignment.

You can model giving commands and delivering consequences (Barkley, 1997). The parents will observe you giving specific directions in a firm yet calm voice. If the child complies, an opportunity for you to demonstrate proper reinforcement follows. When the youth does not comply, you should use the opportunity to show the appropriate use of time-out or response cost strategies. Either way, you seize the chance to model the strategy being discussed. Similarly, coaching and reinforcing parents for appropriately making requests and rewarding their children is recommended.

Just as these techniques may be quite novel to parents, the child may also require an adjustment period for receiving directions. Thus, some youth may initially rebel against these strategies as a way of testing limits. Forewarning parents of this possibility will help them to problem solve and plan for maintaining consistency in the face of these protests by the child. Mrs. Prepared predicted that Allen would initially respond to directions to clean up the dirty clothes in his room with opposition. Thus, she planned and informed him of the consequences. "You will not be allowed to watch *Power Rangers* today if your clothes aren't picked up before it comes on. If you get all of your dirty clothes picked up and in the hamper, you may watch *Power Rangers*."

LINKING CHILD BEHAVIOR TO PARENTAL CONSEQUENCES: CONTINGENCY MANAGEMENT

Carol's mother stated that Carol's biggest problem is that she does not follow through with her chores and her mom's requests. When discussing the possibility of rewarding Carol for compliance, her mother stated, "But she should *want* to help out around the house and to contribute to the family." Be this as it may, Carol doesn't appear to have that intrinsic motivation, and thus an external motivator may be needed.

Contingency management is a specific utilization of the principle of reinforcement. Its purpose is to provide the sometimes needed external motivation for children to comply with certain requests (Anastopoulos, 1998). The process involves positively reinforcing target behaviors on a set schedule. Thus, youth essentially earn rewards by engaging in particular behaviors for a set number of responses or a set amount of time.

To start, parents must decide what behaviors will be part of the contingency management plan. They may reinforce homework completion or washing the dishes after dinner. Whatever the chosen behavior, the plan must be discussed with the youth so that parental expectations are clear. Listing and posting the parental expectations visually will also help. Anastopoulos (1998) recommends having a dialogue with parents about the difference between rights and privileges as a way of facilitating the listing process and to determine if parents have been treating child privileges as rights. Consider Ms. Lenient's belief that she had already removed most of 14-year-old Lauren's privileges. Asking Ms. Lenient what things were necessary for her daughter (e.g., food, clothing, schooling) and what things she could "live without" (e.g., Internet, telephone), helped identify privileges that had always been given to Lauren regardless of her behavior.

Making a contingency chart and putting it on the refrigerator or on a bulletin board will serve as a visual reminder to the youth. For younger children, using pictures of the expected behaviors may make the chart more meaningful and understandable. Similarly, the reinforcer should be clearly identified. Including the child in the decision of specifying a reinforcer as much as possible is preferred. The reinforcer should be named ahead of time so the youth knows what he/she is working for.

Points or tokens are useful for tracking progress toward the reward. Points are assigned for each privilege and each reward. When the behavior is completed, the child earns the preset number of points. The youth can exchange the points for rewards whenever the amount needed for a specific award has accumulated. Eight-year-old Alex wanted more Poke'mon cards and a new Nintendo game. Through a contingency management plan, Alex earned points for picking up his toys, clearing the dishes, and taking his bath when asked. By the end of the week, Alex had earned enough points for a pack of Poke'mon cards. He knew that if he "kept up the good work" he would have enough points at the end of the month to earn a Nintendo game.

We recommend that parents first select behaviors that are relatively less difficult to improve and reward the completion of the target behavior with a moderately rewarding reinforcer selected by the youngster (Barkley et al., 1999). For example, 9-year-old Aaron was rewarded for making his bed four out of seven times a week by treating him at his favorite ice cream parlor on Friday night. The success of this practice will depend in part upon parents' ability to consistently enforce their plan. That is, the youth must not have access to the reward unless he/she completes the target request. If the youth is able to enjoy the reward—be it a special activity, food treat, or video—without completing the assigned task, he/she will have no motivation to follow the plan and the contingency plan will fail. Thus, Aaron's parents had to be sure not to take him to the ice cream parlor unless he met his goal of making his bed at least four times in the preceding week.

Contingency plans come in many shapes and sizes! The specifics of the plan should match the child's cognitive maturity and the family's needs. In general, the child earns some type of reward for completing desired behaviors. He/she earns small rewards in the short term, and larger rewards for long-term improvement. Each day, Lindsey was able to earn the privilege of choosing a special dessert after dinner. At the end of the week, if she met the set goal every day, she was taken to a movie or to McDonald's. After a month's success with her daily goal, Lindsey earned a new computer game. Points, stickers, pennies, or tokens can be awarded immediately when a target behavior occurs. A set number of points, stickers, or tokens is chosen to be exchanged for a larger reward (e.g., 100 points for a special toy, 30 points for an ice cream snack). Younger children respond well to stickers. They are visually appealing, and reinforcing in and of themselves. Further, young children often become invested in placing the stickers on a chart and displaying them on the refrigerator or some other public space. Adolescents will likely see stickers as immature and will probably benefit more from a point system. Barkley et al. (1999) recommend a "checkbook" to keep a running tally of points. Depending on the difficulty of achieving a desired behavior, different amounts of points are awarded. The points can then be traded in for specific reinforcers.

Initially, we recommend only *awarding* points. That is, desirable behavior will *earn* points, stickers, and so on. Undesirable behavior will generally be ignored or dealt with using one of the other strategies presented later in this chapter. Parents are often quick to "take away" points. This can lead to children ending up "in debt" and owing their parents, which is counterproductive. Mr. Debt took 5 points from Teddy when he threw his coat on the floor. Teddy became so upset he began to throw a tantrum. Mr. Debt told Teddy he would take away 5 more points for every minute the coat was on the floor. By the time the tantrum was over 10 minutes later, Teddy had lost 55 points, which meant he owed his parents 35 points! He would have to behave perfectly for one and a half days just to get back to zero. Putting a child in such a position is unmotivating to the child, creates frustration, and will be less effective in changing behavior. For these reasons, it is more beneficial to create success and excitement around the contingency plan by making the child earn rewards, but not lose them. Later, once the strategy is in place, points may be taken away as punishment when specified rules are violated (Anastopoulos, 1998; Barkley et al., 1999). This is called "response cost." Barkley et al. (1999) point out the importance of the penalty matching the violation that has occurred. Thus, noncompliance with day-to-day chores is more appropriately punished with the loss of points, whereas more serious infractions, such as breaking curfew, call for more serious punishments, such as grounding. When 17-year-old Patricia left the dirty dinner dishes in the sink, she lost 10 points. When she was 30 minutes late coming home and had not called, she was grounded for the next evening.

Behavioral contracts between teens and their parents also work well (Barkley et al., 1999). Such contracts should state the behavior the teen is expected to engage in, as well as the consequences of not doing so. Sixteen-year-old Kristen and her parents agreed to the following contract: "I, Kristen, will come straight home after school unless I have called and talked to Mom about doing otherwise. If I do not, I will not be permitted to go to any evening events over the weekend." The contract can then be displayed in the adolescent's room or on the refrigerator.

Parents' beliefs can compromise their contingency management. For instance, Ms. Indulgent thought that "being a good parent means giving my son everything he asks for." Thus, making her plentiful rewards contingent upon young Jeremy's appropriate behavior was quite difficult for her to do. You would need to use cognitive therapy tools to help her evaluate the accuracy of this belief (e.g., "What's the evidence for and against this assumption?"; "What are the advantages and disadvantages of holding onto this belief?" "Is it possible to be a good parent while still limiting your child?").

Parental overprotectiveness and overinvolvement can also influence how the parent implements a contingency management program (Chorpita & Barlow, 1998; Kendall et al., 1991; Silverman & Kurtines, 1996). Chorpita and Barlow (1998) define *overprotection* as "excessive parental involvement in controlling the child's environment to minimize aversive experiences for the child" (p. 12). Parents may think being a good parent means rescuing their child from any discomfort. In truth, these parents are being "too helpful" to their children. For example, whenever 14-year-old Jimmy panicked while working on a science project, his dad stepped in and finished it for him. Dad thought, "This is what fathers are for." Working with Dad to teach him how he is unwittingly robbing Jimmy of the opportunity to cope with his own anxiety and develop a hardy self-concept would be necessary in this instance. Asking Dad "How can fathers help sons build the confidence that they can do difficult things?" might be a useful Socratic question.

Lack of parental follow-through, inattentiveness, and inconsistency are yet other problems that can limit contingency management. Some parents may think, "Why do I have to do this? He should be able to manage his own behavior!" Others may say, "Keeping track of all these points and stars is too much work for me!" Addressing these beliefs requires a gentle, patient, Socratic approach. Consider Mr. and Mrs. Surf who agreed to follow a contingency management plan with their 12-year-old daughter, Mallory. Unfortunately the Surfs never wrote anything down and did not keep track of whether they rewarded Mallory or not. Not surprisingly, the contingency plan was a dismal failure. What would you do?

We would recommend going back to the basics here. First, address the beliefs that buttress the inconsistency (e.g., "How can we teach Mallory that her behavior counts? How can we help her *see* her progress? What would be a simple way to remind Mallory and yourselves that her behavior counts? . . . "). Next, simplify the recording process so it is easy to complete. Use a checkmark or sticker system. If writing is interfering with the process, you might suggest using buttons, marbles, or paperclips as tokens. Each time Mallory did her chores, her parents could simply drop a paperclip into an envelope. Then they could count the paperclips at the end of the week. You could have the family practice the system in session to demonstrate that the program is not time-consuming.

HELPING PARENTS DEAL WITH THEIR CHILD'S UNDESIRABLE BEHAVIORS

Using attention and differential reinforcement, effectively giving directions, and contingency management plans will all increase desirable behaviors. These techniques allow parents to proactively head off problems before they start. However, as many parents tell us, that is not enough! We need to prepare parents for those times when they have to react to children's undesirable behaviors. These are the "defensive" plays of discipline. In this section, we have provided techniques for dealing with misbehavior, acting out, and noncompliance.

Ignoring/Extinction

As previously mentioned, parental attention is a powerful reinforcer. Unfortunately, parents may unwittingly reinforce children's undesirable behaviors. For instance, sometimes children act out in order to get adults' attention. When they get that attention, their acting-out behavior has been rewarded. Ignoring is a parenting technique in which the adult withholds or withdraws attention. Teaching parents to ignore an undesirable act while reinforcing more desirable behavior is a powerful strategy.

Ignoring a child's misbehavior includes removing all attention. Eye contact between parent and child should be avoided. The parent should not respond to the child's behavior, arguments, or whining. For example, Sheila's mother worked on ignoring Sheila's whining. She went about her own work as if nothing was happening, and did not look at or talk to Sheila. As soon as Sheila stopped whining, her mother looked at her, smiled, and complimented her improved behavior.

Disruptive children can appear to be relentless attention seekers. Talking back, arguing, name calling, and complaining are potential attention grabbers. Seven-year-old Warren bugged his mom when she was talking on the phone. It seemed to her that he unleashed his most obnoxious habits when she had the most important phone calls. He would pull the cat's tail, turn the TV volume up louder, chase his sister with spaghetti strands, and yell "Hey, Mom," incessantly. The more his mom attended to these behaviors, the more they increased in intensity, frequency, and duration.

When you teach parents to ignore their children's attention-seeking behaviors, you must keep several things in mind. First, parents need to be sure *they can ignore* the behavior. For example, behavior that is dangerous and destructive should never be ignored. In such cases, other parenting strategies should be employed. Second, in order to extinguish the behavior, parents must be able to ignore the full intensity of the behavior. Mrs. Highstrung dutifully ignored Tammy's screaming and tantrum throwing until her screaming reached its highest pitch. She then responded, "Tammy, you are making me lose my hearing. Stop it!" Mrs. Highstrung had just taught Tammy to scream louder to gain her attention. Third, parents have to be prepared for an *extinction burst* (Spiegler & Guevremont, 1998). This means that when you start to ignore the problem behavior, it is probably going to get worse before it gets better. For example, when 7-year-old Frank's parents ignored his tantrum throwing, he "upped the stakes" and intensified his ear-piercing screaming. His parents needed to ride out this last burst of intensity before he quieted down.

Time-Out

Time-out is one of the most used and misused parenting techniques. When used appropriately and consistently, time-out produces many positive results. However, when misapplied, time-out can lead to increased behavior problems as well as to frustration on the parts of the parents, the child, and the therapist. Reviewing when and how to utilize time-out, as well as modeling or role playing the steps of time-out, is helpful. Problem solving with the parent ways to deal with noncompliance with and resistance to the time-out process is also warranted. Providing psychoeducation about time-out should be routine with any parent who is seeking help managing a child's behavior by using time-out. Often, parents state that they already use time-out or have tried time-out in the past. You should not assume the parent has used time-out properly. Frequently, parents are calling their technique "time-out" when they are not following the basic principles of the intervention.

Mr. Skeptical rolled his eyes, "I don't believe in that time-out. I've already tried it and it doesn't work. My kids talk back, argue, name call, and complain." These behaviors are not easily ignored and all serve as ways of increasing attention and sometimes avoiding punishment. When parents engage in these exchanges with children, they are aiding the children in avoiding the punishment *and* providing them with the attention they seek. The longer Mr. Skeptical and his child argue about the child being in time-out, the more time that passes before the child has to sit in time-out. Mr. Skeptical eventually tired of the conflict and gave up, allowing the child to avoid punishment. When time-out is used properly, it is the child who tires and changes behavior.

Time-out removes a youngster from a reinforcing situation. In fact, Spiegler and Guevremont (1998) call it "time out from generalized reinforcers" (p. 141). The removal is temporary and is intended to serve as a learning tool. Following the brief removal, the youth is permitted to return to the situation. If appropriate behavior is exhibited, the child is reinforced by being allowed to continue in the preferred, desirable activities. If the youngster again engages in inappropriate behavior, he/she is again removed, and thus punished for the behavior.

Parents must be cautioned to "pick their battles" when deciding what limits to set with time-out. Once a decision has been made to address a behavior, the parent must be willing to follow the discipline through. Particularly in the beginning, firm limits and consistency by parents will be met with resistance by children. You must adequately prepare parents for the idea that their child's behavior will likely worsen before it gets better. Outlining basic behavioral principles and the likely consequences of "giving in" may increase parental compliance and consistent implementation.

Parents should begin the time-out process by identifying behaviors they will target. Next, they need to designate a time-out chair or room. The location should include minimal distractions and no reinforcers.

Then the parents must explain the process of time-out with the child. When implemented, the length of time-out should coincide with the child's age. Generally, 1 minute per year of the child's age is generally appropriate (e.g., 7 minutes for a 7-year-old). When the child engages in a misbehavior and parent decides to use time-out, the parent tells the child, "Go to time-out for 5 minutes." The parent may need to walk the child to the time-out chair or room. If the child sits in the chair for the designated length of time, time-out is over and he/she can get up. If the time-out resulted from noncompliance with a request, the child must then complete the request. If he/she does not, then he/she returns to time-out.

Five-year-old Vickie often left the time-out chair without permission. Her mother was unsure about how to handle this behavior. We taught her to immediately return Vickie to the chair and tell her that if she got up again, she would have to sit for an extra 2 minutes. If Vickie got up, her mother would again immediately walk her back to the chair. If she still refused to stay in the chair, Vickie's mother was instructed to sit with her or to hold her on her lap if necessary. It was important to ensure that while she was holding Vickie, she was providing as little reinforcement as possible. Thus, she was not to talk to, sing to, yell at, or cuddle her. Rather, she simply held her in time-out. Vickie soon learned that getting out of time-out no longer allowed her to avoid punishment, but actually prolonged the punishment. After a few trials, she began staying in time-out on her own.

Spiegler and Guevremont (1998) nicely summarize some important general points about time-out. First, the child should be given the reason for and told the duration of time-out. Second, time-outs should be brief. Third, parents should never deliver any reinforcements during the time-out. Fourth, parents need to keep the child in time-out until the time-out is over. If the child is screaming and/or getting up from the time-out chair, the parent must clearly state, "Time-out begins when you are sitting on the chair and quiet." Fifth, time-out should end only when the child is behaving appropriately. Last, but certainly not least, time-outs should not provide a secondary gain for the child by letting the child avoid unpleasant responsibilities. When 8-year-old Beth was put in time-out for refusing to put her shoes away, her mother rightly followed through and made sure that Beth put her shoes away after time-out.

Five-year-old Eddy's mother reported increased frustration with his frequent anger and aggression in the home. She listed several problematic behaviors that she believed Eddy was using to get attention from her. She reported using time-out to deal with the behaviors but admittedly had seen no benefits. When she described her use of time-out, she noted that Eddy became very upset when she sent him to time-out and he cried. Thus, she usually sat in time-out with him, held him in her lap, and sang to him. Although Eddy's mom was choosing an effective strategy and applying it at an appropriate time, she was inadvertently rewarding Eddy's behavior by giving him a great deal of attention. We discussed the importance of removing all reinforcement during time-out with Eddy's mom, as well as ways she could use alone time with Eddy to *reinforce appropriate behavior*. Eddy was then prepared for the "new" time-out with the use of role plays. We told Eddy's mom that it might take some time for both of them to adjust to this new strategy. Initially, Eddy's tantrums in time-out worsened as he sought comfort and attention from his mother. However, he quickly learned that appropriate behavior rather than tantrums would earn him alone time with his mom.

Removal of Rewards and Privileges

Removal of rewards and privileges is a common way to decrease children's undesirable behavior. Like time-out, many parents already use removal of rewards and privileges to manage their children's behavior. However, we encourage you to help parents refine these strategies.

When we teach parents to make the removal of rewards and privileges contingent on misbehavior, we coach them on tying the removal to the value of the misbehavior. For instance, 9-year-old Billy ignored his mother's request to come in the house. He was "too busy" riding his bike around the neighborhood. The proper consequence here would be loss of bike riding for 1 day. Consider another example. Fifteen-year-old Teresa continually pushed the envelope regarding her phone privileges, spending hours on the line with her friends. What is a logical consequence? Removing phone privileges for a day is a punishment directly connected to the misbehavior.

As mentioned previously, choice is a major reward and privilege for children. As family executives, parents can remove this reward as well as grant it. Indeed, sometimes removing a reward like choice is more powerful than removing a tangible privilege such as bike riding or telephone time. For example, on the way to dinner with their parents, Janet and Bob were arguing, yelling, and taunting each other in the back of the car. They were warned, but they relentlessly continued their bickering. The parents then informed them, "Since you ignored us telling you to stop bickering you lost your opportunity to choose where we will eat tonight."

Specifying for how long the privilege or reward is lost is important. Several guidelines are useful. First, losing something for a long period of time is rarely effective (e.g., "You can't play with your sled until next winter!"). Simply, the youngster will forget about the sled and habituate to its absence. Second, removing routine privileges is preferred to removing major life-event-type rewards (e.g., attendance at a birthday party, the prom, the "big game"). We are reminded of an episode of *Leave it to Beaver* in which the parents, Ward and June, were trying to help their son Beaver learn to enjoy eating brussel sprouts. Beaver refused to eat them and his parents warned him that unless he ate his brussel sprouts the next time, he could not go to the football game with them. Then at dinner the night before the game, guess what was served? Brussel sprouts! The Cleavers had boxed themselves into a corner. Not even Ward and June Cleaver, the parental icons, could follow through with this impossible contingency.

Many times parents may be tempted to remove a "big" reward. In our experience, this is due to high levels of emotion associated with the misbehavior. In these instances, we find it helpful to work through these emotions with the parent using the cognitive techniques presented earlier in the book. Think about this example. Ten-year-old Ellie had been hiding her poor school papers from her parents and goofing off at school. Exasperated and desperate, her parents threatened to cancel her birthday party. How would you intervene with this family?

First, we would work with the parents' beliefs ("Ellie's out of control. As a parent, I must regain control by severely punishing her."). Second, we would use some of our cognitive-behavioral skills to help the parents evaluate (e.g., "What are the advantages and disadvantages?"; "What's an alternative way of looking at this?"; "How will you feel in 2 weeks after canceling her birthday party?"; "What are your trying to teach Ellie?"; "How certain are you that extreme punishment is an effective way to teach Ellie to be honest with you and gain greater control?").

Grounding is a parental strategy that includes elements of both time-out and removal of rewards and privileges. Grounding should involve the removal of reinforcers or withholding participation in desired activities (Barkley et al., 1999). Barkley and colleagues point out common pitfalls parents fall into when misusing grounding. Specifically, they may ground the child for a week and then allow him/her to attend a special event, or they may not allow the child out of the house yet permit him to use the TV, Sony PlayStation, and Internet. Other times parents ground children but are unable to monitor the grounding. Sometimes parents ground children for a week at a time, with the child accumulating weeks' worth of grounding in just a few days. Thus, Barkley and colleagues recommend keeping grounding short, from a few hours to 2 days at the most. This punishment includes removal of all privileges, as well as possibly the requirement of some additional chores. As with other punishments, if parents plan out ahead of time how they will handle situations, their own anger will not be as likely to lead to overreaction (Barkley et al., 1999).

CONCLUSION

Parent–child relational issues often impact the presentation and maintenance of affective distress and behavioral acting out in youth. Therefore parental involvement in treatment is a logical component that must not be minimized. Parents are often the holders of reinforcement in much of their children's environment. By providing information to parents and collaboratively working with them to identify target behaviors and skills, therapists can teach parents to provide positive reinforcement and support to their child that generalizes outside the therapy sessions. Doing so should increase the frequency of youngsters' appropriate behaviors. In addition, parents can provide valuable observations of children's behaviors between therapy sessions. Overall, parents are generally attempting to act in their child's best interest. Whatever discipline and parenting strategies they are using, their purpose is to improve the child's behavior. Sharing with them the strategies presented in this chapter will give them specific game plans for doing so.

References

Abramson, L. Y., Seligman, M. E. P., & Teasdale, J. D. (1978). Learned helplessness in humans: Critique and reformulation. *Journal of Abnormal Psychology, 87,* 49–74.

Achenbach, T. M. (1991a). *Integrative guide to the 1991 CBCL, YSR, and TRF profiles.* Burlington: University of Vermont, Department of Psychiatry.

Achenbach, T. M. (1991b). *Manual for the Child Behavior Checklist/4–18 and 1991 profile.* Burlington: University of Vermont, Department of Psychiatry.

Achenbach, T. M. (1991c). *Manual for the Teacher's Report Form and 1991 profile.* Burlington: University of Vermont, Department of Psychiatry.

Achenbach, T. M., & Edelbrock, C. S. (1983). *Manual for the Child Behavior Checklist and Child Behavior Profile.* Burlington: University of Vermont, Department of Psychiatry.

Achenbach, T. M., McConaughy, S. H., & Howell, C. T. (1987). Child/adolescent behavioral and emotional problems: Implications of cross-informant correlations for situational specificity. *Psychological Bulletin, 101,* 212–232.

Alford, B. A., & Beck, A. T. (1997). *The integrative power of cognitive therapy.* New York: Guilford Press.

Allen, J. (1998). Personality assessment with American Indians and Alaska Natives: Instrument considerations and service delivery style. *Journal of Personality Assessment, 70,* 17–42.

American Psychiatric Association (1994). *Diagnostic and statistical manual of mental disorders* (4th ed.). Washington, DC: Author.

Anastopoulos, A. D. (1998). A training program for children with attention-deficit/hyperactivity disorder. In J. M. Briesmeister & C. E. Schaefer (Eds.), *Handbook of parent training: Parents as co-therapists for children's behavior problems* (2nd ed., pp. 27–60). New York: Wiley.

Bandura, A. (1977). *Social learning theory.* Englewood Cliffs, NJ: Prentice-Hall.

Bandura, A. (1986). *Social foundations of thought and action: A social-cognitive theory.* Englewood Cliffs, NJ: Prentice-Hall.

Barkley, R. A. (1997). *Defiant children: A clinician's manual for assessment and parent training* (2nd ed.). New York: Guilford Press.

Barkley, R. A., Edwards, G. H., & Robin, A. L. (1999). *Defiant teens: A clinician's manual for assessment and family intervention.* New York: Guilford Press.

Barlow, D. H. (1994, November). *The scientist–practitioner and practice guidelines in a managed care environment.* Address presented at the annual meeting of the Association for Advancement of Behavior Therapy, San Diego, CA.

Baylor, B. (1976). *Hawk, I am your brother.* New York: Scribners.

Beal, D., Kopec, A. M., & DiGiuseppe, R. (1996). Disputing patients' irrational beliefs. *Journal of Rational-Emotive and Cognitive-Behavioral Therapy, 14,* 215–229.

Beardslee, W. R., Salt, P., Porterfield, K., Rothberg, P. C., vande Velde, P., Swatling, S., Hoke, L., Moilanen, D. L., & Wheelock, I. (1993). Comparison of preventive interventions for families with parental affective disorder. *Journal of the American Academy of Child and Adolescent Psychiatry, 32,* 254–263.

Beck, A. T. (1976). *Cognitive therapy and the emotional disorders.* New York: International Universities Press.

Beck, A. T. (1978). *Beck hopelessness scale.* San Antonio, TX: Psychological Corporation.

Beck, A. T. (1985). Cognitive therapy, behavior therapy, psychoanalysis, and pharmacotherapy: A cognitive continuum. In M. J. Mahoney & A. Freeman (Eds.), *Cognition and psychotherapy* (pp. 325–347). New York: Plenum Press.

Beck, A. T. (1990). *Beck anxiety inventory.* San Antonio, TX: Psychological Corporation.

Beck, A. T. (1993). Cognitive therapy: Past, present, and future. *Journal of Consulting and Clinical Psychology, 61,* 194–198.

Beck, A. T. (1996). *Beck depression inventory–II.* San Antonio, TX: Psychological Corporation.

Beck, A. T., & Clark, D. A. (1988). Anxiety and depression: An information processing perspective. *Anxiety Research, 1,* 23–36.

Beck, A. T., Emery, G., & Greenberg, R. L. (1985). *Anxiety disorders and phobias: A cognitive perspective.* New York: Plenum Press.

Beck, A. T., Freeman, A., & Associates. (1990). *Cognitive therapy of personality disorders.* New York: Guilford Press.

Beck, A. T., Rush, A. J., Shaw, B. F., & Emery, G. (1979). *Cognitive therapy of depression.* New York: Guilford Press.

Beck, J. S. (1995). *Cognitive therapy: Basics and beyond.* New York: Guilford Press.

Becker, W. C. (1971). *Parents are teachers.* Champaign, IL: Research Press.

Beidel, D. C., & Turner, S. M. (1998). *Shy children, phobic adults.* Washington, DC: American Psychological Association.

Beidel, D. C., Turner, S. M., & Morris, T. L. (1995). A new inventory to assess childhood social anxiety and phobia: The Social Phobia and Anxiety Inventory for Children. *Psychological Assessment, 7,* 73–79.

Beidel, D. C., Turner, S. M., & Trager, K. N. (1994). Test anxiety and childhood anxiety disorders in African American and white school children. *Journal of Anxiety Disorders, 8,* 169–179.

Bellak, L. (1993). *The TAT, CAT, and SAT in clinical use.* Needham Heights, MA: Allyn & Bacon.

Bellak, L., & Bellak, S. (1949). *The Children's Apperception Test.* New York: C.P.S.

Bell-Dolan, D., & Wessler, A. E. (1994). Attributional style of anxious children: Extensions from cognitive theory and research on adult anxiety. *Journal of Anxiety Disorders, 8,* 79–96.

Berg, B. (1986). *The assertiveness game.* Dayton, OH: Cognitive Counseling Resources.

Berg, B. (1989). *The anger control game.* Dayton, OH: Cognitive Counseling Resources.

Berg, B. (1990a). *The anxiety management game.* Dayton, OH: Cognitive Counseling Resources.

Berg, B. (1990b). *The depression management game.* Dayton, OH: Cognitive Counseling Resources.

Berg, B. (1990c). *The self-control game.* Dayton, OH: Cognitive Counseling Resources.

Bernal, M. E., Saenz, D. S., & Knight, G. P. (1991). Ethnic identity and adaptation of Mexican-American youths in school settings. *Hispanic Journal of Behavioral Sciences, 13,* 135–154.

Bernard, M. E., & Joyce, M. R. (1984). *Rational-emotive therapy with children and adolescents.* New York: Wiley.

Berry, J. (1995). *Feeling scared.* New York: Scholastic Press.

Berry, J. (1996). *Feeling sad.* New York: Scholastic Press.

Beutler, L. E., Brown, M. T., Crothers, L., Booker, K., & Seabrook, M. K. (1996). The dilemma of factitious demographic distinctions in psychological research. *Journal of Consulting and Clinical Psychology, 64,* 892–902.

Biederman, J., Faraone, S. V., Mick, E., Williamson, S., Wilens, T. E., Spencer, T. S., Weber, W., Jetton, J., Kraus, I., Pert, J., & Zallen, B. (1999). Clinical correlates of ADHD in females: Findings from a large group of girls ascertained from pediatric and psychiatric referral sources. *Journal of the American Academy of Child and Adolescent Psychiatry, 38,* 966–975.

Birleson, P. (1981). The validity of depressive disorder in childhood and the development of a self-rating scale: A research report. *Journal of Child Psychology and Psychiatry and Allied Disciplines, 22,* 73–88.

Birmaher, B., Ryan, N. D., Williamson, D. E., Brent, D. A., Kaufman, J., Dahl, R. E., Perel, J., & Nelson, B. (1996). Childhood and adolescent depression: A review of the past 10 years, Part 1. *Journal of the American Academy of Child and Adolescent Psychiatry, 35,* 1427–1439.

Blos, P. (1979). *The adolescent passage: Development issues.* New York: International Universities Press.

Bode, J. (1989). *New kids on the block: Oral histories of immigrant teens.* New York: Franklin Waters.

Brandell, J. R. (1986). Using children's autogenic stories to assess therapeutic progress. *Journal of the American Academy of Child and Adolescent Psychiatry, 3,* 285–292.

Brehm, J. W. (1966). *A theory of psychological reactance.* New York: Academic Press.

Brems, C. M. (1993). *A comprehensive guide to child psychotherapy.* Boston: Allyn & Bacon.

Brondolo, E., DiGiuseppe, R., & Tafrate, R. C. (1997). Exposure-based treatment for anger problems: Focus on the feeling. *Cognitive and Behavioral Practice, 4,* 75–98.

Bunting, E. (1994). *Smoky night.* San Diego, CA: Harcourt, Brace.

Burns, D. D. (1980). *Feeling good: The new mood therapy.* New York: Signet.

Burns, D. D. (1989). *The feeling good handbook.* New York: William Morrow.

Butcher, J. N., Williams, C. L., Graham, J. R., Archer, R. P., Tellegen, A., Ben-Porath, J. S., & Kaemmer, B. (1992). *MMPI-A: Manual for administration, scoring, and interpretation.* Minneapolis: University of Minnesota Press.

Callow, G., & Benson, G. (1990). Metaphor technique (storytelling) as a treatment option. *Educational and Child Psychology, 7,* 54–60.

Canino, I. A., & Spurlock, J. (2000). *Culturally diverse children and adolescents: Assessment, diagnosis, and treatment* (2nd ed.). New York: Guilford Press.

Cantwell, D. P. (1996). Attention deficit disorder: A review of the past 10 years. *Journal of the American Academy of Child and Adolescent Psychiatry, 35,* 978–987.

Carter, M. M., Sbrocco, T., & Carter, C. (1996). African-Americans and anxiety disorders research: Development of a testable theoretical framework. *Psychotherapy, 33,* 449–463.

Cartledge, G. C., & Feng, H. (1996a). Asian Americans. In G. C. Cartledge & J. F. Milburn (Eds.), *Cultural diversity and social skills instruction: Understanding ethnic and gender differences* (pp. 87–132). Champaign, IL: Research Press.

Cartledge, G. C., & Feng, H. (1996b). The relationship of culture and social behavior. In G. C. Cartledge & J. F. Milburn (Eds.), *Cultural diversity and social skills instruction: Understanding ethnic and gender differences* (pp. 13–44). Champaign, IL: Research Press.

Cartledge, G. C., & Middleton, M. B. (1996). African-Americans. In G. C. Cartledge & J. F. Milburn (Eds.), *Cultural diversity and social skills instruction: Understanding ethnic and gender differences* (pp. 133–203). Champaign, IL: Research Press.

Cartledge, G. C., & Milburn, J. F. (Eds.). (1996). *Cultural diversity and social skills instruction: Understanding ethnic and gender differences.* Champaign, IL: Research Press.

Castellanos, D., & Hunter, T. (1999). Anxiety disorders in children and adolescents. *Southern Medical Journal, 92,* 946–954.

Castro-Blanco, D. (1999, November). *STAND-UP: Cognitive-behavioral inter-*

vention for high-risk adolescents. Workshop presented at the annual meeting of the Association for Advancement of Behavior Therapy, Toronto, Canada.

Chorpita, B. F., & Barlow, D. H. (1998). The development of anxiety: The role of control in the early environment. *Psychological Bulletin, 124,* 3–21.

Clark, D. A., Beck, A. T., & Alford, B. A. (1999). *Scientific foundations of cognitive theory and therapy of depression.* New York: Wiley.

Clark, D. M., & Beck, A. T. (1988). Cognitive approaches. In C. G. Last & M. Hersen (Eds.), *Handbook of anxiety disorders* (pp. 362–385). Elmsford, NY: Pergamon Press.

Cochran, L. L., & Cartledge, G. (1996). Hispanic Americans. In G. C. Cartledge & J. F. Milburn (Eds.), *Cultural diversity and social skills training: Understanding ethnic and gender differences* (pp. 245–296). Champaign, IL: Research Press.

Cole, D. A., Martin, J. M., Peeke, A., Henderson, A., & Harwell, J. (1998). Validation of depression and anxiety measures in white and black youths: Multitrait–multimethod analyses. *Psychological Assessment, 10,* 261–276.

Conners, C. K. (1990). *Conners Rating Scales manual.* North Tonawanda, NY: MultiHealth Systems.

Cosby, B. (1997). *The meanest thing to say.* New York: Scholastic Press.

Costantino, G., & Malgady, R. G. (1996). Culturally sensitive treatment: Cuento and hero/heroine modeling therapies for Hispanic children and adolescents. In E. D. Hibbs & P. S. Jensen (Eds.), *Psychosocial treatment for child and adolescent disorders: Empirically-based strategies for clinical practice* (pp. 639–669). Washington, DC: American Psychological Association.

Costantino, G., Malgady, R. G., & Rogler, L. H. (1994). Storytelling through pictures: Cultural sensitive psychotherapy for Hispanic children and adolescents. *Journal of Clinical Child Psychology, 23,* 13–20.

Craske, M. G., & Barlow, D. H. (2001). Panic disorder and agoraphobia. In D. H. Barlow (Ed.), *Clinical handbook of psychological disorders: A step-by-step treatment manual* (3rd ed., pp. 1–59). New York: Guilford Press.

Crick, N. R., & Grotpeter, J. K. (1995). Relational aggression, gender, and social-psychological adjustment. *Child Development, 66,* 710–722.

Cuellar, I. (1998). Cross-cultural psychological assessment of Hispanic Americans. *Journal of Personality Assessment, 70,* 71–86.

Daleiden, E. L., Vasey, M. V., & Brown, L. M. (1999). Internalizing disorders. In W. K. Silverman & T. H. Ollendick (Eds.), *Developmental issues in the clinical treatment of children* (pp. 261–278). Boston: Allyn & Bacon.

Dattilio, F. M., & Padesky, C. A. (1990). *Cognitive therapy with couples.* Sarasota, FL: Professional Resource Exchange.

Davis, N. (1989). The use of therapeutic stories in the treatment of abused children. *Journal of Strategic and Systemic Therapies, 8,* 18–23.

Deblinger, E. (1997, November). *Therapeutic interventions for sexually abused children and their non-offending parents.* Workshop presented at the annual meeting of the Association for Advancement of Behavior Therapy, Miami, FL.

DeRoos, Y., & Allen-Measures, P. (1998). Application of Rasch analysis: Exploring differences in depression between African-American and white children. *Journal of Social Service Research, 23,* 93–107.

DiGiuseppe, R., Tafrate, R., & Eckhardt, C. (1994). Critical issues in the treatment of anger. *Cognitive and Behavioral Practice, 1,* 111–132.

Dishion, T. J., French, D. C., & Patterson, G. R. (1995). The development and ecology of antisocial behavior. In D. Cicchetti & D. J. Cohen (Eds.), *Developmental psychopathology: Vol. 2. Risk, disorder, and adaptation* (pp. 421–471). New York: Wiley.

Dodge, K. A. (1985). Attributional bias in aggressive children. In P. C. Kendall (Ed.), *Advances in cognitive-behavioral research and therapy* (Vol. 4, pp. 73–110). New York: Academic Press.

D'Zurilla, T. J. (1986). *Problem-solving therapy: A social competence approach to clinical intervention.* New York: Springer.

Eisen, A. R., & Silverman, W. K. (1993). Should I relax or change my thoughts?: A preliminary examination of cognitive therapy, relaxation, and their combination with overanxious children. *Journal of Cognitive Psychotherapy, 1,* 265–279.

Elliott, J. (1991). Defusing conceptual fusions: The "just because" technique. *Journal of Cognitive Psychotherapy, 5,* 227–229.

Ellis, A. (1962). *Reason and emotion in psychotherapy.* New York: Lyle Stuart.

Ellis, A. (1979). Rational-emotive therapy as a new theory of personality and therapy. In A. Ellis & J. M. Whiteley (Eds.), *Theoretical and empirical foundations of rational-emotive therapy* (pp. 1–6). New York: Brooks/Cole.

Exner, J. E., Jr. (1986). *The Rorschach: A comprehensive system: Vol. 1. Basic foundations* (2nd ed.). New York: Wiley.

Eyberg, S. (1974). *Eyberg Child Behavior Inventory.* (Available from S. Eyberg, Department of Clinical and Health Psychology, Box 100165 HSC, University of Florida, Gainesville, FL 32610)

Eyberg, S. (1992). Parent and teacher behavior inventories for the assessment of conduct problem behaviors in children. In L. VandeCreek, S. Knapp, & T. L. Jackson (Eds.), *Innovations in clinical practice: A source book* (Vol. 11, pp. 261–266). Sarasota, FL: Professional Resource Press.

Eyberg, S. M., & Boggs, S. R. (1998). Parent–child interaction therapy. A psychosocial intervention for the treatment of young conduct-disordered children. In J. M. Briesmeister & C. E. Schaefer (Eds.), *Handbook of parent training: Parents as co-therapists for children's behavior problems* (2nd ed., pp. 61–97). New York: Wiley.

Eyberg, S. M., & Ross, A. W. (1978). Assessment of child behavior problems: The validation of a new inventory. *Journal of Clinical Child Psychology, 7,* 113–116.

Feindler, E. L. (1991). Cognitive strategies in anger control interventions for children and adolescents. In P. C. Kendall (Ed.), *Child and adolescent therapy: Cognitive and behavioral procedures* (pp. 66–97). New York: Guilford Press.

Feindler, E. L., & Ecton, R. B. (1986). *Adolescent anger control: Cognitive-behavioral techniques.* New York: Pergamon Press.

Feindler, E. L., & Guttman, J. (1994). Cognitive-behavioral anger control training. In C. W. LeCroy (Ed.), *Handbook of child and adolescent treatment manuals* (pp. 170–199). New York: Lexington Books.

Fennell, M. J. V (1989). Depression. In K. Hawton, P. M. Salkovskis, J. Kirk, & D. M. Clark (Eds.), *Cognitive-behavior therapy for psychiatric problems: A practical guide* (pp. 169–234). Oxford, England: Oxford Medical.

Fiske, S. T., & Taylor, S. E. (1991). *Social cognition*. New York: McGraw-Hill.

Forehand, R. L., & Kotchick, B. A. (1996). Cultural diversity: A wake-up call for parent training. *Behavior Therapy, 27,* 187–206.

Forehand, R. L., & McMahon, R. J. (1981). *Helping the non-compliant child: A clinician's guide to parent training*. New York: Guilford Press.

Francis, G., & Gragg, R. A. (1995, November). *Assessment and treatment of obsessive-compulsive disorder in children and adolescents*. Workshop presented at the annual meeting of the Association for Advancement of Behavior Therapy, Washington, DC.

Freeman, A., & Dattilio, F. M. (1992). Cognitive therapy in the year 2000. In A. Freeman & F. M. Dattilio (Eds.), *Comprehensive case book of cognitive therapy* (pp. 375–379). New York: Plenum Press.

Frey, D., & Fitzgerald, T. (2000). *Chart your course*. Dayton, OH: Mandalay.

Friedberg, R. D. (1993). Inpatient cognitive therapy: Games cognitive therapists play. *Behavior Therapist, 16,* 41–42.

Friedberg, R. D. (1994). Storytelling and cognitive therapy with children. *Journal of Cognitive Therapy, 8,* 209–217.

Friedberg, R. D. (1995). Confessions of a cognitive therapist. *Behavior Therapist, 18,* 120–121.

Friedberg, R. D., & Crosby, L. E. (2001). *Therapeutic exercises for children: A professional guide*. Sarasota, FL: Professional Resource Press.

Friedberg, R. D., & Dalenberg, C. J. (1991). Attributional processes in young children: Theoretical, methodological, and clinical considerations. *Journal of Rational-Emotive and Cognitive-Behavioral Therapy, 9,* 173–183.

Friedberg, R. D., Fidaleo, R. A., & Mason, C. A. (1992). *Switching channels: A cognitive-behavioral work journal for adolescents*. Sarasota, FL: Psychological Assessment Resources.

Friedberg, R. D., Friedberg, B. A., & Friedberg, R. J. (2001). *Therapeutic exercises for children: Guided self-discovery through cognitive-behavioral techniques*. Sarasota, FL: Professional Resource Press.

Fristad, M. A., Emery, B. L., & Beck, S. J. (1997). Use and abuse of the Children's Depression Inventory. *Journal of Consulting and Clinical Psychology, 65,* 699–702.

Garcia, E. J., & Pellegrini, N. (1974). *Homer the homely hound dog*. New York: Institute for Rational Living.

Gardner, R. A. (1970). The mutual storytelling technique: Use in the treatment of a child with post-traumatic neurosis. *American Journal of Psychotherapy, 24,* 419–439.

Gardner, R. A. (1971). *Therapeutic communication with children: The mutual storytelling technique*. New York: Science House.

Gardner, R. A. (1972). Once upon a time there was a doorknob and everybody used to make him all dirty with fingerprints. *Psychology Today, 10,* 67–71, 91.

Gardner, R. A. (1975). Techniques for involving the child with MBD in meaningful psychotherapy. *Journal of Learning Disabilities, 8,* 16–26.

Gardner, R. A. (1986). *The psychotherapeutic techniques of Richard Gardner.* Cresskill, NJ: Creative Therapeutics.

Gibbs, J. T. (1998). African-American adolescents. In J. T. Gibbs, L. N. Huang, & Associates (Eds.), *Children of color: Psychological interventions with culturally diverse youth* (pp. 143–170). San Francisco: Jossey-Bass.

Gillham, J. E., Reivich, K. J., Jaycox, L. J., & Seligman, M. E. P. (1995). Prevention of depressive symptoms in school children: Two-year follow-up. *Psychological Science, 6,* 343–351.

Ginsburg, G. S., & Silverman, W. K. (1996). Phobic and anxiety disorders in Hispanic and Caucasian youth. *Journal of Anxiety Disorders, 10,* 517–528.

Gluhoski, V. L. (1995). Misconceptions of cognitive therapy. *Psychotherapy, 31,* 594–600.

Godin, J., & Oughourlian, J. M. (1994). The transitional gap in metaphor and therapy: The essence of the story. In J. K. Zeig (Ed.), *Ericksonian methods: The essence of the story* (pp. 182–191). New York: Brunner/Mazel.

Goldfried, M. R., & Davison, G. R. (1976). *Clinical behavior therapy.* New York: Holt, Rinehart, & Winston.

Goldstein, A. (1973). Behavior therapy. In R. Corsini (Ed.), *Current psychotherapies* (pp. 207–250). Itasca, IL: Peacock.

Goldstein, A. P., Glick, B., Reiner, S., Zimmerman, D., & Coultry, T. M. (1987). *Aggression replacement training: A comprehensive intervention for aggressive youth.* Champaign, IL: Research Press.

Goncalves, O. F. (1994). Cognitive narrative psychotherapy: The hermeneutic construction of alternative meanings. In M. J. Mahoney (Ed.), *Cognitive and constructive psychotherapies theory, research, and practice* (pp. 139–162). New York: Springer.

Goodyer, I. M., Herbert, J., Secher, S. M., & Pearson, J. (1997). Short-term outcome of Major Depression, Part I: Co-morbidity and severity at presentation as predictors of persistent disorder. *Journal of the American Academy of Child and Adolescent Psychiatry, 36,* 179–187.

Gotlib, I. H., & Hammen, C. L. (1992). *Psychological aspects of depression.* New York: Wiley.

Greenberg, L. (1993). The three little pigs: A new story for families recovering from violence and intimidation. *Journal of Systemic Therapies, 12,* 39–40.

Greenberger, D., & Padesky, C. A. (1995). *Mind over mood: Changing how you feel by changing the way you think.* New York: Guilford Press.

Greenspan, S., & Greenspan, N. T. (1985). *First feelings.* New York: Penguin Books.

Greenspan, S., & Greenspan, N. T. (1989). *The essential partnership.* New York: Penguin Books.

Guidano, V. F., & Liotti, G. (1983). *Cognitive processes and emotional disorders: A structural approach to psychotherapy.* New York: Guilford Press.

Guidano, V. F., & Liotti, G. (1985). A constructionalist foundation for cognitive therapy. In M. J. Mahoney & A. Freeman (Eds.), *Cognition and psychotherapy* (pp. 101–142). New York: Plenum Press.

Hammen, C. (1988). Self-cognitions, stressful events, and the prediction of depression in children of depressed mothers. *Journal of Abnormal Child Psychology, 16,* 347–360.

Hammen, C., & Goodman-Brown, T. (1990). Self-schemas and vulnerability to specific life stress in children at risk for depression. *Cognitive Therapy and Research, 14,* 215–227.

Hammen, C., & Zupan, B. A. (1984). Self-schemas, depression, and the processing of personal information in children. *Journal of Experimental Child Psychology, 37,* 598–608.

Hammond, W. R. (1991). *Dealing with anger: Givin' it, takin' it, workin' it out.* Champaign, IL: Research Press.

Hammond, W. R., & Yung, B. R. (1991). Preventing violence in at-risk African-American youth. *Journal of Health Care for the Poor and Underserved, 2,* 359–373.

Hart, K. J., & Morgan, J. R. (1993). Cognitive-behavioral procedures with children: Historical context and current status. In A. J. Finch, W. M. Nelson, & E. S. Ott (Eds.), *Cognitive-behavioral procedures with children and adolescents* (pp. 1–24). Boston: Allyn & Bacon.

Hicks, D., Ginsburg, G., Lumpkin, P. W., Serafini, L., Bravo, I., Ferguson, C., & Silverman, W. K. (1996, November). *Phobic and anxiety disorders in Hispanic and white youth.* Poster presented at the annual meeting of the Association for Advancement of Behavior Therapy, New York, NY.

Ho, M. K. (1992). *Minority children and adolescents in therapy.* Newbury Park, CA: Sage.

Hoffman, M. (1991). *Amazing Grace.* New York: Dial.

Hope, D. A., & Heimberg, R. G. (1993). Social phobia and social anxiety. In D. H. Barlow (Ed.), *Clinical handbook of psychological disorders* (pp. 99–136). New York: Guilford Press.

Howard, K. A., Barton, C. E., Walsh, M. E., & Lerner, R. M. (1999). Social and contextual issues in interventions with children and families. In S. W. Russ & T. H. Ollendick (Eds.), *Handbook of psychotherapies with children and families* (pp. 45–66). New York: Plenum Press.

Ingram, R. E., & Kendall, P. C. (1986). Cognitive clinical psychology: Implications of an information-processing perspective. In R. E. Ingram (Ed.), *Information processing approaches to clinical psychology* (pp. 3–21). Orlando, FL: Academic Press.

Jacobson, E. (1938). *Progressive relaxation.* Chicago: University of Chicago Press.

Jaycox, L. H., Reivich, K. J., Gillham, J., & Seligman, M. E. P. (1994). Prevention of depressive symptoms in school children. *Behavior Research and Therapy, 32,* 801–816.

Johnson, C. T., Cartledge, G., & Milburn, J. F. (1996). Social skills and the culture of gender. In G. Cartledge & J. F. Milburn (Eds.), *Cultural diversity and social skills instruction: Understanding ethnic and gender differences* (pp. 297–352). Champaign, IL: Research Press.

Johnson, M. E. (1993). A culturally sensitive approach to therapy with children. In C. M. Brems, *A comprehensive guide to child psychotherapy* (pp. 68–93). Boston: Allyn & Bacon.

Jolly, J. B. (1993). A multi-method test of the cognitive content-specificity hypothesis in young adolescents. *Journal of Anxiety Disorders, 7,* 223–233.

Jolly, J. B., & Dykman, R. A. (1994). Using self-report data to differentiate anxious and depressive symptoms in adolescents: Cognitive content specificity and global distress. *Cognitive Therapy and Research, 18,* 25–37.

Jolly, J. B., & Kramer, T. A. (1994). The hierarchical arrangement of internalizing cognitions. *Cognitive Therapy and Research, 18,* 1–14.

Kagan, J. (1986). Rates of change in psychological processes. *Journal of Applied Developmental Psychology, 7,* 125–130.

Kashani, J. H., & Orvaschel, H. (1990). A community study of anxiety in children and adolescents. *American Journal of Psychiatry, 147,* 313–318.

Kaslow, N. J., & Racusin, G. R. (1990). Childhood depression: Current status and future directions. In A. S. Bellack, M. Hersen, & A. E. Kazdin (Eds.), *International handbook of behavior modification and therapy* (pp. 649–667). New York: Plenum Press.

Kaslow, N. J., & Thompson, M. P. (1998). Applying the criteria for empirically supported treatments to studies of psychosocial interventions for child and adolescent depression. *Journal of Clinical Child Psychology, 27,* 146–155.

Kazdin, A. E. (1993). Conduct disorder. In T. O. Ollendick & M. Hersen (Eds)., *Handbook of child and adolescent assessment* (pp. 292–310). Boston: Allyn & Bacon.

Kazdin, A. E. (1994). Antisocial behavior and conduct disorder. In L. W. Craighead, W. E. Craighead, A. E. Kazdin, & M. J. Mahoney (Eds.), *Cognitive and behavioral interventions* (pp. 267–299). Boston: Allyn & Bacon.

Kazdin, A. E. (1996). Problem-solving and parent management in treating aggressive and anti-social behavior. In E. D. Hibbs & P. S. Jensen (Eds.), *Psychosocial treatments for child and adolescent disorders: Empirically-based strategies for clinical practice* (pp. 377–408). Washington, DC: American Psychological Association.

Kazdin, A. E. (1997). Practitioner review: Psychosocial treatments for conduct disorder in children. *Journal of Child Psychology and Psychiatry, 38,* 161–178.

Kazdin, A. E., Rodgers, A., & Colbus, D. (1986). The Hopelessness Scale for Children: Psychometric characteristics and concurrent validity. *Journal of Consulting and Clinical Psychology, 54,* 241–245.

Kearney, C. A., & Albano, A. M. (2000). *Therapist's guide for school refusal behavior.* San Antonio, TX: Psychological Corporation.

Kendall, P. C. (1988). *The stop and think workbook.* Philadelphia, PA: Temple University.

Kendall, P. C. (1990). *The coping cat workbook.* Philadelphia, PA: Temple University.

Kendall, P. C., Chansky, T. E., Friedman, F. M., & Siqueland, L. (1991). Treating anxiety disorders in children and adolescents. In P. C. Kendall (Ed.), *Child and adolescent therapy: Cognitive-behavioral procedures* (pp. 131–164). New York: Guilford Press.

Kendall, P. C., Chansky, T. E., Kane, M. T., Kim, R. S., Kortlander, E., Ronan, K. R., Sessa, F. M., & Siqueland, L. (1992). *Anxiety disorders in youth: Cognitive-behavioral interventions.* Boston: Allyn & Bacon.

Kendall, P. C., Flannery-Schroeder, E., Panichelli-Mindell, S. M., Southam-Gerow, M., Henin, A., & Warman, M. (1997). Therapy for youths with anxiety disorders: A second randomized clinical trial. *Journal of Consulting and Clinical Psychology, 65,* 366–380.

Kendall, P. C., & MacDonald, J. P. (1993). Cognition in the psychopathology of youth and implications for treatment. In K. S. Dobson & P. C. Kendall (Eds.), *Psychopathology and cognition* (pp. 387–427). San Diego, CA: Academic Press.

Kendall, P. C., & Treadwell, K. R. H. (1996). Cognitive-behavioral treatment for childhood anxiety disorders. In E. D. Hibbs & P. S. Jensen (Eds.), *Psychosocial treatments for child and adolescent disorders: Empirically-based strategies for clinical practice* (pp. 23–42). Washington, DC: American Psychological Association.

Kershaw, C. J. (1994). Restorying the mind: Using therapeutic narrative in psychotherapy. In J. K. Zeig (Ed.), *Ericksonian methods: The essence of the story* (pp. 192–206). New York: Brunner/Mazel.

Kestenbaum, C. J. (1985). The creative process in child psychotherapy. *American Journal of Psychotherapy, 39,* 479–489.

Kimball, W., Nelson, W. M., & Politano, P. M. (1993). The role of developmental variables in cognitive-behavioral interventions with children. In A. J. Finch, W. M. Nelson, & E. S. Ott (Eds.), *Cognitive-behavioral procedures with children and adolescents* (pp. 25–67). Boston: Allyn & Bacon.

Knell, S. M. (1993). *Cognitive-behavior play therapy.* Northvale, NJ: Jason Aronson.

Koeppen, A. S. (1974). Relaxation training for children. *Journal of Elementary School Guidance and Counseling, 9,* 14–21.

Kottman, T., & Stiles, K. (1990). The mutual storytelling technique: An Adlerian application in child therapy. *Individual Psychology, 46,* 148–156.

Kovacs, M. (1992). *Children's Depression Inventory.* North Tonawanda, NY: Multi-Health Systems.

Kovacs, M., Feinberg, T. L., Crouse-Novak, M., Paulauskas, S. L., & Finkelstein, R. (1984). Depressive disorders in childhood, Part 2: Longitudinal prospective study of characteristics and recovery. *Archives of General Psychiatry, 41,* 229–237.

Kovacs, M., Feinberg, T. L., Crouse-Novak, M., Paulauskas, S. L., Pollock, M., & Finkelstein, R. (1984). Depressive disorders in childhood, Part 2: A longitudinal study of risk for a subsequent major depression. *Archives of General Psychiatry, 41,* 643–649.

Kovacs, M., Gatsonis, C., Paulauskas, S. L., & Richards, C. (1989). Depressive disorders in childhood, Part 4: A longitudinal study of co-morbidity with and risk for anxiety disorders. *Archives of General Psychiatry, 46,* 776–782.

Kovacs, M., & Goldston, D. (1991). Cognitive and social cognitive development of depressed children and adolescents. *Journal of the American Academy of Child and Adolescent Psychiatry, 30,* 388–392.

Kovacs, M., Goldston, D., & Gatsonis, C. (1993). Suicidal behaviors and childhood-onset depressive disorders: A longitudinal investigation. *Journal of the American Academy of Child and Adolescent Psychiatry, 32,* 8–20.

Kronenberger, W. G., & Meyer, R. G. (1996). *The child clinician's handbook.* Needham Heights, MA: Allyn & Bacon.

LaFramboise, T. D., & Low, K. G. (1998). American Indian children and adolescents. In J. T. Gibbs & L. N. Huang, & Associates (Eds.), *Children of color: Psychological interventions with culturally diverse youth* (pp. 112–142). San Francisco: Jossey-Bass.

Laurent, J., & Stark, K. D. (1993). Testing the cognitive content-specificity hypothesis with anxious and depressed youngsters. *Journal of Abnormal Psychology, 102,* 226–237.

Lawson, D. M. (1987). Using therapeutic stories in the counseling process. *Elementary School Guidance and Counseling, 22,* 134–142.

Lazarus, A. A. (1984). *In the mind's eye: The power of imagery for personal enrichment.* New York: Guilford Press.

LeCroy, C. W. (1994). Social skills training. In C. W. LeCroy (Ed.), *Handbook of child and adolescent treatment manuals* (pp. 126–169). New York: Lexington Books.

Lee, J. W., & Cartledge, G. (1996). Native Americans. In G. Cartledge & J. F. Milburn (Eds.), *Cultural diversity and social skills instruction: Understanding ethnic and gender differences* (pp. 205–244). Champaign, IL: Research Press.

Lerner, J., Safren, S. A., Henin, A., Warman, M., Heimberg, R. G., & Kendall, P. C. (1999). Differentiating anxious and depressive self-statements in youth: Factor structure of the Negative Affect Self-Statement Questionnaire among youth referred to an anxiety disorders clinic. *Journal of Clinical Child Psychology, 28,* 82–93.

Leve, R. M. (1995). *Child and adolescent psychotherapy: Process and integration.* Boston: Allyn & Bacon.

Lewinsohn, P. M., Clarke, G. N., Rohde, P., Hops, H., & Seeley, J. R. (1996). A course in coping: A cognitive-behavioral approach to the treatment of adolescent depression. In E. D. Hibbs & P. S. Jensen (Eds.), *Psychosocial treatments for child and adolescent disorders: Empirically-based strategies for clinical practice* (pp. 105–135). Washington, DC: American Psychological Association.

Liotti, G. (1987). The resistance to change of cognitive structures: A counter proposal to psychoanalytic metapsychology. *Journal of Cognitive Psychotherapy, 1,* 87–104.

Lord, B. B (1984). *In the year of the boar and Jackie Robinson.* Baltimore: Harper Collins.

March, J. (1997). *MASC: Multidimensional Anxiety Scale for Children technical manual.* New York: Multi-Health Systems.

Masters, J. C., Burish, T. G., Hollon, S. D., & Rimm, D. C. (1987). *Behavior ther-*

apy: Techniques and empirical findings (2nd ed.). San Diego, CA: Harcourt Brace Jovanovich.

Mayer, M. (1999). *Shibumi and the kitemaker.* Tarrytown, NY: Marshall Cavendish.

McArthur, D., & Roberts, G. (1982). *Roberts Apperception Test for Children: Manual.* Los Angeles: Western Psychological Services.

Meichenbaum, D. H. (1985). *Stress inoculation training.* New York: Pergamon Press.

Messer, S. C., Kempton, T., Van Hasselt, V. B., Null, J. A., & Bukstein, O. G. (1994). Cognitive distortions and adolescent affective disorder: Validity of the CNCEQ in an inpatient sample. *Behavior Modification, 18,* 339–351.

Mills, J. C., Crowley, R. J., & Ryan, M. O. (1986). *Therapeutic metaphors for children and the child within.* New York: Brunner/Mazel.

Mischel, W. (1981). Metacognition and the rules of delay. In J. H. Flavell & L. Ross (Eds.), *Social cognitive development: Frontiers and possible futures* (pp. 240–271). Cambridge, England: Cambridge University Press.

Morris, R. J., & Kratochwill, T. R. (1998). Childhood fears and phobias. In R. J. Morris & T. R. Kratochwill (Eds.), *The practice of child therapy* (3rd ed., pp. 91–132). Boston: Allyn & Bacon.

Morris, T. L. (1999, November). *The development of social anxiety: Current knowledge and future directions.* Paper presented at the annual meeting of the Association for Advancement of Behavior Therapy, Toronto, Canada.

Munn, A. E., Sullivan, M. A., & Romero, R. T. (1999, November). *The use of the Revised Children's Manifest Anxiety Scale (RCMAS) with Caucasian and highly acculturated Native American children.* Poster presented at the annual meeting of the Association for Advancement of Behavior Therapy, Toronto, Canada.

Murray, H. (1943). *Thematic Apperception Test.* Cambridge, MA: Harvard University Press.

Myers, W. D. (1975). *Fast Sam, cool Clyde, and stuff.* New York: Viking Press.

Myers, W. D. (1981). *Hoops.* New York: Dell.

Myers, W. D. (1988). *Scorpions.* Cambridge, MA: Harper & Row.

Nagata, D. K. (1998). The assessment and treatment of Japanese American children and adolescents. In J. T. Gibbs, L. N. Huang, & Associates. (Eds.), *Children of color: Psychological interventions with culturally diverse youth* (pp. 215–239). San Francisco: Jossey-Bass.

Neal, A. M., Lilly, R. S., & Zakis, S. (1993). What are African-American children afraid of? *Journal of Anxiety Disorders, 1,* 129–139.

Nettles, S. M., & Pleck, J. H. (1994). Risk, resilience, and development: The multiple ecologies of black adolescents in the United States. In R. J. Haggerty, L. R. Sherrod, N. Garmezy, & M. Rulter (Eds.), *Stress and resilience in children and adolescents* (pp. 147–181). New York: Cambridge University Press.

Nolen-Hoeksema, S., & Girgus, J. (1995). Explanatory style, achievement, depression, and gender differences in childhood and early adolescence. In G. M. Buchanan & M. E. P. Seligman (Eds.), *Explanatory style* (pp. 57–70). Hillsdale, NJ: Erlbaum.

Nolen-Hoeksema, S., Girgus, J. S., & Seligman, M. E. P. (1996). Predictors and consequences of childhood depressive symptoms: A 5–year longitudinal study. *Journal of Abnormal Psychology, 101,* 405–422.

Ollendick, T. H. (1983). Reliability and validity of the Revised Fear Schedule for Children (FSSC-R). *Behaviour Research and Therapy, 21,* 685–692.

Ollendick, T. H., & Cerny, J. A. (1981). *Clinical behavior therapy with children.* New York: Plenum Press.

Ollendick, T. H., & King, N. J. (1998). Empirically supported treatments for children with phobic and anxiety disorders: Current status. *Journal of Clinical Child Psychology, 27,* 156–167.

Ollendick, T. H., King, N. J., & Frary, R. B. (1989). Fears in children and adolescents: Reliability and generalizability across gender, age, and nationality. *Behaviour Research and Therapy, 27,* 19–26.

Overholser, J. C. (1993a). Elements of the Socratic method, Part 1: Systematic questioning. *Psychotherapy, 30,* 67–74.

Overholser, J. C. (1993b). Elements of the Socratic method, Part 2: Inductive reasoning. *Psychotherapy, 30,* 75–85.

Overholser, J. C. (1994). Elements of the Socratic method, Part 3: University definitions. *Psychotherapy, 31,* 286–293.

Padesky, C. A. (1986, September). *Cognitive therapy approaches for treating depression and anxiety in children.* Paper presented at the 2nd International Conference on Cognitive Psychotherapy, Umea, Sweden.

Padesky, C. A. (1988). *Intensive training series in cognitive therapy.* Workshop series presented at Newport Beach, CA.

Padesky, C. A. (1994). Schema change processes in cognitive therapy. *Clinical Psychology and Psychotherapy, 1,* 267–278.

Padesky, C. A., & Greenberger, D. (1995). *Clinician's guide to mind over mood.* New York: Guilford Press.

Patterson, G. R. (1976). *Living with children: New methods for parents and teachers-revised.* Champaign, IL: Research Press.

Persons, J. B. (1989). *Cognitive therapy in practice.* New York: Norton.

Persons, J. B. (1995, November). *Cognitive-behavioral case formulation.* Workshop presented at the annual meeting of the Association for Advancement of Behavior Therapy, Washington, DC.

Pitts, P. (1988). *Racing the sun.* New York: Avon Books.

Poznanski, E. O., Grossman, J. A., Buchsbaum, Y., Bonegas, M., Freeman, L., & Gibbons, R. (1984). Preliminary studies of the reliability and validity of the Children's Depression Rating Scale. *Journal of the American Academy of Child Psychiatry, 23,* 191–197.

Pretzer, J. L., & Beck, A. T. (1996). A cognitive theory of personality disorders. In J. F. Clarkin & M. F. Lenzenweger (Eds.), *Major theories of personality disorder* (pp. 36–105). New York: Guilford Press.

Quiggle, N. L., Garber, J., Panak, W. F., & Dodge, K. A. (1992). Social information processing in aggressive and depressed children. *Child Development, 63,* 1305–1320.

Ramirez, O. (1998). Mexican-American children and adolescents. In J. T. Gibbs, L. N. Huang, & Associates (Eds.), *Children of color: Psychological interven-*

tions with culturally diverse youth (pp. 215–239). San Francisco, CA: Jossey-Bass.

Reinecke, M. A., Ryan, N. E., & DuBois, D. L. (1998). Cognitive-behavioral therapy of depression and depressive symptoms during adolescence: A review and meta-analysis. *Journal of the American Academy of Child and Adolescent Psychiatry, 37,* 26–34.

Reynolds, C. R., & Richmond, B. O. (1985). *Revised Children's Manifest Anxiety Scale.* Los Angeles: Western Psychological Services.

Reynolds, W. M., Anderson, G., & Bartell, N. (1985). Measuring depression in children: A multimethod assessment investigation. *Journal of Abnormal Child Psychology, 13,* 513–526.

Roberts, R. E. (1992). Manifestation of depressive symptoms among adolescents: A comparison of Mexican Americans with the majority and other minority populations. *Journal of Nervous and Mental Disease, 180,* 627–633.

Roberts, R. E. (2000). Depression and suicidal behaviors among adolescents: The role of ethnicity. In I. Cuellar & F. A. Paniqua (Eds.), *Handbook of multicultural mental health* (pp. 359–388). San Diego: Academic Press.

Robins, C. J., & Hayes, A. M. (1993). An appraisal of cognitive therapy. *Journal of Consulting and Clinical Psychology, 61,* 205–214.

Ronen, T. (1997). *Cognitive developmental therapy for children.* New York: Wiley.

Ronen, T. (1998). Linking developmental and emotional elements into child and family cognitive-behavioral therapy. In P. Graham (Ed.), *Cognitive-behaviour therapy for children and families* (pp. 1–17). Cambridge, England: Cambridge University Press.

Rotter, J. B. (1982). *The development and application of social learning theory.* New York: Praeger.

Russell, R. L., Van den Brock, P., Adams, S., Rosenberger, K., & Essig, T. (1993). Analyzing narratives in psychotherapy: A formal framework and empirical analyses. *Journal of Narrative and Life History, 3,* 337–360.

Rutter, J. G., & Friedberg, R. D. (1999). Guidelines for the effective use of Socratic dialogue in cognitive therapy. In L. VandeCreek, S. Knapp, & T. L. Jackson (Eds.), *Innovations in clinical practice: A sourcebook* (Vol. 17, pp. 481–490). Sarasota, FL: Professional Resource Press.

Sanders, D. E., Merrell, K. W., & Cobb, H. C. (1999). Internalizing symptoms and affect of children with emotional and behavioral disorders: A comparative study with an urban African-American sample. *Psychology in the Schools, 36,* 187–197.

Santiango, D. (1983). *Famous all over town.* New York: Simon & Schuster.

Scherer, M. W., & Nakamura, C. Y. (1968). A Fear Survey Schedule for Children (FSS-C): A factor analytic comparison with manifest anxiety. *Behaviour Research and Therapy, 6,* 173–182.

Schwartz, J. A. J., Gladstone, T. R. G., & Kaslow, N. J. (1998). Depressive disorders. In T. H. Ollendick & M. Hersen (Eds.), *Handbook of child psychopathology* (3rd ed., pp. 269–289). New York: Plenum Press.

Seligman, M. E. P., Reivich, K., Jaycox, L., & Gillham, J. (1995). *The optimistic child.* Boston: Houghton Mifflin.

340 References

Shirk, S. R. (1999). Integrated child psychotherapy: Treatment ingredients in search of a recipe. In S. W. Russ & T. H. Ollendick (Eds.), *Handbook of psychotherapies with children and families* (pp. 369–385). New York: Plenum Press.

Silverman, W. K., & Kurtines, W. M. (1996). *Anxiety and phobic disorders: A pragmatic approach.* New York: Plenum Press.

Silverman, W. K., & Kurtines, W. M. (1997). Theory in child psychosocial treatment research: Have it or had it? *Journal of Abnormal Child Psychology, 25,* 359–366.

Silverman, W. K., LaGreca, A. M., & Wasserstein, S. (1995). What do children worry about?: Worries and their relation to anxiety. *Child Development, 66,* 671–686.

Silverman, W. K., & Ollendick, T. H. (Eds.). (1999). *Developmental issues in the clinical treatment of children.* Boston: Allyn & Bacon.

Sokoloff, R. M., & Lubin, B. (1983). Depressive mood in adolescent, emotionally disturbed females: Reliability and validity of an adjective checklist (C-DACL). *Journal of Abnormal Child Psychology, 11,* 531–536.

Sommers-Flanagan, J., & Sommers-Flanagan, R. (1995). Psychotherapeutic techniques with treatment-resistant adolescents. *Psychotherapy, 32,* 131–140.

Speier, P. L., Sherak, D. L., Hirsch, S., & Cantwell, D. P. (1995). Depression in children and adolescents. In E. E. Beckham & W. R. Leber (Eds.), *Handbook of depression* (2nd ed., pp. 467–493). New York: Guilford Press.

Spiegler, M. D., & Guevremont, D. C. (1995). *Contemporary behavior therapy.* Pacific Grove, CA: Brooks/Cole.

Spiegler, M. D., & Guevremont, D. C. (1998). *Contemporary behavior therapy* (3rd ed.). Pacific Grove, CA: Brooks/Cole.

Stahl, N. D., & Clarizio, H. F. (1999). Conduct disorder and co-morbidity. *Psychology in the Schools, 36,* 41–50.

Stanek, M. (1989). *I speak English for my mom.* Niles, IL: Whitman.

Stark, K. D. (1990). *Childhood depression: School-based intervention.* New York: Guilford Press.

Stark, K. D., Rouse, L. W., & Livingstone, R. (1991). Treatment of depression during childhood and adolescence: Cognitive-behavior procedures for individual and family. In P. C. Kendall (Ed.), *Child and adolescent therapy: Cognitive-behavioral procedures* (pp. 165–206). New York: Guilford Press.

Stirtzinger, R. M. (1983). Storytelling: A creative therapeutic technique. *Canadian Journal of Psychiatry, 28,* 561–565.

Sue, S. (1998). In search of cultural competence in psychotherapy and counseling. *American Psychologist, 53,* 440–448.

Sutter, J., & Eyberg, S. (1984). *Sutter–Eyberg Student Behavior Inventory.* (Available from S. Eyberg, Department of Clinical and Health Psychology, Box 100165 HSC, University of Florida, Gainesville, FL 32610)

Taylor, L., & Ingram, R. E. (1999). Cognitive reactivity and depressotypic information processing in children of depressed mothers. *Journal of Abnormal Psychology, 108,* 202–210.

Tharp, R. G. (1991). Cultural diversity and treatment of children. *Journal of Consulting and Clinical Psychology, 59,* 799–812.

Thompson, M., Kaslow, N. J., Weiss, B., & Nolen-Hoeksema, S. (1998). Children's Attributional Style Questionnaire—Revised. *Psychological Assessment, 10*, 166–190.

Trad, P. V., & Raine, M. J. (1995). The little girl who wouldn't walk: Exploring the narratives of preschoolers through previewing. *Journal of Psychotherapy Practice and Research, 4*, 224–236.

Treadwell, K. R. H., Flannery-Schroeder, E. D., & Kendall, P. C. (1995). Ethnicity and gender in relation to adaptive functioning, diagnostic status, and treatment outcome in children from an anxiety clinic. *Journal of Anxiety Disorders, 9*, 373–384.

Tsubakiyama, M. H. (1999). *Mei-Mei loves the morning.* Morton Grove, IL: Whitman.

Turner, J. E., & Cole, D. A. (1994). Developmental differences in cognitive diatheses for child depression. *Journal of Abnormal Child Psychology, 22*, 15–32.

U.S. Surgeon General. (1999). *Mental health: A report of the Surgeon General* [online]. Available: www.surgeongeneral.gove./library/mentalhealth.

Vasey, M. W. (1993). *Development and cognition in childhood anxiety.* In T. H. Ollendick & R. J. Prinz (Eds.), *Advances in clinical child psychology* (Vol. 15, pp. 1–39). New York: Plenum Press.

Vernon, A. (1989a). *Thinking, feeling, and behaving: An emotional educational curriculum for children (Grades 1–6).* Champaign, IL: Research Press.

Vernon, A. (1989b). *Thinking, feeling, and behaving: An emotional education curriculum for children (Grades 7–12).* Champaign, IL: Research Press.

Vernon, A. (1998). *The passport program: A journey through emotional, social, cognitive, and self-development (Grades 1–5).* Champaign, IL: Research Press.

Viorst, J. (1972). *Alexander and the terrible, horrible, no good, very bad day.* New York: Atheneum.

Warfield, J. R. (1999). Behavioral strategies for helping hospitalized children. In L. VandeCreek, S. Knapp, & T. L. Jackson (Eds.), *Innovations in clinical practice: A source book* (Vol. 17, pp. 169–182). Sarasota, FL: Professional Resource Press.

Waters, V. (1979). *Color us rational.* New York: Institute for Rational Living.

Waters, V. (1980). *Rational stories for children.* New York: Institute for Rational-Emotive Therapy.

Webster-Stratton, C., & Hancock, L. (1998). Training for parents of young children with conduct problems: Content, methods, and therapeutic processes. In J. M. Briesmeister & C. E. Schaefer (Eds.), *Handbook of parent training: Parents as co-therapists for children's behavior problems* (2nd ed., pp. 98–152). New York: Wiley.

Wellman, H. M., Hollander, M., & Schult, C. A. (1996). Young children's understanding of thought bubbles and of thought. *Child Development, 67,* 768–788.

Wexler, D. B. (1991). *The PRISM workbook: A program for innovative self-management.* New York: Norton.

Wolpe, J. (1958). *Psychotherapy by reciprocal inhibition.* Stanford, CA: Stanford University Press.

Woodward, L. J., & Ferguson, D. M. (1999). Early conduct problems and later risk of teenage pregnancy in girls. *Development and Psychopathology, 11,* 127–141.

Wright, J. H., & Davis, D. D. (1994). The therapeutic relationship in cognitive-behavioral therapy: Patient perceptions and therapist responses. *Cognitive and Behavioral Practice, 1,* 47–70.

Young, J. E. (1990). *Cognitive therapy for personality disorders: A schema-focused approach.* Sarasota, FL: Professional Resource Exchange.

Young, J. E., Weinberger, A., & Beck, A. T. (2001). Cognitive therapy for depression. In D. H. Barlow (Ed.), *Clinical handbook of psychological disorders: A step-by-step treatment manual* (3rd ed., pp. 264–308). New York: Guilford Press.

Zayas, L. H., & Solari, F. (1994). Early childhood socialization in Hispanic families: Context, culture, and practice implications. *Professional Psychology: Research and Practice, 25,* 200–206.

Zupan, B. A., Hammen, C., & Jaenicke, C. (1987). The effects of current mood and prior depressive history on self-schematic processing in children. *Journal of Experimental Child Psychology, 43,* 149–158.

Index